Extractable and Non-Extractable Antioxidants

Extractable and Non-Extractable Antioxidants

Special Issue Editors
Alessandra Durazzo
Massimo Lucarini

MDPI • Basel • Beijing • Wuhan • Barcelona • Belgrade

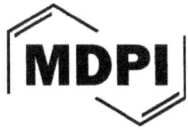

Special Issue Editors
Alessandra Durazzo
CREA-Research Centre for Food and Nutrition
Italy

Massimo Lucarini
CREA-Research Centre for Food and Nutrition
Italy

Editorial Office
MDPI
St. Alban-Anlage 66
4052 Basel, Switzerland

This is a reprint of articles from the Special Issue published online in the open access journal *Molecules* (ISSN 1420-3049) from 2017 to 2019 (available at: https://www.mdpi.com/journal/molecules/special_issues/extract_antioxidants)

For citation purposes, cite each article independently as indicated on the article page online and as indicated below:

LastName, A.A.; LastName, B.B.; LastName, C.C. Article Title. *Journal Name* **Year**, *Article Number*, Page Range.

ISBN 978-3-03921-437-2 (Pbk)
ISBN 978-3-03921-438-9 (PDF)

© 2019 by the authors. Articles in this book are Open Access and distributed under the Creative Commons Attribution (CC BY) license, which allows users to download, copy and build upon published articles, as long as the author and publisher are properly credited, which ensures maximum dissemination and a wider impact of our publications.

The book as a whole is distributed by MDPI under the terms and conditions of the Creative Commons license CC BY-NC-ND.

Contents

About the Special Issue Editor vii

Alessandra Durazzo and Massimo Lucarini
Extractable and Non-Extractable Antioxidants
Reprinted from: *molecules* **2019**, *24*, 1933, doi:10.3390/molecules24101933 1

Daniela Thomas da Silva, Rene Herrera, Berta Maria Heinzmann, Javier Calvo and Jalel Labidi
Nectandra grandiflora By-Products Obtained by Alternative Extraction Methods as a Source of Phytochemicals with Antioxidant and Antifungal Properties
Reprinted from: *molecules* **2018**, *23*, 372, doi: 5

Andrea Nemes, Erzsébet Szőllősi, László Stündl, Attila Biró, Judit Rita Homoki, Mária Magdolna Szarvas, Péter Balogh, Zoltán Cziáky and Judit Remenyik
Determination of Flavonoid and Proanthocyanidin Profile of Hungarian Sour Cherry
Reprinted from: *molecules* **2018**, *23*, 3278, doi:10.3390/molecules23123278 21

Didier Fraisse, Alexandra Degerine-Roussel, Alexis Bred, Samba Fama Ndoye, Magali Vivier, Catherine Felgines and François Senejoux
A Novel HPLC Method for Direct Detection of Nitric Oxide Scavengers from Complex Plant Matrices and Its Application to *Aloysia triphylla* Leaves
Reprinted from: *molecules* **2018**, *23*, 1574, doi:10.3390/molecules23071574 41

Jenny R. Rodriguez-Jimenez, Carlos A. Amaya-Guerra, Juan G. Baez-Gonzalez, Carlos Aguilera-Gonzalez, Vania Urias-Orona and Guillermo Nino-Medina
Physicochemical, Functional, and Nutraceutical Properties of Eggplant Flours Obtained by Different Drying Methods
Reprinted from: *molecules* **2018**, *23*, 3210, doi:10.3390/molecules23123210 49

Edith Espinosa-Páez, Ma. Guadalupe Alanis-Guzmán, Carlos E. Hernández-Luna, Juan G. Báez-González, Carlos A. Amaya-Guerra and Ana M. Andrés-Grau
Increasing Antioxidant Activity and Protein Digestibility in *Phaseolus vulgaris* and *Avena sativa* by Fermentation with the *Pleurotus ostreatus* Fungus
Reprinted from: *molecules* **2017**, *22*, 2275, doi: 62

Jana Šic Žlabur, Nadica Dobričević, Stjepan Pliestić, Ante Galić, Daniela Patricia Bilić and Sandra Voća
Antioxidant Potential of Fruit Juice with Added Chokeberry Powder (*Aronia melanocarpa*)
Reprinted from: *molecules* **2017**, *22*, 2158, doi: 73

Alessandra Durazzo, Massimo Lucarini, Antonello Santini, Emanuela Camilli, Paolo Gabrielli, Stefania Marconi, Silvia Lisciani, Altero Aguzzi, Loretta Gambelli, Ettore Novellino and Luisa Marletta
Antioxidant Properties of Four Commonly Consumed Popular Italian Dishes
Reprinted from: *molecules* **2019**, *24*, 1543, doi:10.3390/molecules24081543 84

Massimo Lucarini, Alessandra Durazzo, Annalisa Romani, Margherita Campo, Ginevra Lombardi-Boccia and Francesca Cecchini
Bio-Based Compounds from Grape Seeds: A Biorefinery Approach
Reprinted from: *molecules* **2018**, *23*, 1888, doi:10.3390/molecules23081888 97

Anna Maria Posadino, Grazia Biosa, Hatem Zayed, Haissam Abou-Saleh, Annalisa Cossu, Gheyath K. Nasrallah, Roberta Giordo, Daniela Pagnozzi, Maria Cristina Porcu, Luca Pretti and Gianfranco Pintus
Protective Effect of Cyclically Pressurized Solid–Liquid Extraction Polyphenols from *Cagnulari* Grape Pomace on Oxidative Endothelial Cell Death
Reprinted from: *molecules* **2018**, 23, 2105, doi:10.3390/molecules23092105 109

Wojciech Koch, Wirginia Kukula-Koch and Łukasz Komsta
Black Tea Samples Origin Discrimination Using Analytical Investigations of Secondary Metabolites, Antiradical Scavenging Activity and Chemometric Approach
Reprinted from: *molecules* **2018**, 23, 513, doi: 121

Chinedu Anokwuru, Muendi Sigidi, Marlaine Boukandou, Peter Tshisikhawe, Afsatou Traore and Natasha Potgieter
Antioxidant Activity and Spectroscopic Characteristics of Extractable and Non-Extractable Phenolics from *Terminalia sericea* Burch. ex DC.
Reprinted from: *molecules* **2018**, 23, 1303, doi:10.3390/molecules23061303 133

Huairong Zhong, Yong Xue, Xiaoyuan Lu, Qiang Shao, Yuelei Cao, Zhaoxia Wu and Gao Chen
The Effects of Different Degrees of Procyanidin Polymerization on the Nutrient Absorption and Digestive Enzyme Activity in Mice
Reprinted from: *molecules* **2018**, 23, 2916, doi:10.3390/molecules23112916 150

Zoriţa Diaconeasa
Time-Dependent Degradation of Polyphenols from Thermally-Processed Berries and Their In Vitro Antiproliferative Effects against Melanoma
Reprinted from: *molecules* **2018**, 23, 2534, doi:10.3390/molecules23102534 161

Alessandra Durazzo, Laura D'Addezio, Emanuela Camilli, Raffaela Piccinelli, Aida Turrini, Luisa Marletta, Stefania Marconi, Massimo Lucarini, Silvia Lisciani, Paolo Gabrielli, Loretta Gambelli, Altero Aguzzi and Stefania Sette
From Plant Compounds to Botanicals and Back: A Current Snapshot
Reprinted from: *molecules* **2018**, 23, 1844, doi:10.3390/molecules23081844 179

Qing Li, Shihua Yang, Yongqiang Li, Xiaofeng Xue, Yonghua Huang, Hengguo Luo, Yiming Zhang and Zhichao Lu
Comparative Evaluation of Soluble and Insoluble-Bound Phenolics and Antioxidant Activity of Two Chinese Mistletoes
Reprinted from: *molecules* **2018**, 23, 359, doi: 190

Shujing Li, Li Yuan, Yong Chen, Wei Zhou and Xinrui Wang
Studies on the Inclusion Complexes of Daidzein with β-Cyclodextrin and Derivatives
Reprinted from: *molecules* **2017**, 22, 2183, doi: 202

Munkhtugs Davaatseren, Yeon-Ji Jo, Geun-Pyo Hong, Haeng Jeon Hur, Sujin Park and Mi-Jung Choi
Studies on the Anti-Oxidative Function of *trans-* Cinnamaldehyde-Included β-Cyclodextrin Complex
Reprinted from: *molecules* **2017**, 22, 1868, doi: 213

About the Special Issue Editors

Alessandra Durazzo was awarded her Master's degree in Chemistry and Pharmaceutical Technology cum laude in 2003, and PhD in Horticulture in 2010. Durazzo has been Researcher at the CREA-Research Centre for Food and Nutrition since her appointment in 2005. The core of her research is the study of chemical, nutritional, and bioactive components of food, with particular regard to the wide spectrum of substances classes and their nutraceutical features. For several years, she was involved in national and international research projects on the evaluation of several factors (agronomic practices, processing, etc.) that affect food quality, the levels of bioactive molecules and total antioxidant properties as well as on their possible impact on human physiology resulting from the biological roles of bioactive components. Her research activities also involve the development, management, and updating of the Food Composition Database, as well as Bioactive Compounds and Food Supplements databases; particular attention is given towards the harmonization of analytical procedures and classification and codification of food preparation and food supplements.

Massimo Lucarini received his Master's Degree in Industrial Chemistry cum laude from the University of Rome "La Sapienza", Italy (1992), where he was also awarded his PhD in Chemistry. His main research activities are in the evaluation of nutrient content, molecules with biological and antinutrient activity in foods and diets, stability studies with regards to technological treatments of food products and using specific process markers. Particular interest is focused on the evaluation of the nutritional quality of foods, the bioavailability of nutrients and bioactive components and their interaction with the food matrix (using in vitro models and cellular models), and to applications in the nutraceutical field; recent attention has also been given to the exploitation of waste from the agri-food industry, with a view toward sustainable agri-food production. In relation to the study of bioactive molecules, the experience gained in this field is wide ranging: from carotenoids to phenolic substances, and from caseinophosphopeptides (CPP) to the components of dietary fiber. An integral part of the research is linked to institutional activity, including Food Composition Tables, Guidelines for Healthy Nutrition, and evaluation of fraud risk in the agri-food system. In relation to food production, the effects of technological treatments on molecules of nutritional interest are also evaluated. Lucarini is also interested in using natural substances with strong antioxidant properties to improve the shelf-life of food products. His research is also aimed at the development of new analytical methods, the exchange of scientific information, and the acquisition of new skills both at national and international level through training courses, participation in congresses, and seminars. The dissemination activity is carried out through the production of scientific articles, interviews released in national journals and broadcasting systems, creation of web pages, participation in congresses, and educational and informative activities.

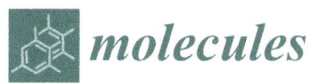

Editorial

Extractable and Non-Extractable Antioxidants

Alessandra Durazzo * and Massimo Lucarini *

CREA Research Centre for Food and Nutrition, Via Ardeatina 546, 00178 Rome, Italy
* Correspondence: alessandra.durazzo@crea.gov.it (A.D.); massimo.lucarini@crea.gov.it (M.L.);
Tel.: +30-065-149-4430 (A.D.); +30-065-149-4446 (M.L.)

Received: 14 May 2019; Accepted: 16 May 2019; Published: 20 May 2019

In addition to documented scientific interest on antioxidant phytochemicals (plant secondary metabolites) [1], the entire scientific community agrees on the importance of determination of extractable and non-extractable antioxidants [2–4]. In this context, the delineation and exploitation of extractable and non-extractable antioxidants in the main food groups as well as by-products [5–13] was the main focus of this Special Issue. This Special Issue was addressed towards the description and update of the methodological approach of antioxidant compounds in a multidisciplinary and innovative design. Conventional procedures and advanced extraction technologies, as well as analytical techniques, were considered, with particular regard to green procedures. It is worth mentioning the study of Da Silva et al. [14] on the effect of three different extraction methods—conventional (CE), ultrasound-assisted (UAE), and microwave-assisted (MAE)—on *Nectandra grandiflora* leaf extracts (NGLE) chemical yields, phenolic and flavonoid composition, physical characteristics, as well as antioxidant and antifungal properties: CE achieves the highest extraction phytochemical yield (22.16%), but with similar chemical composition to that obtained by UAE and MAE. Moreover, the authors added that CE also provided a superior thermal stability of NGLE [14].

Another example was given by Nemes et al. [15] that proposed a new process for extracting non-extractable procyanidins bound to the membrane, proteins, and fibers. Fraisse et al. [16] proposed a novel HPLC method for direct detection of nitric oxide scavengers from complex plant matrices and its application to *Aloysia triphylla* leaves.

On the other hand, Rodriguez-Jimenez et al. [17] studied physicochemical, functional, and nutraceutical properties of eggplant flours obtained by different drying methods: the drying oven flour results as a potential ingredient for the preparation of foods with functional properties, since it is rich in phenolic compounds and antioxidants. Espinosa-Páez et al. [18] reported increasing antioxidant activity and protein digestibility in *Phaseolus vulgaris* and *Avena sativa* by fermentation with the *Pleurotus ostreatus* fungus. Šic Žlabur, [19] by evaluating the possibility of using chokeberry powder as a supplement in apple juice to increase the nutritional value of the final product, showed a positive correlation between vitamin C content, total phenols, flavonoids, and anthocyanins content and antioxidant capacity in juice samples with added chokeberry powder treated with high intensity ultrasound. Durazzo et al. [20] reported the antioxidant properties of four commonly consumed popular Italian dishes our popular dishes, in terms of extractable and non-extractable antioxidants.

Particular attention was given to the studies of extractable and non-extractable antioxidants on food waste, in line with the concepts of circular economy and biorefineries. In this regard, it is worth mentioning the study of Lucarini et al. [21] on bio-based compounds from grape seeds, by giving the main lines of a biorefinery approach. Posadino et al. [22] concluded that the Naviglio extraction, as a green technology process, can be used to exploit wine waste to obtain antioxidants which can be used to produce enriched foods and nutraceuticals high in antioxidants.

The combination of emerging analytical techniques and the application of statistical methods, i.e., infrared spectroscopy, multielemental analysis, isotopic ratio mass spectrometry, and nanotechnologies coupled with chemometrics were taken into account. For instance, in the work of Kock et al. [23]

on black tea samples origin discrimination using analytical investigations of secondary metabolites, antiradical scavenging activity and chemometric approach, the applied principal component analysis (PCA) and ANOVA revealed several correlations between the level of catechins in tea infusions. Anokwuru et al. [24] studied antioxidant activity and spectroscopic characteristics of extractable and non-extractable phenolics from *Terminalia sericea* Burch. ex DC.: This study demonstrated that extractable phenolics contributed more to the antioxidant activities compared to the non-extractables.

Indeed, the potential effects of extractable and non-extractable antioxidants were investigated. In this regard, the study of Zhong et al. [25] studied the effects of different degrees of procyanidin polymerization on nutrient absorption and digestive enzyme activity in mice and concluded that in the process of food production, the anti-nutritional properties of polyphenols could be minimized by reducing the degree of polymerization of proanthocyanidins. Diaconeasa et al. [26], in a study on time-dependent degradation of polyphenols from thermally-processed berries, revealed that when processed and stored in time, the bioactive compounds from berry jams are degrading, but they still exert antioxidant and antiproliferative potential.

The utilization of extractable and non-extractable antioxidants in the nutraceuticals field [3,4,27–35] was another focal point of this Special Issue: extracts, fractions, purified, and semi-purified substances, used alone or in combination with other ingredients as dietary supplements or functional foods. This field needs to be explored using rigorous science approaches, considering a combination of studies from different fields (nutrition, food chemistry, medicine, etc.) is increasing.

In this regard, Durazzo et al. [35] have given an updated picture of the strict interaction between main plant biologically active compounds and botanicals, by underlying actual possibilities of study approach and research strategies. Li et al. [36], by studying soluble- and insoluble-bound phenolics and antioxidant activity of two Chinese mistletoes, indicated it as source of antioxidants in human healthcare. On the other hand, Li et al. [37], by studying the inclusion complexes of daidzein with β-cyclodextrin and derivatives, showed that the antioxidant performance of the inclusion complexes was enhanced in comparison to that of the native daidzein. Moreover, Davaatseren et al. [38] evaluated the anti-inflammatory and antioxidant effects of trans-Cinnamaldehyde self-included in β-cyclodextrin complexes (CIs) in lipopolysaccharide (LPS)-treated murine RAW 264.7 macrophages: CIs may have strong anti-inflammatory and antioxidant effects, similar to those of trans-Cinnamaldehyde when used alone.

We would like to acknowledge the efforts of the authors of the publications in this Special Issue.

Funding: This research received no external funding.

Conflicts of Interest: The authors declare no conflict of interest.

References

1. Yeung, A.W.K.; Tzvetkov, N.T.; El-Tawil, O.S.; Bungau, S.G.; Abdel-Daim, M.M.; Atanasov, A.G. Antioxidants: Scientific Literature Landscape Analysis. *Oxid. Med. Cell. Longev.* **2019**, *2019*, 8278454. [CrossRef]
2. Durazzo, A. Study Approach of Antioxidant Properties in Foods: Update and Considerations. *Foods* **2017**, *6*, 17. [CrossRef]
3. Durazzo, A. Extractable and Non-extractable polyphenols: An overview. In *Non-Extractable Polyphenols and Carotenoids: Importance in Human Nutrition and Health*; Saura-Calixto, F., Pérez-Jiménez, J., Eds.; Royal Society of Chemistry: London, UK, 2018; pp. 1–37.
4. Durazzo, A.; Lucarini, M. A Current shot and re-thinking of antioxidant research strategy. *Braz. J. Anal. Chem.* **2018**, *5*, 9–11. [CrossRef]
5. Pérez-Jiménez, J.; Torres, J.L. Analysis of non-extractable phenolic compounds in foods: The current state of the art. *J. Agric. Food Chem.* **2011**, *59*, 12713–12724. [CrossRef] [PubMed]
6. Durazzo, A.; Turfani, V.; Azzini, E.; Maiani, G.; Carcea, M. Phenols, lignans and antioxidant properties of legume and sweet chestnut flours. *Food Chem.* **2013**, *140*, 666–671. [CrossRef] [PubMed]
7. Durazzo, A.; Turfani, V.; Narducci, V.; Azzini, E.; Maiani, G.; Carcea, M. Nutritional characterisation and bioactive components of commercial carobs flours. *Food Chem.* **2014**, *153*, 109–113. [CrossRef] [PubMed]

8. Pérez-Jiménez, J.; Díaz-Rubio, M.E.; Saura-Calixto, F. Non-extractable polyphenols, a major dietary antioxidant: Occurrence, metabolic fate and health effects. *Nutr. Res. Rev.* **2013**, *26*, 118–129. [CrossRef]
9. Camelo-Méndez, G.A.; Bello-Pérez, L.A. Antioxidant capacity of extractable and bon-extractable polyphenols of pigmented maize. *Food Biotechnol.* **2014**, *4*, 6–13.
10. Durazzo, A.; Gabrielli, P.; Manzi, P. Qualitative study of functional groups and antioxidant properties of soy-based beverages compared to cow milk. *Antioxidants* **2015**, *4*, 523–532. [CrossRef] [PubMed]
11. Durazzo, A.; Casale, G.; Melini, V.; Maiani, G.; Acquistucci, R. Total polyphenol content and antioxidant properties of Solina (*Triticum aestivum* L.) and derivatives thereof. *It. J. Food Sci.* **2016**, *28*, 221.
12. Turfani, V.; Narducci, V.; Durazzo, A.; Galli, V.; Carcea, M. Technological, nutritional and functional properties of wheat bread enriched with lentil or carob flours. *LWT Food Sci. Technol.* **2017**, *78*, 361. [CrossRef]
13. Durazzo, A.; Lisciani, S.; Camilli, E.; Gabrielli, P.; Marconi, S.; Gambelli, L.; Aguzzi, A.; Lucarini, M.; Maiani, G.; Casale, G.; et al. Nutritional composition and antioxidant properties of traditional Italian dishes. *Food Chem.* **2017**, *218*, 70–77. [CrossRef]
14. Da Silva, D.T.; Herrera, R.; Heinzmann, B.M.; Calvo, J.; Labidi, J. *Nectandra grandiflora* by-products obtained by alternative extraction methods as a source of phytochemicals with antioxidant and antifungal properties. *Molecules* **2018**, *23*, 372. [CrossRef]
15. Nemes, A.; Szőllősi, E.; Stündl, L.; Biró, A.; Homoki, J.R.; Szarvas, M.M.; Balogh, P.; Cziáky, Z.; Remenyik, J. Determination of flavonoid and proanthocyanidin profile of hungarian sour cherry. *Molecules* **2018**, *23*, 3278. [CrossRef]
16. Fraisse, D.; Degerine-Roussel, A.; Bred, A.; Ndoye, S.F.; Vivier, M.; Felgines, C.; Senejoux, F. A Novel HPLC method for direct detection of nitric oxide scavengers from complex plant matrices and its application to *Aloysia triphylla* Leaves. *Molecules* **2018**, *23*, 1574. [CrossRef]
17. Rodriguez-Jimenez, J.R.; Amaya-Guerra, C.A.; Baez-Gonzalez, J.G.; Aguilera-Gonzalez, C.; Urias-Orona, V.; Nino-Medina, G. Physicochemical, functional, and nutraceutical properties of eggplant flours obtained by different drying methods. *Molecules* **2018**, *23*, 3210. [CrossRef]
18. Espinosa-Páez, E.; Alanis-Guzmán, M.G.; Hernández-Luna, C.E.; Báez-González, J.G.; Amaya-Guerra, C.A.; Andrés-Grau, A.M. Increasing antioxidant activity and protein digestibility in *Phaseolus vulgaris* and *Avena sativa* by fermentation with the *Pleurotus ostreatus* Fungus. *Molecules* **2017**, *22*, 2275. [CrossRef]
19. Šic Žlabur, J.; Dobričević, N.; Pliestić, S.; Galić, A.; Bilić, D.P.; Voća, S. Antioxidant potential of fruit juice with added chokeberry powder (*Aronia melanocarpa*). *Molecules* **2017**, *22*, 2158. [CrossRef]
20. Durazzo, A.; Lucarini, M.; Santini, A.; Camilli, E.; Gabrielli, P.; Marconi, S.; Lisciani, S.; Aguzzi, A.; Gambelli, L.; Novellino, E.; et al. Antioxidant properties of four commonly consumed popular Italian dishes. *Molecules* **2019**, *24*, 1543. [CrossRef]
21. Lucarini, M.; Durazzo, A.; Romani, A.; Campo, M.; Lombardi-Boccia, G.; Cecchini, F. Bio-based compounds from grape seeds: A biorefinery approach. *Molecules* **2018**, *23*, 1888. [CrossRef]
22. Posadino, A.M.; Biosa, G.; Zayed, H.; Abou-Saleh, H.; Cossu, A.; Nasrallah, G.K.; Giordo, R.; Pagnozzi, D.; Porcu, M.C.; Pretti, L.; et al. Protective effect of cyclically pressurized solid–liquid extraction polyphenols from Cagnulari grape pomace on oxidative endothelial cell death. *Molecules* **2018**, *23*, 2105. [CrossRef] [PubMed]
23. Koch, W.; Kukula-Koch, W.; Komsta, Ł. Black tea samples origin discrimination using analytical Investigations of Secondary Metabolites, Antiradical Scavenging Activity and Chemometric Approach. *Molecules* **2018**, *23*, 513. [CrossRef]
24. Anokwuru, C.; Sigidi, M.; Boukandou, M.; Tshisikhawe, P.; Traore, A.; Potgieter, N. Antioxidant activity and spectroscopic characteristics of extractable and non-extractable phenolics from *Terminalia sericea* Burch. ex DC. *Molecules* **2018**, *23*, 1303. [CrossRef]
25. Zhong, H.; Xue, Y.; Lu, X.; Shao, Q.; Cao, Y.; Wu, Z.; Chen, G. The effects of different degrees of Procyanidin Polymerization on the Nutrient Absorption and Digestive Enzyme Activity in Mice. *Molecules* **2018**, *23*, 2916. [CrossRef]
26. Diaconeasa, Z. Time-dependent degradation of polyphenols from thermally-processed berries and their in vitro antiproliferative effects against melanoma. *Molecules* **2018**, *23*, 2534. [CrossRef]
27. Andrew, R.; Izzo, A.A. Principles of pharmacological research of nutraceuticals. *Br. J. Pharmacol.* **2017**, *174*, 1177–1194. [CrossRef] [PubMed]

28. Santini, A.; Novellino, E.; Armini, V.; Ritieni, A. State of the art of Ready-to-Use Therapeutic Food: A tool for nutraceuticals addition to foodstuff. *Food Chem.* **2013**, *140*, 843–849. [CrossRef]
29. Santini, A.; Novellino, E. To Nutraceuticals and Back: Rethinking a Concept. *Foods* **2017**, *6*, 74. [CrossRef]
30. Santini, A.; Tenore, G.C.; Novellino, E. Nutraceuticals: A paradigm of proactive medicine. *Eur. J. Pharm. Sci.* **2017**, *96*, 53–61. [CrossRef] [PubMed]
31. Santini, A.; Novellino, E. Nutraceuticals: Shedding light on the grey area between pharmaceuticals and food. *Expert Rev. Clin. Pharmacol.* **2018**, *11*, 545–547. [CrossRef]
32. Santini, A.; Cammarata, S.M.; Capone, G.; Ianaro, A.; Tenore, G.C.; Pani, L.; Novellino, E. Nutraceuticals: Opening the debate for a regulatory framework. *Br. J. Clin. Pharmacol.* **2018**, *84*, 659–672. [CrossRef]
33. Daliu, P.; Santini, A.; Novellino, E. From pharmaceuticals to nutraceuticals: Bridging disease prevention and management. Expert Rev. *Clin. Pharmacol.* **2018**, *28*, 1–7.
34. Daliu, P.; Santini, A.; Novellino, E. A decade of nutraceutical patents: Where are we now in 2018? *Expert Opin. Ther. Patents* **2018**, *28*, 875–882. [CrossRef]
35. Durazzo, A.; D'Addezio, L.; Camilli, E.; Piccinelli, R.; Turrini, A.; Marletta, L.; Marconi, S.; Lucarini, M.; Lisciani, S.; Gabrielli, P.; et al. From Plant Compounds to Botanicals and Back: A Current Snapshot. *Molecules* **2018**, *23*, 1844. [CrossRef]
36. Li, Q.; Yang, S.; Li, Y.; Xue, X.; Huang, Y.; Luo, H.; Zhang, Y.; Lu, Z. Comparative evaluation of soluble and insoluble-bound phenolics and antioxidant activity of two Chinese mistletoes. *Molecules* **2018**, *23*, 359. [CrossRef]
37. Li, S.; Yuan, L.; Chen, Y.; Zhou, W.; Wang, X. Studies on the inclusion complexes of daidzein with β-cyclodextrin and derivatives. *Molecules* **2017**, *22*, 2183. [CrossRef]
38. Davaatseren, M.; Jo, Y.-J.; Hong, G.-P.; Hur, H.J.; Park, S.; Choi, M.-J. Studies on the anti-oxidative function of trans-cinnamaldehyde-included β-cyclodextrin complex. *Molecules* **2017**, *22*, 1868. [CrossRef]

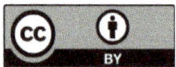

© 2019 by the authors. Licensee MDPI, Basel, Switzerland. This article is an open access article distributed under the terms and conditions of the Creative Commons Attribution (CC BY) license (http://creativecommons.org/licenses/by/4.0/).

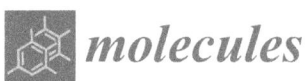

Article

Nectandra grandiflora By-Products Obtained by Alternative Extraction Methods as a Source of Phytochemicals with Antioxidant and Antifungal Properties

Daniela Thomas da Silva [1], Rene Herrera [2], Berta Maria Heinzmann [3], Javier Calvo [4] and Jalel Labidi [2,*]

1. Center of Rural Sciences, Federal University of Santa Maria, Ave. Roraima 1000, Santa Maria 97105-900, Brazil; dthomasdasilva@gmail.com
2. Biorefinery Processes Research Group, Department of Chemical and Environmental Engineering, University of the Basque Country (UPV/EHU), Plaza Europa 1, 20018 Donostia, Spain; renealexander.herrera@ehu.eus
3. Department of Industrial Pharmacy, Federal University of Santa Maria, Ave. Roraima 1000, Santa Maria 97105-900, Brazil; berta.heinzmann@gmail.com
4. Chromatography and Mass Spectrometry Platform, CIC BiomaGUNE, Paseo Miramon 182, 20009 San Sebastian, Spain; jcalvo@cicbiomagune.es
* Correspondence: jalel.labidi@ehu.es; Tel.: +34-94301-7178

Received: 26 December 2017; Accepted: 6 February 2018; Published: 9 February 2018

Abstract: *Nectandra grandiflora* Nees (Lauraceae) is a Brazilian native tree recognized by its durable wood and the antioxidant compounds of its leaves. Taking into account that the forest industry offers the opportunity to recover active compounds from its residues and by-products, this study identifies and underlines the potential of natural products from *Nectandra grandiflora* that can add value to the forest exploitation. This study shows the effect of three different extraction methods: conventional (CE), ultrasound-assisted (UAE) and microwave-assisted (MAE) on *Nectandra grandiflora* leaf extracts (NGLE) chemical yields, phenolic and flavonoid composition, physical characteristics as well as antioxidant and antifungal properties. Results indicate that CE achieves the highest extraction phytochemical yield (22.16%), but with similar chemical composition to that obtained by UAE and MAE. Moreover, CE also provided a superior thermal stability of NGLE. The phenolic composition of NGLE was confirmed firstly, by colorimetric assays and infrared spectra and then by chromatographic analysis, in which quercetin-3-*O*-rhamnoside was detected as the major compound (57.75–65.14%). Furthermore, the antioxidant capacity of the NGLE was not altered by the extraction methods, finding a high radical inhibition in all NGLE (>80% at 2 mg/mL). Regarding the antifungal activity, there was observed that NGLE possess effective bioactive compounds, which inhibit the *Aspergillus niger* growth.

Keywords: forest residues; phenolic compounds; natural antioxidants; quercitrin; value-added by-products

1. Introduction

Innovative and environmental-friendly approaches are the key to increase the profitability, economic viability and sustainability in the forest industry by optimizing the process in order to obtain high-valued products (bio/chemicals and biomaterials). Forest residues (bark, foliage, branches) represent a renewable feedstock that has been used for many years as a combustible material, however, the development of by-products is an essential path for forest valorization [1]. Tree bark and foliage constitute a little explored but promising source of natural compounds or phytochemicals (in the form of pure or as mixtures/extracts) that could be used as active ingredients for agronomic, cosmetic, food additives, pharmaceutical and in nutraceutical formulations [1,2]. Several techniques have been described for extracting active natural compounds from low-cost raw material [3]. These procedures include the so-called heating systems, such as traditional Soxhlet and heat reflux extraction [4,5], ultrasound-assisted extraction [6,7] and microwave-assisted extraction [8,9], as well as supercritical fluid and pressurized extraction [10,11] or the combination of these extraction techniques [12].

Conversely, many natural matrix products are thermally unstable and may degrade under thermal extraction conditions [12]. Moreover, large consumption of solvents, energy and lengthy extraction time are some drawbacks that should also be taken into account. The ideal extraction procedure has to retain the maximum of the bioactive constituents in a shortest processing time with low economic costs [13] and low environmental impact [14]. Additionally, the extraction methods should be simple, safer for users and with a level of automation for industrial application [14,15]. In general, the selection of an appropriate extraction procedure depends on the type of compound to be extracted, as well as the development of the technique [16]. Several studies reported the efficiency of microwave-assisted extraction (MAE) and ultrasound-assisted extraction (UAE) for increasing the content of polyphenols [9,17]. In MAE, the microwave energy is used to heat the polar solvents in contact with solid samples and thus, recovering the target compounds [18]. Likewise, the UAE involves a superficial disrupt of plant tissue, allowing the penetration of solvent into cell walls through the acoustic cavitation [19].

It is worth noting that the Brazilian flora is a rich source of phytochemicals, aromas and bioactive compounds of medicinal and pharmaceutical importance, as well the fine chemicals segment [20]. *Nectandra* is one of the largest genera of Lauraceous family that includes ca. 120 tree species and more than 190 reported different types of natural substances with several therapeutic applications [21]. *Nectandra grandiflora* Nees, commonly known as "canela-amarela" or "canela-fedida", is a medium-sized tree (10–15 m) endemic of Brazilian Atlantic forest and Cerrado biomes [22]. This species presents a moderately heavy and naturally durable wood recommended for timbering and furniture [23]. On the other hand, there are not enough scientific studies regarding the environmental-friendly and cost-effective technologies to recover phytochemicals (e.g., phenolic compounds) from *Nectandra grandiflora* leaves. Ribeiro et al. [24] extracted flavonoid glycosides (natural antioxidants) and neoliganans from the tree foliage by conventional heating processing (Soxhlet). On these grounds, the present study aims to address the unexplored potential of *Nectandra grandiflora* co-products describing the phenolic composition, thermal behavior, antioxidant and antifungal properties of its leaf extracts obtained by alternative green processes (MAE and UAE).

2. Results and Discussion

2.1. Extraction Yields and Phytochemicals Contents

Extraction yield refers to the percentage of ethanolic extract obtained from a dried plant sample through an extraction technique [17]. The three extraction methods applied on *Nectandra grandiflora* leaves showed significantly different yields of phytochemicals (Table 1).

The conventional Soxhlet (CE) method presented the highest yield (22.16 g DW/100 g dried plant), followed by ultrasound-assisted (UAE) and microwave-assisted extraction (MAE). The highest yield achieved by conventional extraction compared to ultrasound- and microwave-assisted methods can be explained by the application of heat for a longer period. However, the processing time used in ultrasound and microwave heating methods was significantly shorter (30 min) than for the conventional one and taking the energy consumption into account, UAE and MAE appear as favorable extraction methods for *Nectandra grandiflora* leaves. Our findings are in accordance with Mustapa et al. [25], who reported a superior yield of *Clinacanthus nutans* extracts by CE compared to MAE. According to Chirinos et al. [26], after 60 min, increasing extraction time did not significantly improve the phytochemical yield and may increasing the risk of phenolic oxidation (alterations in color, aroma and product quality).

Table 1. Effect of extraction method on the phytochemical yields, total phenolic (TPC) and flavonoid (FLC) contents of *Nectandra grandiflora* Nees leaf extracts.

Extraction Method	Yield (g DW/100g Dried Plant)	TPC (mg GaE/g DW)	FLC (mg QE/g DW)
CE	22.16 ± 1.18 [a]	279.00 ± 7.32 [a]	150.85 ± 0.71 [a]
UAE	13.99 ± 2.58 [b]	254.94 ± 7.58 [b]	114.50 ± 0.71 [b]
MAE	8.21 ± 2.74 [c]	229.62 ± 1.85 [c]	123.83 ± 3.60 [b]
F	28.32	62.55	22.40
p	<0.001	<0.001	0.002
MSD	2.28	10.18	5.47

Lower case letters indicate significant differences among the extraction methods for the same column by Tukey test ($p < 0.05$). CE: Conventional Soxhlet extraction; UAE: Ultrasound-assisted extraction; MAE: Microwave-assisted extraction; DW: Extract based on dried weight; GaE: Equivalent gallic acid; QE: Equivalent quercetin; MSD: Minimum Significant Difference.

In this work, the three evaluated extraction methods were able to recover high contents of total phenolic compounds, flavonoid and condensed tannins. However, we detected that the values determined in the extracts depended significantly on the process applied (Table 1). The CE extract presented higher values of total phenolic and flavonoid contents (279 mg GaE/g DW and 150.85 mg QE/g DW, respectively) than UAE and MAE extracts. Considering the composition of natural sources of polyphenols and flavonoid compounds, as well as their chemical structures and properties, an universal extraction procedure is not feasible and a specific method must be optimized for each natural bioactive compound [27,28]. Currently, some alternative techniques such as extraction under pressure (N_2) or enzymatic extraction in combination with UAE and MAE have been applied to increase phenolic yields from plant matrices [29,30].

2.2. FTIR Analysis

Leaf extracts exhibited similar absorption bands in FTIR spectra but with slight differences in the extract obtained by CE. The spectra profiles are presented in Figure 1 and the assignments are given in Table S1.

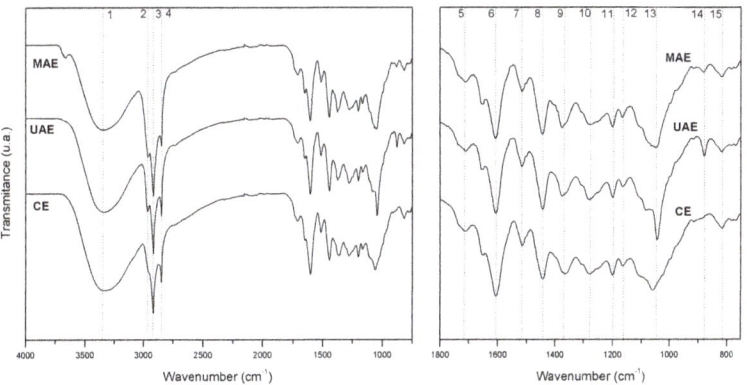

Figure 1. FTIR spectra of leaf extracts obtained from *Nectandra grandiflora*, by conventional Soxhlet extraction (CE), ultrasound-assisted extraction (UAE) and microwave-assisted extraction (MAE). Wavenumber range 4000–800 cm^{-1} (**Left**) and fingerprint region 1800–750 cm^{-1} (**Right**); band assignments are shown in Table S1.

Analysis of the FTIR spectra ranging from 3400 to 3200 cm^{-1} shows the sum of different vibrational bands of –OH groups. The elongated U shape around this region is characteristic of alcoholic and phenolic compounds [31,32]. The region of 2945–2845 cm^{-1} is composed by the overlapping of the CH$_2$, and CH$_3$ stretching asymmetric and symmetric vibrations; possibly derived from carbohydrates [33].

However, these first regions analysed do not present conclusive features to identify the nature of the phytochemicals. Several authors have described the FTIR spectra fingerprinting region (1800–750 cm^{-1}) because the target functional groups appear primarily in this range [25]. The weak peak at 1709 cm^{-1} shows the presence of the carbonyl group, possibly due to dimeric saturated acids [31]. The signals detected in the range 1615–1440 cm^{-1} (peaks 6–8) are assigned to aromatic ring stretching vibrations. A strong and intense peak at 1606 cm^{-1} corresponds to within-ring skeletal stretching, alongside with the stretching of the C=C–C aromatic bond that appears at 1515 cm^{-1}.

The peak in the region of 1375–1361 cm^{-1} is assigned to the hydroxyl in-plane bending of primary and secondary alcohols [31,34]. Furthermore, *Nectandra grandiflora* extracts also show bands in the 1277–1271 cm^{-1} region, which correspond to the C–O asymmetrical stretching vibration arising from the pyran-derived ring structure of flavonoids [33]. The peak around 1200 cm^{-1} is associated with phenol C–OH stretches.

The 1154–1046 cm^{-1} region (peak 13) can be assigned to the C–H in-plane deformation of aromatic compounds [33]. The extract obtained by UAE exhibited a strong and intense peak, while the other extracts only exhibit shoulders in this region. Finally, the aromatic C–H out-of-plane bending vibration region between 920 and 750 cm^{-1} mostly shows signals of low intensity [32]. The extract obtained by ultrasound technique shows a medium-intensity signal at 878 cm^{-1} corresponding to the deformation of the C–H bond in a substituted *meta*-diaromatic compound [35]. This signal was lower for the MAE extract and did not appear at all in the CE extract. Another low-intensity peak at 816 cm^{-1} can be seen in the FTIR spectra of all extracts.

The presence of peaks due to hydroxyl and carbonyl vibrations indicates that there are some polar compounds in the *Nectandra grandiflora* foliage extracts, such as flavonoids, neolignans and phenolic acids. These results are in agreement with those found by the total phenolic and flavonoid contents in this study and other scientific studies [24,36].

2.3. LC-UV/ESI-HR-MS and MALDI/MS/MS Analysis

In the LC-MS and MALDI/MS/MS analysis of *Nectandra grandiflora* leaf extracts, six compounds were detected based on their retention time, UV (wavelength of maximum absorbance) and mass spectra and MS fragmentation parameters. The molecular mass of the compounds was obtained from their positive ion electrospray mass spectra (ESI-MS), which showed the corresponding protonated pseudomolecular ions as well as the sodium adduct ions (parent ions). Table 2 lists the major (>5%) compounds detected in *Nectandra grandiflora* extracts.

Table 2. Phenolic compounds detected in the leaf extracts obtained from *Nectandra grandiflora* Nees by LC-UV/ESI-HR-MS in the positive mode.

CE							
Proposed Compound	Peak	t$_R$ (min)	λ$_{max}$ (nm)	MW	[M + Na]$^+$ (m/z)	Fragment Ions (m/z)	Peak Area (%)
Myricetin-rhamnoside	1	10.17	256.93; 351.93	464	487.1861	319.1163; 273.2263	11.26
Quercetin-rhamnoside	2	11.72	255.93; 349.93	448	471.1797	303.1064; 325.1030	65.32
Kaempferol-rhamnoside	3	12.96	263.93	432	455.1926	218.2257; 287.1182; 304.2944	5.13
Unidentified	6	19.98	253.93	250	273.2414	219.3682; 149.1013; 137.0943	15.57
Total identified							81.71
MAE							
Proposed Compound	Peak	t$_R$ (min)	λ$_{max}$ (nm)	MW	[M + Na]$^+$ (m/z)	Fragment Ions (m/z)	Peak Area (%)
Myricetin-rhamnoside	1	10.14	258.93; 352.93	464	487.1981	319.1164; 273.2266; 341.1031	9.95

Table 2. Cont.

Proposed Compound	Peak	t_R (min)	λ_{max} (nm)	MW	[M + Na]$^+$ (m/z)	Fragment Ions (m/z)	Peak Area (%)
MAE							
Quercetin-rhamnoside	2	11.69	255.93; 340.93	448	471.1819	**303.1085**; 325.1035	62.54
Kaempferol-rhamnoside	3	12.93	263.93	432	455.1905	**287.1170**; 218.2304; 309.1042	5.50
Unidentified	6	19.98	254.93	250	273.2419	**219.3695**; 149.1015	19.58
Total identified							77.99
UAE							
Proposed Compound	Peak	t_R (min)	λ_{max} (nm)	MW	[M + Na]$^+$ (m/z)	Fragment Ions (m/z)	Peak Area (%)
Myricetin-rhamnoside	1	10.14	256.93; 348.93	464	487.1881	**319.1158**; 273.2258; 341.1027	9.77
Quercetin-rhamnoside	2	11.69	255.93; 349.93	448	471.1833	**303.1102**; 325.1038	61.18
Kaempferol-rhamnoside	3	12.93	263.93	432	455.1806	**287.1170**; 218.2305; 304.2939	5.11
Unidentified	6	19.98	255.00	250	273.2429	**220.2213**; 149.1024; 137.0951	20.83
Total identified							76.06

The base peaks are in bold; CE: Conventional Soxhlet extraction; UAE: Ultrasound-assisted extraction; MAE: Microwave-assisted extraction.

All extracts presented a similar phenolic profile (Figure 2) with some differences in the estimated percentages of the compounds. More than 76% of the total chemical composition was established, achieving 81.71% in the conventional method. The compounds identified are glycosylated flavonols, of which quercetin rhamnoside (quercitrin) was the most abundant in the extract obtained by the conventional method (65.32%). Kaempferol rhamnoside (afzelin) (11.26–9.77%) and myricetin rhamnoside (myricitrin) (<6%) were also detected. Figure S2 shows the MS fragmentation of the peaks 1, 2 and 3 obtained through MALDI/MS/MS analysis, where is possible to see the fragmentation of glycosides by loss of the mass corresponding to rhamnose (≈146 Da).

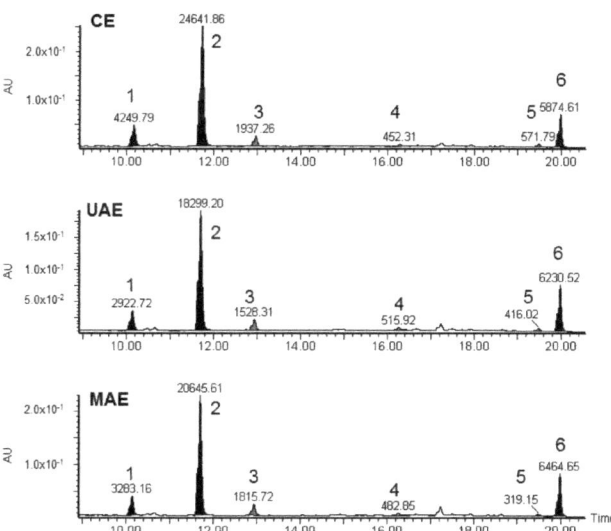

Figure 2. LC-UV chromatograms at 280 nm of the *Nectandra grandiflora* extracts obtained by conventional Soxhlet extraction (CE), ultrasound-assisted extraction (UAE) and microwave-assisted extraction (MAE). For peak identification, see Table 2.

The peak numbers 4–6 were not identified by the LC-MS and MALDI/MS/MS techniques, but taking into account the UV spectrum of peak 6 (maximum absorbance in the 251–255 nm range) and MW data (250 MW), we hypothesized that this peak could correspond to a low molecular weight substance, such as a polyalcohol or a phenolic acid. Besides, according to Rijke et al. [37], flavonoids display a typical UV spectrum with a first absorbance maximum in the 240–285 nm range and a second one in the 300–550 nm range, as exhibited by quercitrin and myricitrin.

In previous studies, the compounds quercitrin and afzelin were identified in the ethanolic leaf extract from a *Nectandra grandiflora* specimen collected in São Paulo, Brazil [24,36]. Moreover, Ribeiro et al. [24] found protocatechuic acid, a naturally occurring phenolic acid, as constituent of *Nectandra grandiflora* leaves. Other phenolic compounds such as neolignan licarin B [38] and burchellin [24] were isolated from *Nectandra grandiflora* leaves and fruits, respectively.

2.4. TG/DTG Profiles

Thermal analysis was carried out as a first step to characterize the decomposition stages and thermal stability of *Nectandra grandiflora* extracts in the absence of parallel reactions. The TG/DTG curves of all extracts exhibited similar decomposition patterns, as displayed in Figure 3.

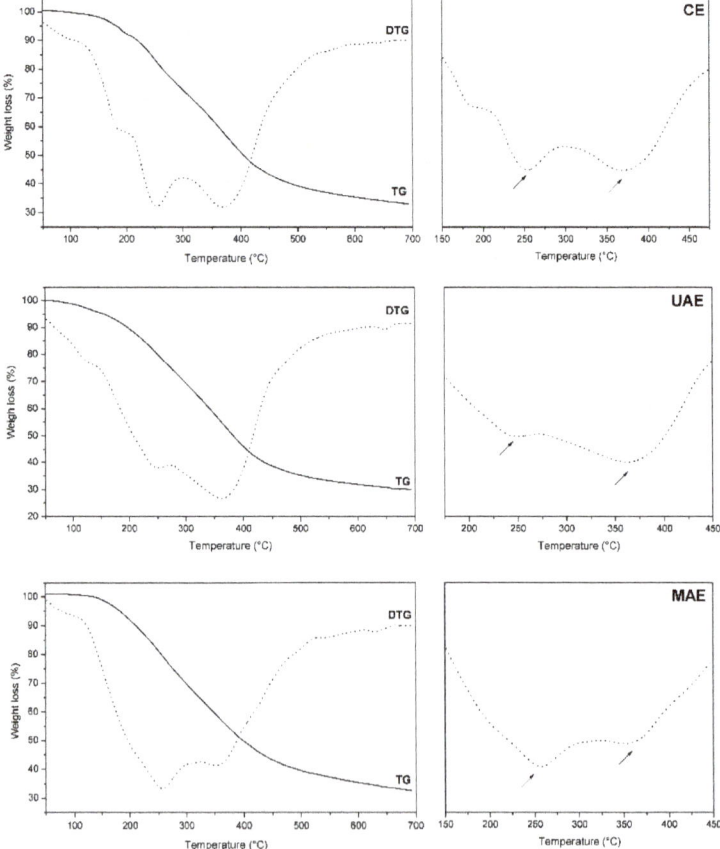

Figure 3. TG/DTG profiles of *Nectandra grandiflora* extracts obtained by different techniques. CE: Conventional Soxhlet extraction; UAE: Ultrasound-assisted extraction; MAE: Microwave-assisted extraction. The arrows indicate the temperatures where the greatest mass loss occurred.

During the extraction process, several bioactive substances from different class can be recovered from the plant raw material. Besides phenolic compounds, polar solvents (such as ethanol) can also extract lipids, fats, terpenoids, sugars and chlorophylls [36].

DTG curves from all extracts showed a slight mass loss within the temperature range 50–180 °C, which was mainly caused by water desorption [39] and decomposition of terpenoid derivatives (volatile compounds) [40]. All thermograms showed two main degradation peaks indicating the main organic matter losses [41]. The first one was between 240 and 270 °C (peak 1), and the second between 340 and 380 °C (peak 2). Peak 1 may be attributed to thermal breakdown of aliphatic structures and glycosylated aromatic compounds (such as quercetin-3-O-rhamnoside detected by the LC-MS technique), and peak 2 was associated with the degradation of more stable compounds [39–44].

At the end of the TG process (about 700 °C), the solid residues for CE, UAE and MAE were 32.76, 29.85 and 31.88%, respectively. The percentage of residual mass in the CE sample can be attributed to the higher presence of phenolic substances (78.66% estimated by LC-MS), which tend to become fixed carbon during the pyrolysis process [45].

2.5. Solubility Results

The solubility of the obtained extracts was evaluated using an organic solvent and then analysing the optical images formed by the solutions (Figure S1). We detected similar physical characteristics (solubility) of the obtained extracts. The solution prepared with CE sample presented an average concentration of 3.98 × 106 particles/µL, while UAE sample presented 3.49 × 106 particles/µL and MAE, 3.31 × 106 particles/µL. No pronounced variation in the average diameter of the undissolved particles was observed among the extract solutions, only a slight variation between MAE and CE samples was detected (4.9 µm and 5.1 µm, respectively). The applied method is a novel fast assessment that provides useful information such as particle size and organic solubilization, which are important characteristics in the natural materials subject and regarding environmental issues [46].

2.6. Antioxidant Activity

Regarding the antioxidant activities, *Nectandra grandiflora* leaf extracts were able to inhibit both DPPH and ABTS free radicals, in comparison with quercetin, used as positive control. The antioxidant effect in a concentration-response relationship was verified in all samples and the corresponding equations are displayed in Figure 4.

All ethanolic extracts showed good scavenging activities to reduce the stable radical DPPH to yellow-colored 2,2-diphenyl-1-picrylhydrazine. Besides, the results indicate that there are no significant differences between the *Nectandra grandiflora* extract samples at the same tested concentration. At the highest concentration (2 mg/mL), the DPPH radical inhibition reached 85.59% with CE and UAE, and 82.39% with MAE. Quercetin reached 86.85% of inhibition at 2 mg/mL, significantly different in all *Nectandra grandiflora* samples. In the ABTS radical cation decoloration assay, the leaf extracts have a similar inhibition rate to that found against DPPH radical. No statistical differences among any of the samples were detected at 2 mg/mL (Figure 4B). At the lowest concentration, UAE presented better values than the CE and MAE procedures; however, these values were lower than those achieved by the positive control was. Considering the R^2 values among the tests, the observed differences can be due to the reaction environment (alcoholic or hydro-alcoholic), the solubility of the main compounds in each reaction medium as well as the variable activity of antioxidants in reducing the pre-formed radical cation radical ($ABTS^{\bullet+}$) to ABTS [47].

Our findings illustrate the antioxidant capacity of *Nectandra grandiflora* leaves was weakly affected by the extraction protocol [17]. The positive results detected can be assigned to the phytochemicals present in the leaf extracts. Probably the most active natural phytochemicals in the *Nectandra grandiflora* extracts are from the flavonoid chemical class, since they present specific structural characteristics that promote antioxidant activity. The o-catechol group on the B-ring as occurs in quercetin derivatives, the major phytochemicals detected in this study, is the most important of them [48]. Moreover, the same partial structure appears in protocatechuic acid [49], already described in *Nectandra grandiflora* [24]. Other flavonoids with chemical characteristics can contribute the antioxidant properties, such as the three hydroxyl groups on the B-ring (present in myricetin derivatives) and the α,β-unsaturated carbonyl system on the C-ring [45]. These characteristics confer great stability to the phenolic radical as soon it is formed after one H radical donation to DPPH [24,50,51].

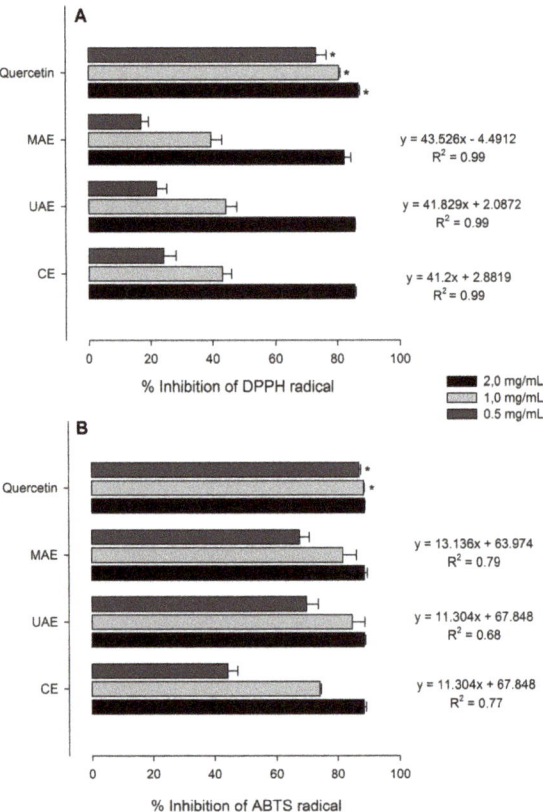

Figure 4. Antioxidant capacities on DPPH (**A**) and ABTS (**B**) free radicals of leaf extracts obtained from *Nectandra grandiflora*. * Indicate significant differences among the extraction methods and quercetin for the same concentration by Tukey test ($p < 0.05$). CE: Conventional Soxhlet extraction; UAE: Ultrasound-assisted extraction; MAE: Microwave-assisted extraction; Quercetin: Positive control.

2.7. Antifungal Activity

The methods used to measure the antifungal effect of the extracts were designed to determine both the efficacy of compounds to prevent fungal growth and as a method to assess the susceptibility of the growth of molds to impregnated materials. Results from exposure of *Aspergillus. niger* to various concentrations of *Nectandra grandiflora* extracts are displayed in Figure 5, which in turn were contrasted with a positive control (amphotericin B) and with a negative control (without product).

As indicated in Figure 5, the leaf extracts did not inhibit fungal growth dose-dependently according to the evaluated methods. In Figure 5A, all extracts tested at 100 mg/mL of concentration were effective in controlling the fungal growth (growth intensity = 1), by visual assessment (without contact with the center of the dish).

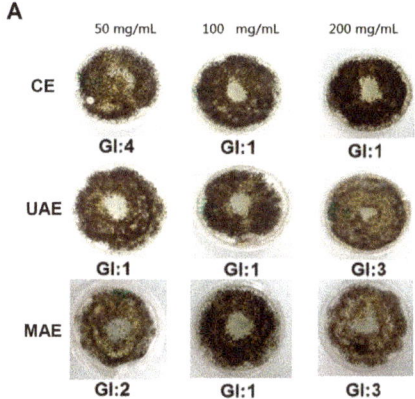

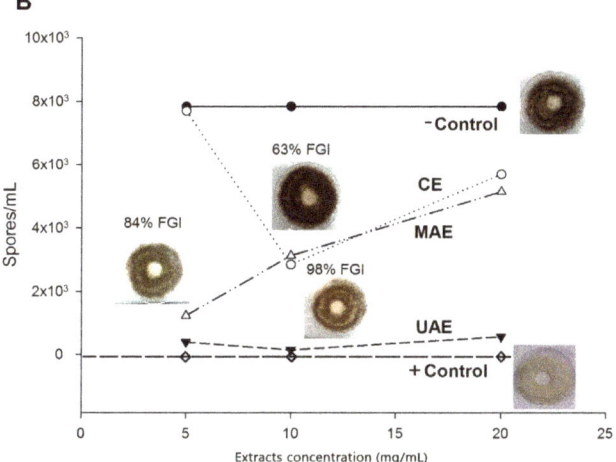

Figure 5. Antifungal activity of *Nectandra grandiflora* extracts against *Aspergillus niger* by the potato dextrose agar method (**A**) and cellulose pellets method (**B**). GI: Growth intensity; FGI: Fungal growth inhibition; CE: Conventional Soxhlet extraction; UAE: Ultrasound-assisted extraction; MAE: Microwave-assisted extraction.

At 200 mg/mL, the samples of CE were more efficient than those samples from UAE and MAE (growth intensity = 3). A similar trend of fungal growth inhibition was observed with the second method (cellulose pellets; Figure 5B). The CE sample at 100 mg/mL inhibited 63% of fungal growth and UAE extract reached to a maximum of 98% at the final concentration of 100 mg/mL, compared to non-treated control. Regarding the MAE sample, higher fungal inhibition (84%) was achieved at a concentration of 50 mg/mL.

To the best of our knowledge, there are no reports regarding the inhibitory potential of *Nectandra grandiflora* against *Aspergillus niger*. Previously, the antifungal activity of the *Nectandra grandiflora* leaf essential oil against wood-rot fungi was reported [40], where it was able to inhibit *Pycnoporus sanguineus* and *Gloeophyllum trabeum* growth at a concentration of 5 µl/mL. From these findings and from Magro et al.'s study [52], which examined the *Anthemis nobilis* leaf extract and found an inhibitory effect at 920 mg/mL against *Aspergillus niger*, we can affirm that the *Nectandra grandiflora* leaves possess potential antifungal constituents.

3. Materials and Methods

3.1. Plant Material

Aerial parts of *Nectandra grandiflora* were collected from a natural habitat in Jaguari County, in the South of Brazil (29°26' S and 54°40' W), in December 2013. Leaves were separated from the branches and fractionated in order to achieve the ethanolic extracts. A voucher specimen, identified by Solon Jonas Longhi, is archived under number 13162 at the Herbarium of Biology Department (SMDB, Federal University of Santa Maria, Brazil).

3.2. Preparation of Ethanolic Extracts

Leaves were air-dried at room temperature (25 °C), milled (Willey mill, Swedesboro, NJ, USA) and then extracted with ethanol 96%, which is regarded as a generally recognized as safe (GRAS) solvent, at a raw material: solvent ratio of 1:20, by means of ultrasound-assisted extraction (UAE), microwave-assisted extraction (MAE) or conventional solvent extraction (CE) [17]. The extraction procedures were as follows: the UAE was carried out using an ultrasonic cleaner (Elmasonic S 70H, Elma Schmidbauer GmbH, Singen, Germany) at a power of 750 W and 50 °C and MAE was done with a CEM Discover microwave (CEM Corporation, Matthews, NC, USA) at 50 °C and power controlled by the equipment. Both UAE and MAE were performed for 30 min using ca. 5 g per replicate ($n = 3$). The CE was performed using a Soxhlet apparatus (Hermanos Álamo, Madrid, Spain) (ca. 15 g per replicate; $n = 3$) until the total exhaustion of the plant material (24 h). After the extraction period, the ethanolic extracts were cooled to room temperature and filtered. The solvent was removed at 50 °C under reduced pressure on a rotary evaporator and then the extraction yields were calculated by weighing the extracts obtained per each 100 grams of dried plant based on dried weight (DW).

3.3. Total Phenolic Content

The total phenolic content of *Nectandra grandiflora* leaf extracts was measured spectrophotometrically (Jasco V-630 spectrophotometer, Jasco Deutschland GmbH, Hamburg, Germany) by the Folin-Ciocalteu's method, as described by Cândido et al. [53], with some modifications. Dried extracts were solubilized in methanol (0.5 mg/mL), aliquots of these samples (0.25 mL) were mixed with 2.5 mL of distilled water, and 0.25 mL of the Folin-Ciocalteu reagent (previously diluted 1:10 with distilled water). After 5 min, 0.25 mL of sodium carbonate (75 mg/mL in aqueous solution) was added and adjusted to 10 mL with distilled water. The mixtures were kept at room temperature for 60 min and the absorbance was measured at 725 nm. Gallic acid (0–0.2 mg/mL) was used for calibration of a standard curve. The calibration curve was linear at $R^2 = 0.99$, and the results were expressed as mg of gallic acid equivalents per gram of dried weight (mg GaE/g DW). Triplicate measurements were taken and data were presented as mean ± standard deviation.

3.4. Flavonoid Content

The flavonoid content of the extracts was determined by the $AlCl_3$ technique [54] using a spectrophotometer (Jasco V-630). The results were expressed as mg of quercetin equivalents (QE) per g DW from a standard calibration curve (0–0.1 mg/mL; $R^2 = 0.99$).

3.5. Infrared Analysis

In order to determine the functional groups presents in CE, UAE and MAE samples, Fourier Transform Infrared (FTIR) analysis was applied. Infrared spectra were recorded in a Perkin Elmer spectrophotometer (Waltham, MA, USA) at a resolution of 4 cm^{-1} over the 700–4000 cm^{-1} range using milled samples [55].

3.6. LC-UV/ESI-HR-MS Analysis

LC-UV/ESI-HR-MS analysis was carried out on a UPLC system (Waters ACQUITY UPLC System, Milford, MA, USA) equipped with a UV-Vis photodiode array detector and coupled to a mass spectrometer. UV spectra were recorded between 200 and 500 nm and the UV detection was measured at 280 nm (100% correspond to sum of area of six detected peaks in each sample). An Acquity C_{18} column (100 × 2.1 mm i.d., 1.7 µm) at 40 °C was used to chromatography separation. The mobile phase was constituted by two solvents: water-formic acid (0.1%, A) and methanol (B), and the gradient elution had the following profile: 0–25 min 95% A, 25–27.7 min 1% A and 27.7–30 min 5% A at a flow rate of 300 µL/min. Extract samples were prepared at 200 µg/mL in methanol:water (1:1) and 10 µL aliquots were injected for analysis.

Mass spectra were acquired using a LCT Premier XE (Waters) equipped with an electrospray ionization (ESI) source operated in the positive W mode. The experimental parameters were set as follows: the capillary voltage was 750 V; cone voltage was 50 V; and ions were recorded in the range of m/z 100–1000. In order to obtain exact mass measurements, leukine-enkephalin was used as lockmass reference compound (m/z 556.2771). Data acquisition and analysis were performed using Waters MassLynx 4.1 software (Waters Corporation, Milford, MA, USA).

3.7. MALDI-TOF/TOF MS Analysis

MALDI-TOF/TOF mass analysis were performed on an Ultraflextreme III time-of-flight mass spectrometer equipped with a pulsed Nd:YAG laser (355 nm) and controlled by FlexControl 3.3 software (Bruker Daltonics, Bremen, Germany). The acquisitions (total of 4000–5000) were carried out in positive reflector ion mode with pulse duration of 70 ns, laser fluence of 35% and laser frequency of 1 kHz. Laser intensity was set marginally above the threshold of ionization to avoid fragmentation (less than 10% for all the cases). Fragmentation of the molecules were performed with a LIFT cell voltage of 19 kV and a final acceleration voltage set at 29.3 kV and the parent mass ions were assigned manually (monoisotopic peak M + Na). Ion source 1, 2 and lens voltages were set at 7.56, 6.86 and 3.52. 5 µL of sample (extract at 200 µg/mL in Water/MeOH) was mixed with 10 µL of α-Cyano-4-hydroxycinnamic acid matrix solution (10 mg/mL in Methanol Water 1/1). 1 µL of the analyte/matrix mixture was deposited onto the polished stainless-steel MALDI target plate and was allowed to dry.

All the peaks were detected as sodium/potassium adducts. The acquired data was processed (baseline substraction and normalized) using the Bruker FlexAnalysis 3.3 software (Bruker Daltonics, Bremen, Germany).

3.8. Thermogravimetric Analysis

Thermal behavior of *Nectandra grandiflora* extracts (CE, UAE and MAE) was measured in a nitrogen atmosphere using a TGA/SDTA RSI analyser (Mettler Toledo, L'Hospitalet de Llobregat, Barcelona, Spain) according to Herrera et al. [55]. For the quantitative calculations, the response factors between the weight gain (TG) and the mass loss rate (DTG) were determined.

3.9. Solubility Measurement of Extracts

To investigate the extracts solubility in organic solvents, CE, UAE and MAE samples were diluted in dimethyl sulfoxide (DMSO) at a concentration of 10 mg/mL and the solubility was analyzed by a Cellometer® Mini Vision equipment (Nexcelom Bioscience LLC, Lawrence, MA, USA). Each extract solution was precisely pipetted (0.02 mL) into a Nexcelom disposable counting chamber to determinate the concentration of undissolved extracts (particles/µL) and the particles sizes (average size from 1 to 35 µm) by the Cellometer® Mini Counter Software (Nexcelom Bioscience LLC, Lawrence, MA, USA, Software version 1.2.3.3).

3.10. Antioxidant Activities

3.10.1. DPPH Assay

The DPPH (2,2-diphenyl-1-picrylhydrazyl) radical scavenging activity of the extracts was carried out according to Dudonné et al. [56] on a Jasco V-630 Spectrophotometer. An aliquot (0.02 mL) of leaf extracts at different concentrations was added to 2 mL of DPPH methanolic solution (0.06 mM) and kept at room temperature for 30 min. The absorbance was measured at 517 nm and quercetin was utilized as positive control.

3.10.2. ABTS Assay

The antioxidant capacity was also evaluated by ABTS spectrophotometric assay [47]. Extract samples were diluted in methanol at different concentrations and an aliquot (0.04 mL) was added to 2 mL of ABTS radical solution. This solution was prepared by mixing ABTS (7 mM) and potassium persulfate (2.45 mM) in water for 12–16 h at room temperature in a light-free environment. Then, the absorbance of radical solution was adjusted to 0.60 ± 0.02 at 734 nm in ethanol: water (1:1). Each extract sample was measured between 1 and 6 min.

3.11. Determination of Antifungal Activity against Aspergillus niger

The fungus *Aspergillus niger* (Tiegh MB284309 CBS-KNAW, Utrecht, The Netherlands) was cultured on potato dextrose agar (PDA) for 7 days at $27 \pm 1.5\ °C$ and used in this assay. Extracts samples were diluted in DMSO at final concentrations of 50, 100 and 200 mg/mL, and then evaluated by two methods: (1) extracts pipetted directly in PDA medium and inoculated with fungal strain; and (2) extracts impregnated in cellulose pellets and exposed to fungal strain in PDA.

In the first method, an aliquot (40 µL) of each extract was pipetted to the center of a Petri dish filled with PDA, and around that was inoculated a fungal strain. The Petri dishes were sealed and incubated at $27 \pm 1.5\ °C$ (Selecta Medilow climatic chamber, JP Selecta S.A., Barcelona, Spain) for 7 days. After incubation time, we determined the growth intensity (GI) by visual assessment using a numerical scale according to ISO 846, as displayed in Table 3. Three repetitions of each extracts and control (without extracts) were prepared.

Table 3. Visual assessment of growth intensity according to ISO 846.

Growth Intensity (GI)	Evaluation
0	No growth apparent under magnification
1	No visible growth but visible under magnification
2	Visible growth up to 25% coverage
3	Visible growth up to 50% coverage
4	Visible growth up to 75% coverage
5	Heavy growth covering more than 75% of the studied area

In parallel, cellulose pellets (ø = 10 mm) were soaked with 5 µL of each extract set and placed on Petri dishes with PDA (10 mL) and 0.4% streptomycin. Each PDA dish was inoculated with a spore suspension (1×10^6 spores/mL) and incubated at $27 \pm 1.5\ °C$ for 7 days. Subsequently, pellets were removed from Petri dishes and washed with sterile Ringer's solution (Sigma-Aldrich-96724, St. Louis, MI, USA). The solution was stained (Lactophenol blue) and homogenized to count the spores concentration on the pellets with a Cellometer® Mini automated cell counter by placing 20 µL of each spore solution inside counting chambers and using Cellometer® Mini software for the analysis. The fungal growth inhibition (FGI %) was calculated as concentration of spores (conidia) per mL, according to the following Equation (1):

$$\text{FGI (\%)} = \frac{Cg - Tg}{Cg} \times 100 \qquad (1)$$

where, *Cg* is the average spores concentration in the control sample and *Tg* is the average concentration in the treated one [57].

3.12. Statistical Procedure

The results are expressed as the mean of three measurements ± standard deviation. Normality (Shapiro-Wilk) and Equal Variance (Levene) tests were performed before the statistical approach. Analysis of variance (ANOVA) was conducted for the values of total phenolic, flavonoid and tannin contents, as well as for antioxidants data, followed by Tukey test. The differences with $p < 0.05$ were considered significant.

4. Conclusions

The experimental results indicated that ultrasound- and microwave-assisted extraction techniques were effective to recover bioactive compounds from *Nectrandra grandiflora* leaves. Despite the fact that higher phytochemical contents were achieved by conventional extraction, the chemical composition, thermal stability and antioxidant activity did not present great differences to that found with the alternative green techniques. Besides, microwave- and ultrasound-assisted are timesaving extraction processes with lower energy consumption comparing to the Soxhlet method; however, it is necessary to optimize the ultrasound and microwave process conditions to increase the phytochemical yields. Furthermore, *Nectandra grandiflora* by-products could be an interesting source of active compounds for the natural antioxidants and antifungal market.

Supplementary Materials: The Supplementary Materials are available online.

Acknowledgments: This research was financially supported by the Department of Education of Basque Government (IT1008-16) and by Conselho Nacional de Desenvolvimento Científico e Tecnológico (CNPq process 454447/2014-0). Authors would like to thanks the CNPq for research grants received by Berta Maria Heinzmann, Ph.D. scholarship (process 203796/2014-4) granted to Daniela Thomas da Silva and the Basque Government for scholarship of young researchers training granted to Rene Herrera.

Author Contributions: Daniela Thomas da Silva, Berta Maria Heinzmann and Jalel Labidi conceived and designed the experiments; Daniela Thomas da Silva prepared the ethanolic extracts and analyzed the total phenolic content and antioxidant capacity; Javier Calvo prepared the LC-UV/ESI-HR-MS and MALDI-TOF/TOF MS analysis; Rene Herrera determined the antifungal activity; Daniela Thomas da Silva and Rene Herrera analyzed the TGA, FT-IR and solubility; Daniela Thomas da Silva and Rene Herrera wrote the article.

Conflicts of Interest: The authors declare no conflict of interest.

References

1. Devappa, R.K.; Rakshit, S.K.; Dekker, R.F.H. Forest biorefinery: Potential of poplar phytochemicals as value-added co-products. *Biotechnol. Adv.* **2015**, *33*, 681–716. [CrossRef] [PubMed]
2. Romani, A.; Pinelli, P.; Ieri, F.; Bernini, R. Sustainability, innovation, and green chemistry in the production and valorization of phenolic extracts from *Olea europaea* L. *Sustainability* **2016**, *8*, 1002–1012. [CrossRef]
3. Balasundram, N.; Sundram, K.; Samman, S. Phenolic compounds in plants and agri-industrial by-products: Antioxidant activity, occurrence, and potential uses. *Food Chem.* **2006**, *99*, 191–203. [CrossRef]
4. Yang, Y.; Chen, H.; Lin, C.; Chu, W.; Lo, H. Species distribution and drug susceptibilities of *Candida* isolates in TSARY 2010. *Diagn. Microbiol. Infect. Dis.* **2013**, *76*, 182–186. [CrossRef] [PubMed]
5. Pan, X.; Niu, G.; Liu, H. Comparison of microwave-assisted extraction and conventional extraction techniques for the extraction of tanshinones from *Salvia miltiorrhiza bunge*. *Biochem. Eng. J.* **2002**, *12*, 71–77. [CrossRef]
6. Hemwimol, S.; Pavasant, P.; Shotipruk, A. Ultrasound-assisted extraction of anthraquinones from roots of *Morinda citrifolia*. *Ultrason. Sonochem.* **2006**, *13*, 543–548. [CrossRef] [PubMed]

7. Rodríguez-Pérez, C.; Quirantes-Piné, R.; Fernández-Gutiérrez, A.; Segura-Carretero, A. Optimization of extraction method to obtain a phenolic compounds-rich extract from *Moringa oleifera* Lam leaves. *Ind. Crops Prod.* **2015**, *66*, 246–254. [CrossRef]
8. Zhang, B.; Yang, R.; Liu, C. Microwave-assisted extraction of chlorogenic acid from flower buds of *Lonicera japonica* Thunb. *Sep. Purif. Technol.* **2008**, *62*, 480–483. [CrossRef]
9. Dahmoune, F.; Nayak, B.; Moussi, K.; Remini, H.; Madani, K. Optimization of microwave-assisted extraction of polyphenols from *Myrtus communis* L. leaves. *Food Chem.* **2015**, *166*, 585–595. [CrossRef] [PubMed]
10. Castro-Vargas, H.I.; Rodríguez-Varela, L.I.; Ferreira, S.R.; Parada-Alfonso, F. Extraction of phenolic fraction from guava seeds (*Psidium guajava* L.) using supercritical carbon dioxide and co-solvents. *J. Supercrit. Fluids* **2010**, *51*, 319–324. [CrossRef]
11. Monrad, J.K.; Howard, L.R.; King, J.W.; Srinivas, K.; Mauromoustakos, A. Subcritical solvent extraction of anthocyanins from dried red grape pomace. *J. Agric. Food Chem.* **2010**, *58*, 2862–2868. [CrossRef] [PubMed]
12. Wei, M.; Yang, Y.; Chiu, H.; Hong, S. Development of a hyphenated procedure of heat-reflux and ultrasound-assisted extraction followed by RP-HPLC separation for the determination of three flavonoids content in *Scutellaria barbata* D. Don. *J. Chromatogr. B* **2013**, *940*, 126–134. [CrossRef] [PubMed]
13. Wang, J.; Lu, H.D.; Muḥammad, U.; Han, J.Z.; Wei, Z.H.; Lu, Z.X.; Bie, X.M.; Lu, F.X. Ultrasound-assisted extraction of polysaccharides from *Artemisia selengensis* Turcz and its antioxidant and anticancer activities. *J. Food Sci. Technol.* **2016**, *53*, 1025–1034. [CrossRef] [PubMed]
14. Vilkhu, K.; Mawson, R.; Simons, L.; Bates, D. Applications and opportunities for ultrasound assisted extraction in the food industry—A review. *Innov. Food Sci. Emerg. Technol.* **2008**, *9*, 161–169. [CrossRef]
15. Zhang, Z.; Wang, X.; Li, J.; Wang, G.; Mao, G. Extraction and free radical scavenging activity of polysaccharide from 'Anji Baicha' (*Camellia sinensis* (L.) O. Kuntze). *Int. J. Biol. Macromol.* **2016**, *84*, 161–165. [CrossRef] [PubMed]
16. Wijngaard, H.; Hossain, M.B.; Rai, D.K.; Brunton, N. Techniques to extract bioactive compounds from food by-products of plant origin. *Food Res. Int.* **2012**, *46*, 505–513. [CrossRef]
17. Nguyen, V.T.; Bowyer, M.C.; Vuong, Q.V.; Altena, I.A.; Scarlett, C.J. Phytochemicals and antioxidant capacity of Xao tam phan (*Paramignya trimera*) root as affected by various solvents and extraction methods. *Ind. Crops Prod.* **2015**, *67*, 192–200. [CrossRef]
18. Delazar, A.; Nahar, L.; Hamedeyazdan, S.; Sarker, S.D. Microwave-assisted extraction in natural products isolation. *Methods Mol. Biol.* **2012**, *864*, 89–115. [PubMed]
19. Wang, L.; Li, D.; Bao, C.; You, J.; Wang, Z.; Shi, Y.; Zhang, H. Ultrasonic extraction and separation of anthraquinones from *Rheum palmatum* L. *Ultrason. Sonochem.* **2008**, *15*, 738–746. [CrossRef] [PubMed]
20. Vieira, R.F.; Bizzo, H.R.; Deschamps, C. Genetic resources of aromatic plants from Brazil. *Isr. J. Plant Sci.* **2010**, *58*, 263–271. [CrossRef]
21. Grecco, S.S.; Lorenzi, H.; Tempone, A.G.; Lago, J.H.G. Update: Biological and chemical aspects of *Nectandra* genus (Lauraceae). *Tetrahedron Asymmetry* **2016**, *27*, 793–810. [CrossRef]
22. Lorenzi, H. *Árvores Brasileiras: Manual de Identificação e Cultivo de Plantas Arbóreas Nativas do Brasil*, 2nd ed.; Instituto Plantarum: Nova Odessa, Brazil, 2002.
23. Lorenzi, H. *Árvores Brasileiras: Manual de Identificação e Cultivo de Plantas Arbóreas Nativas do Brasil*, 3rd ed.; Instituto Plantarum: Nova Odessa, Brazil, 2009.
24. Ribeiro, A.B.; Bolzani, V.D.S.; Yoshida, M.; Santos, L.S.; Eberlin, M.N.; Silva, D.H.S. A new neolignan and antioxidant phenols from *Nectandra grandiflora*. *J. Braz. Chem. Soc.* **2005**, *16*, 526–530. [CrossRef]
25. Mustapa, A.N.; Martin, Á.; Mato, R.B.; Cocero, M.J. Extraction of phytocompounds from the medicinal plant *Clinacanthus nutans* Lindau by microwave-assisted extraction and supercritical carbon dioxide extraction. *Ind. Crops Prod.* **2015**, *74*, 83–94. [CrossRef]
26. Chirinos, R.; Rogez, H.; Campos, D.; Pedreschi, R.; Larondelle, Y. Optimization of extraction conditions of antioxidant phenolic compounds from mashua (*Tropaeolum tuberosum* Ruíz & Pavón) tubers. *Sep. Purif. Technol.* **2007**, *55*, 217–225.
27. Madja, M.H.; Rajaei, A.; Bashi, D.S.; Mortazavi, S.A.; Bolourian, S. Optimization of ultrasonic-assisted extraction of phenolic compounds from bovine pennyroyal (*Phlomidoschema parviflorum*) leaves using response surface methodology. *Ind. Crops Prod.* **2014**, *57*, 195–202.

28. Vuong, Q.V.; Hiruna, S.; Roach, P.D.; Bowyer, M.C.; Phillips, P.A.; Scarlett, C.J. Effect of extraction conditions on total phenolic compounds and antioxidant activities of *Carica papaya* leaf aqueous extracts. *J. Herb. Med.* **2013**, *3*, 104–111. [CrossRef]
29. Jacotet-Navarro, M.; Rombaut, N.; Fabiano-Tixier, A.-S.; Danguien, M.; Bil, A.; Chemat, F. Ultrasound versus microwave as green processes for extraction of rosmarinic, carnosic and ursolic acids from rosemary. *Ultrason. Sonochem.* **2015**, *27*, 102–109. [CrossRef] [PubMed]
30. Wu, D.; Gao, T.; Yang, H.; Du, Y.; Li, C.; Wei, L.; Zhou, T.; Lu, J.; Bi, H. Simultaneous microwave/ultrasonic-assisted enzymatic extraction of antioxidant ingredients from *Nitraria tangutorun* Bobr. Juice by-products. *Ind. Crops Prod.* **2015**, *66*, 229–238. [CrossRef]
31. Ajuong, E.; Redington, M. Fourier transform infrared analyses of bog and modern oak wood (*Quercus petraea*) extractives. *Wood Sci. Technol.* **2004**, *38*, 181–190. [CrossRef]
32. Grasel, F.S.; Ferrão, M.F.; Wolf, C.R. Development of methodology for identification the nature of the polyphenolic extracts by FTIR associated with multivariate analysis. *Spectrochim. Acta A Mol. Biomol. Spectrosc.* **2016**, *153*, 94–101. [CrossRef] [PubMed]
33. Ping, L.; Pizzi, A.; Guo, Z.D.; Brosse, N. Condensed tannins from grape pomace: Characterization by FTIR and MALDI TOF and production of environment friendly wood adhesive. *Ind. Crops Prod.* **2012**, *40*, 13–20. [CrossRef]
34. Liu, H.; Shang, J.; Chen, X.; Kamke, F.A.; Guo, K. The influence of thermal-hydro-mechanical processing on chemical characterization of *Tsuga heterophylla*. *Wood Sci. Technol.* **2014**, *48*, 373–392. [CrossRef]
35. Rodríguez-Solana, R.; Daferera, D.J.; Mitsi, C.; Trigas, P.; Polissiou, M.; Tarantilis, P.A. Comparative chemotype determination of Lamiaceae plants by means of GC–MS, FT-IR, and dispersive-Raman spectroscopic techniques and GC-FID quantification. *Ind. Crops Prod.* **2014**, *62*, 22–33. [CrossRef]
36. Ribeiro, A.B.; Silva, D.H.S.; Bolzani, V.S. Antioxidant flavonol glycosides from *Nectandra grandiflora* (Lauraceae). *Eclética Química* **2002**, *27*, 35–44. [CrossRef]
37. De Rijke, E.; Out, P.; Niessen, W.M.; Ariese, F.; Gooijer, C.; Udo, A.T. Analytical separation and detection methods for flavonoids. *J. Chromatogr. A* **2006**, *1112*, 31–63. [CrossRef] [PubMed]
38. Le Quesne, P.W.; Larrahondo, J.E.; Raffauf, R.F. Antitumor plants X Constituents of *Nectandra rigida*. *J. Nat. Prod.* **1980**, *43*, 353–359. [CrossRef] [PubMed]
39. Ross, A.B.; Anastasakis, K.; Kubacki, M.; Jones, J.M. Investigation of the pyrolysis behaviour of brown algae before and after pre-treatment using PY-GC/MS and TGA. *J. Anal. Appl. Pyrolysis* **2009**, *85*, 3–10. [CrossRef]
40. Silva, D.T.; Bianchini, N.H.; Muniz, M.F.B.; Heinzmann, B.M.; Labidi, J. Chemical composition and inhibitory effects of *Nectandra grandiflora* leaves essential oil against wood decay fungi. *Drewno* **2016**, *59*, 1–8.
41. Tenorio, C.; Moy, R. Thermogravimetric characteristics, its relation with extractives and chemical properties and combustion characteristics of ten fast-growth species in Costa Rica. *Thermochim. Acta* **2013**, *563*, 12–21. [CrossRef]
42. Carballo, T.; Gil, M.V.; Gómez, X.; González-Andrés, F.; Morán, A. Characterization of different compost extracts using Fourier-transform infrared spectroscopy (FTIR) and thermal analysis. *Biodegradation* **2008**, *19*, 815–830. [CrossRef] [PubMed]
43. Conceição, M.C.; Junqueira, L.A.; Guedes, S.K.C.; Prado, M.E.T.; de Resende, J.V. Thermal and microstructural stability of a powdered gum derived from *Pereskia aculeata* Miller leaves. *Food Hydrocoll.* **2014**, *40*, 104–114. [CrossRef]
44. Shebani, A.; Van Reenen, A.; Meincken, M. The effect of wood extractives on the thermal stability of different wood species. *Thermochim. Acta* **2008**, *471*, 43–50. [CrossRef]
45. Missio, A.L.; Mattos, B.D.; Gatto, D.A.; De Lima, E.A. Thermal analysis of charcoal from fast-growing eucalypt wood: Influence of raw material moisture content. *J. Wood Chem. Technol.* **2014**, *34*, 191–201. [CrossRef]
46. Martins, C.R.; Lopes, W.A.; Andrade, J.B. Solubilidade das substâncias orgânicas. *Química Nova* **2013**, *36*, 1248–1255. [CrossRef]
47. Re, R.; Pellegrini, N.; Proteggente, A.; Pannala, A.; Yang, M.; Rice-Evans, C. Antioxidant activity applying an improved ABTS radical cation decolorization assay. *Free Radic. Biol. Med.* **1999**, *26*, 1231–1237. [CrossRef]
48. Pietta, P. Flavonoids as antioxidants. *J. Nat. Prod.* **2000**, *63*, 1035–1042. [CrossRef] [PubMed]
49. Kakkar, S.; Bais, S. A review on protocatechuic acid and its pharmacological potential. *ISRN Pharmacol.* **2014**, *2014*, 1–9. [CrossRef] [PubMed]

50. Wu, P.; Ma, G.; Li, N.; Deng, Q.; Yin, Y.; Huang, R. Investigation of in vitro and in vivo antioxidant activities of flavonoids rich extract from the berries of *Rhodomyrtus tomentosa* (Ait.) Hassk. *Food Chem.* **2015**, *173*, 194–202. [CrossRef] [PubMed]
51. Vundać, V.B.; Brantner, A.H.; Plazibat, M. Content of polyphenolic constituents and antioxidant activity of some *Stachys* taxa. *Food Chem.* **2007**, *104*, 1277–1281. [CrossRef]
52. Magro, A.; Carolino, M.; Bastos, M.; Mexia, A. Efficacy of plant extracts against stored products fungi. *Revista Iberoamericana de Micología* **2006**, *23*, 176–178. [CrossRef]
53. Cândido, T.L.N.; Silva, M.R.; Agostini-Costa, T.S. Bioactive compounds and antioxidant capacity of buriti (*Mauritia flexuosa* L.f.) from the Cerrado and Amazon biomes. *Food Chem.* **2015**, *177*, 313–319. [CrossRef] [PubMed]
54. Metrouh-Amir, H.; Duarte, C.M.M.; Maiza, F. Solvent effect on total phenolic contents, antioxidant, and antibacterial activities of *Matricaria pubescens*. *Ind. Crops Prod.* **2015**, *67*, 249–256. [CrossRef]
55. Herrera, R.; Erdocia, X.; Llano-Ponte, R.; Labidi, J. Characterization of hydrothermally treated wood in relation to changes on its chemical composition and physical properties. *J. Anal. Appl. Pyrolysis* **2014**, *107*, 256–266. [CrossRef]
56. Dudonné, S.; Vitrac, X.; Coutière, P.; Woillez, M.; Mérillon, J.M. Comparative study of antioxidant properties and total phenolic content of 30 plant extracts of industrial interest using DPPH, ABTS, FRAP, SOD, and ORAC assays. *J. Agric. Food Chem.* **2009**, *57*, 1768–1774. [CrossRef] [PubMed]
57. Robles, E.; Salaberria, A.M.; Herrera, R.; Fernandes, S.C.; Labidi, J. Self-bonded composite films based on cellulose nanofibers and chitin nanocrystals as antifungal materials. *Carbohydr. Polym.* **2016**, *144*, 41–49. [CrossRef] [PubMed]

Sample Availability: Ethanolic extracts of *Nectarina grandiflora* leaves are available from the authors.

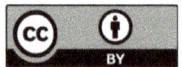

© 2018 by the authors. Licensee MDPI, Basel, Switzerland. This article is an open access article distributed under the terms and conditions of the Creative Commons Attribution (CC BY) license (http://creativecommons.org/licenses/by/4.0/).

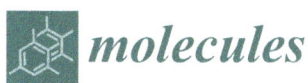

Article

Determination of Flavonoid and Proanthocyanidin Profile of Hungarian Sour Cherry

Andrea Nemes [1], Erzsébet Szőllősi [1], László Stündl [1], Attila Biró [1], Judit Rita Homoki [1], Mária Magdolna Szarvas [1], Péter Balogh [2], Zoltán Cziáky [3] and Judit Remenyik [1,*]

[1] Institute of Food Technology, University of Debrecen, H-4032 Debrecen, Hungary; nemes.andrea@agr.unideb.hu (A.N.); szzsoka83@gmail.com (E.S.); stundl@agr.unideb.hu (L.S.); attila.biro88@gmail.com (A.B.); homoki.judit@agr.unideb.hu (J.R.H.); sebestyen.magdolna@agr.unideb.hu (M.M.S.)

[2] Faculty of Economics and Business, Institute of Sectoral Economics and Methodology, Department of Research Methodology and Statistics, H-4032 Debrecen, Hungary; balogh.peter@econ.unideb.hu

[3] Agricultural and Molecular Research and Service Institute, University of Nyíregyháza, H-4400 Nyíregyháza, Hungary; cziaky.zoltan@nye.hu

* Correspondence: remenyik@agr.unideb.hu

Received: 7 November 2018; Accepted: 7 December 2018; Published: 11 December 2018

Abstract: Hungarian sour cherries (SC) are excellent source of anthocyanin (concentrations (100–300 mg in 100 g fresh fruit) and melatonin (0.15 mg in 100 g fresh fruit), but other flavonoid derivatives also can be isolated by aqueous alcoholic extraction. We have developed a new process for extracting non-extractable procyanidines bound to the membrane, proteins, and fibers. These compounds were seperated with UHPLC-MS methods, and the structure of individual components were identified on the basis of their mass fragmentation spectra. The antioxidant capacity of soluble and non-soluble antioxidants were measured with ferric reducing antioxidant power (FRAP), 1,1-diphenyl-2-picrylhydrazyl radical scavenging activity (DPPH), trolox equivalent antioxidant capacity (TEAC) assays, and compared to the new measurement methods of water-soluble antioxidant capacity (ACW), lipid-soluble antioxidant capacity (ACL). Furthermore, total phenolic content (TPC) and total procyanidin content (PAC) were determinated. As a result of our investigation, we found that the solvent combination, where in the first step is water–ethanol (1:1), then 100% ethanol were suitable for the extraction of the extractable antioxidants. However, the chemiluminescence method that is based on the elimination of the superoxide radical is more accurate than other colorimetric methods which measure antioxidant capacity.

Keywords: sour cherry; anthocyanins; extractable polyphenols; non-extractable polyphenols

---

1. Introduction

Sour cherry (*Prunus cerasus* L.) belongs to the family of Rosaceae, subfamily Prunoideae, to the genus Prunus, subgenus Cerasus. This is the hybrid that is produced by crosses between sweet cherry (*Prunus avium* (L.) L.) and European dwarf cherry (*Prunus fruticosa*) [1]. According to the FAOSTAT, world production of sour cherries in 2016 was 1,378,216 tons. The largest producers of cherries are Russia, Poland, Turkey, and the USA. Hungary is only the eighth, with nearly 70 thousand tons. Furthermore, the Hungarian cultivation of sour cherry has several centuries of history. Because of the geographic and climatic conditions of Hungary and the long breeding work, the Hungarian cultivar assortment and their varieties wiht outstanding nutritional parameters were developed, that are unique in the world. The popularity of the Hungarian varieties is shown by the fact that a Hungarian cultivar 'Újfehértói fürtös' was introduced into the United States in 1984 (in Michigan, Utah, and Wisconsin), that is marketed under the name Balaton and is regarded as a super food [2].

In recent years, clinical trials have shown the positive physiological effects of various components that accumulate in the cherry. Different classes of flavonoids have been shown to increase the expression of the gene encoding the γ-glutamylcysteine synthetase catalytic subunit, a protein reported to be the rate-limiting step in GSH synthesis [3,4]. Cy3G has cytoprotective effects, so it protects cells such as aortic endothelial cells (EC) by reducing hydrogen peroxide (H_2O_2)-induced oxidative stress in vitro and in vivo [5–7]. Youdim et al. (2000) presented for the first time that vascular endothelial cells can incorporate anthocyanins (mainly cyanidin-3-glucoside) into the membrane and cytosol, and the incorporation of anthocyanins by the EC significantly enhanced their resistance to the damaging effects of reactive oxygen species (ROS) [8].

Moreover, flavonoids have anti-oxidative, anti-inflammatory, anti-mutagenic, and anti-carcinogenic properties coupled with their capacity to modulate key cellular enzyme function. Lipoxygenase, xanthine oxidase, and NADPH oxidase enzymes in EC are activated during inflammatory processes. The activity of the NADPH oxidase enzyme can cause endothelial dysfunction in two ways. The activity of the NADPH oxidase enzyme produces oxygen-containing free radicals. The first is that the resulting superoxide anion (O2 •−) directly affects the function of the endothelial nitric oxide synthase (eNOS) enzymes by utilizing the cofactor needed for NO synthesis. It follows that the functioning of the eNOS enzyme is disturbed. The second is that O2 •− reacts with NO and connects to peroxinite. Peroxynitrite damages membrane proteins therefore it causes the disruption of mitochondrial electron transport chain [9].

Anthocyanins and some flavone and flavan-3-ol compounds may contribute to the prevention of hypertension [10]. Furthermore, it was demonstrated that the dietary anthocyanin Cy3G acts as a natural activator of eNOS in EC [11]. It has also been known that many extracellular agents (free fatty acids, H2O2, TNF-α) contribute to insulin resistance [12].

Furthermore, Guo et al. (2008) investigated the effect of Cy3G on H_2O_2- and TNF-α-induced insulin resistance on the 3T3-L1 adipocyte cell culture. Based on their measurements, it has been demonstrated that Cy3G protects adipocytes by inhibiting the kinase activity of the c-Jun NH2 terminal kinases, so the phosphorylation of the insulin receptor protein (IRS1) occurs via tyrosine [13].

The most significant antioxidant compounds in SC are phenol carboxylic acids (hydroxycinnamic acid, chlorogenic acid, neochlorogenic acid, p-coumaroylquinic acid) [14,15], flavanols (catechin, epicatechin, epigallocatechin, gallocatechin), and derivatives [16,17]. The accumulation of melatonin is also significant [18,19]. Polyphenol content in sour cherries and its health effect have been widely studied, for the extractable polyphenols only. Antioxidant capacity is usually measured in food extracts with different combination of organic solvents (e.g., methanol, ethanol, acetone) and water, but these usually do not result complete extraction of antioxidant compounds. This is mainly problem in the case of phenolics compounds, because these compounds are extracted by organic solvents, which probably leaves behind significant other phenolics existing in bound form. Usually, just the amount of extractable fractions were analyzed, the non-extractable compounds (in the solid residue) were ignored and associated with cell wall matrix. Nevertheless, unextractable phenolics from plant foods and their role in health benefits have become increasingly important [14–16].

These non-extractable phenolic compounds are considered to contribute more beneficial effects (gastrointestinal health, cancer, cardiovascular disease) because after gastrointestinal digestion they remain undegraded, and are absorbed into blood plasma after being released by intestinal microflora fermentation [17,18].

Phenolics can be classified as soluble and insoluble-bound form. Thus, the polyphenols that can be extracted from foods with aqueous-organic solvent, called extractable polyphenols (EPP). However, a significant fraction of polyphenols remains in the residue after the extraction; the so-called non-extractable polyphenols (NEPP) [19].

The solid residue contains macromolecules (e.g., high-molecular-weight proanthocyanidins) and single phenolic compounds (e.g., phenolic acids, associated with macromolecules) mainly polysaccharide constituents of dietary fibre and protein. NEPP are generally not included in polyphenol analysis, however, the NEPP content may be much higher than the EPP fraction. With regards to their chemical nature, NEPP mainly include polyphenols such as proanthocyanidins, other flavonoids, phenolic acids, and hydrolysable tannins. Accordingly, the NEPP usually were divided into two groups, hydrolysable tannins and non-extractable proanthocyanidins (NEPA) [18,20].

Acid and alkaline hydrolysis are the most common chemical methods used to extract the NEPP and recently, many other new methods such as enzymatic hydrolysis has been employed for better release of NEPP from cell wall matrices [14,21–23].

Plants contain various chemical compounds and the antioxidant effectiveness is determined by many factors (the heterogeneity and heterophasic nature of the system, the type of lipid substrate, including its physicochemical state and degree of unsaturation, the types of initiators (notably transition metals), other components, and their possible interaction).

Because of these, for assessment of antioxidant potential of endogenous compounds, single assay methods are not sufficient.

Several in vitro methods exist to measure the total antioxidant capacity. The different antioxidant assays differ in terms of assay principle and experimental conditions. Depending on what kind of reaction is involved, these assays can be classified into two groups: assays based on hydrogen atom transfer (HAT) reactions and assays based on electron transfer (ET) [24].

The most widely used procedures are FRAP (ferric reducing antioxidant power), ABTS (2,2′-Azino-bis(3-ethylbenzothiazoline-6-sulfonic acid)) or TEAC (trolox equivalent antioxidant capacity), DPPH (2,2-diphenyl-1-picrylhydrazyl), and oxygen radical absorbance capacity (ORAC). The FRAP, TEAC, and DPPH methods belong to ET methods. Unfortunately, however, they have some disadvanteges and limitations. The main disadvantage of FRAP method is that the measured reducing capacity does not necessarily reflect antioxidant activity. Since the method does not include an oxidisable substrate, no information is provided on the protective properties of antioxidants [25]. DPPH assay is limited because DPPH radicals interact with other radicals (alkyl), and the time response curve to reach the steady state is not linear with different ratios of antioxidant/DPPH [26,27]. The TEAC assay also has several limitations. The ability of an antioxidant to scavenge the artificial ABTS radical may not reflect the antioxidant activity due to other mechanisms effective in complex food lipids or physiologically relevant substrates, including metal chelation and effects of antioxidant partitioning among phases of different polarities [25]. The biological and physiological functions of antioxidants are wide-ranging. The identification and quantitative determination of antioxidants, characterization of antioxidant capacity, and the evaluation of interactions between different food matrices can only be done by examining the entire antioxidant system. In order for it to be compare or examine foods with the same or different matrices, an extraction process have to develop that can efficiently obtaining the active compounds, where the componunds retain their chemical composition. Since it is important to identify the antioxidant compounds, and to determine the antioxidant capacity of the components as accurately as possible. The choice of the right method is also a goal because oxidative stress is well known and studied, but there is antioxidative stress too.

In our opinion, PLC technique (HAT method) can be the best choice to determine the antioxidant capacity, since this method is based on the photo-induced autooxidation inhibition of luminol by antioxidants, mediated from the radical $O_2^{\bullet-}$, which can be found in human body, and is suitable to measure the radical scavenging properties of single antioxidants as well as more complex systems in the nanomolar range.

This study aims at investigating the differences between extraction processes. The first was commonly used combination of methanol, acetone, and water by Saura-Calixto and Goñi [28], and the second was an ethanol extraction that is used by the food and pharmaceutical industry too. During the experiment, not only were the extractable fractions analyzed, but also non-extractable compounds in the solid residue.

2. Results and Discussion

2.1. Extractable Antioxidant Compounds of Sour Cherry

Extracts (1/A + 1/B and 2/A + 2/B), were obtained by the two extraction methods, and analyzed with UHPLC-MS (Table 1). It can be seen that the solution combination 1 and 2 also extracted flavonoids and phenolic components. Among the flavonoids, anthocyanin-glucosides [29] and flavanol-*O*-glycosides [30] occur in large quantitiesin the sour cherry. The combination of solvent 1 has proved to be more effective mainly in the extraction of procyanidin C isomer.

Table 1. Polyphenolic compounds identified by LC-MS in *Prunus cerasus* L. extracts.

No	RT [min]	Compound	Chemical Formula	Measured [M + H]+	Measured [M − H]−	Calculated	Δ ppm	Fragment Ions (relative abundance, %)	Reference [1]
1 [4]	10.37	Neochlorogenic acid	C16H18O9	355.10251		355.10291	−1.13	163.0391 (100); 145.0286 (11); 135.0443 (13)	[31]
2 [4]	12.83	Coumaroylquinic acid isomer [1]	C16H18O8		337.09293	337.09235	1.72	191.0553 (52); 163.0388 (100); 119.0487 (48)	[32]
3 [4]	12.84	Procyanidin B isomer [1]	C30H26O12		577.13531	577.13460	1.23	407.0771 (58); 289.0721 (60); 125.0229 (100)	[31,33]
4 [4]	13.45	Coumaroylquinic acid isomer [2]	C16H18O8		337.09317	337.09235	2.43	191.0555 (10); 163.0388 (100); 119.0487 (44)	[32]
5 [3]	13.92	Procyanidin C isomer 1	C45H38O18		865.19922	865.19799	1.42	407.0771 (23); 289.0729 (30); 125.0229 (100)	[34]
6 [4]	14.12	Catechin [2]	C15H14O6		289.07196	289.07121	2.60	245.0819 (34); 151.0025 (63); 109.0280 (100)	[31,33]
7 [3]	14.77	Procyanidin C isomer [2]	C45H38O18		865.19910	865.19799	1.28	407.0774 (25); 289.0722 (26); 125.0230 (100)	[34]
8 [4]	14.94	Chlorogenic acid [2]	C16H18O9	355.10211		355.10291	−2.25	163.0390 (100); 145.0286 (11); 135.0443 (12)	[31,33]
9 [4]	15.21	Feruloylquinic acid isomer [1]	C17H20O9		367.10304	367.10291	0.35	193.0498 (100); 173.0445 (7); 134.0360 (65)	
10 [4]	15.77	Procyanidin B isomer [2]	C30H26O12		577.13519	577.13460	1.02	407.0768 (62); 289.0719 (64); 125.0230 (100)	[31,33]
11 [3]	16.24	Chryptochlorogenic acid	C16H18O9	355.10223		355.10291	−1.92	163.0390 (100); 145.0285 (12); 135.0443 (12)	
12 [4]	16.32	Coumaroylquinic acid isomer [3]	C16H18O8		337.09201	337.09235	−1.01	191.0554 (16); 173.0444 (100); 163.0388 (19)	[32]
13 [4]	16.42	Feruloylquinic acid isomer [2]	C17H20O9		367.10301	367.10291	0.27	193.0497 (100); 173.0444 (85); 134.0362 (62)	
14 [3]	17.23	Cyanidin-3-O-sophoroside	C27H30O16	611.16071		611.16122	−0.83	287.0552 (100); 213.0545 (4); 137.0226 (3)	[35]
15 [3]	17.41	Procyanidin C isomer [3]	C45H38O18		865.19835	865.19799	0.42	407.0762 (23); 289.0714 (27); 125.0230 (100)	[34]
16 [4]	17.60	Cyanidin-3-O-glucoside [2]	C21H20O11	449.10773		449.10839	−1.47	287.0552 (100); 213.0548 (3); 137.0229 (5)	[35]
17 [3]	17.68	Epicatechin [2]	C15H14O6		289.07175	289.07121	1.87	245.0818 (78); 151.0382 (31); 109.0281 (100)	[31,33]
18 [4]	17.81	Cyanidin-3-O-(2G-glucosyl)-rutinoside	C33H40O20	757.21814		757.21912	−1.29	611.1639 (4); 287.0552 (100); 213.0547 (2)	[35]
19 [4]	18.20	Coumaroylquinic acid isomer [4]	C16H18O8		337.09311	337.09235	2.26	173.0444 (100); 163.0388 (23); 119.0487 (17)	[31,33]
20 [3]	18.47	Cyanidin-3-O-rutinoside	C27H30O15	595.16626		595.16630	−0.07	449.1094 (4); 287.0552 (100); 213.0551 (2)	[35]
21 [4]	18.54	Cyanidin-3-O-(2G-xylosyl)-rutinoside	C32H38O19	727.20795		727.20855	−0.83	581.1515 (3); 287.0553 (100); 213.0545 (2)	[35]
22 [4]	18.80	Pelargonidin-3-O-(2G-glucosyl)rutinoside	C33H40O19	741.22491		741.22420	0.96	271.0602 (100)	[35]
23 [3]	19.41	Cinchonain I isomer [1]	C24H20O9		451.10318	451.10291	0.60	341.0666 (100); 217.0137 (33)	[35]
24 [3]	19.45	Pelargonidin-3-O-rutinoside	C27H30O14	579.17096		579.17138	−0.73	433.1135 (4); 271.0603 (100);	[35]

Table 1. *Cont.*

No	RT [min]	Compound	Chemical Formula	Exact Mass (m/z) Measured [M + H]⁺	Exact Mass (m/z) Measured [M − H]⁻	Exact Mass (m/z) Calculated	Δ ppm	Fragment Ions (relative abundance, %)	Reference [1]
25 [4]	20.05	Peonidin-3-O-rutinoside	C28H32O15	609.18152		609.18195	−0.71	463.1237 (4); 301.0708 (100); 286.0474 (14)	[35]
26 [4]	20.35	Cyanidin-O-pentoside	C20H18O10	419.09750		419.09783	−0.79	287.0554 (100)	
27 [3]	20.36	Quercetin-O-(hexosyl)rutinoside	C33H40O21		771.19940	771.19839	1.31	300.0276 (100); 271.0248 (40); 255.0298 (19)	
28 [4]	20.76	Quercetin-O-(hexosyl)hexoside isomer [1]	C27H30O17		625.14056	625.14048	0.13	300.0276 (100); 271.0251 (37); 255.0305 (20)	
29 [3]	20.96	Quercetin-di-O-hexoside	C27H30O17		625.14111	625.14048	1.01	463.0888 (48); 301.0356 (70); 300.0277 (100)	
30 [4]	21.01	Procyanidin B isomer [3]	C30H26O12		577.13605	577.13460	2.51	407.0768 (31); 289.0724 (53); 125.0229 (100)	[31,33]
31 [3]	21.09	Quercetin-O-rutinoside-O-glucoside	C33H40O21		771.19904	771.19839	0.84	609.1465 (89); 301.0355 (90); 300.0277 (100)	[34]
32 [4]	21.44	Naringenin chalcone-O-hexoside	C21H22O10		433.11380	433.11348	0.74	271.0613 (100); 151.0024 (59); 119.0488 (22)	
33 [3]	21.81	Cinchonain I isomer [2]	C24H20O9		451.10123	451.10291	−3.72	341.0667 (100); 217.0135 (36)	
34 [4]	22.27	Quercetin-O-(hexosyl)hexoside isomer [2]	C27H30O17		625.14001	625.14048	−0.75	300.0277 (100); 271.0244 (33); 255.0288 (18)	
35 [3]	22.81	Cinchonain I isomer [3]	C24H20O9		451.10248	451.10291	−0.95	341.0667 (100); 217.0138 (39)	
36 [4]	22.88	Di-O-caffeoylquinic acid	C25H24O12		515.11914	515.11896	0.35	353.0879 (60); 191.0553 (100); 179.0339 (62)	[36]
37 [4]	22.99	Prunin	C21H22O10		433.11389	433.11348	0.95	271.0612 (100); 151.0024 (41); 119.0487 (26)	
38 [3]	23.55	Isoquercitrin [2]	C21H20O12		463.08810	463.08765	0.97	301.0354 (43); 300.0276 (100); 271.0249 (37)	[31,33]
39 [4]	23.63	Rutin [2]	C27H30O16	611.16071		611.16122	−0.83	465.1029 (3); 303.0500 (100); 85.0289 (16)	[31,33]
40 [3]	23.74	Dihydroxy(iso)flavone-C-glucoside	C21H20O9	417.11816		417.11856	−0.96	399.1080 (33); 381.0978 (25); 297.0760 (100)	
41 [3]	25.34	Astragalin	C21H20O11		447.09348	447.09274	1.66	285.0406 (66); 284.0328 (100); 255.0297 (86)	
42 [4]	25.47	Nicotiflorin	C27H30O15		593.15094	593.15065	0.49	285.0406 (100); 284.0328 (73); 255.0298 (42)	
43 [3]	25.51	Cinchonain I isomer [4]	C24H20O9		451.10400	451.10291	1.35	341.06747 (100); 217.01355 (48)	
44 [4]	25.83	Narcissin	C28H32O16		623.16132	623.16122	0.16	315.0512 (100); 314.0435 (44); 299.0197 (40)	[31,33]
45 [3]	27.30	Quercetin-3-O-(4-coumaroyl)glucoside	C30H26O14		609.12531	609.12444	1.43	463.0896 (41); 300.0279 (100); 271.0247 25)	[31,33]
46 [4]	27.89	Naringenin [2]	C15H12O5		271.06122	271.06065	2.10	177.0182 (17); 151.0024 (100); 119.0488 (80)	[31,33]

[1] Identified compounds in *Prunus cerasus L*. in the literature. [2] Confirmed by standard. [3] Detected only in the ethanol/water extract (1/A + 1/B). [4] Detected in both extracts (1/A + 1/B and 2/a + 2/B).

2.2. Main Anthocyanin Compounds of Sour Cherry

The main anthocyanin components in the 'Újfehértói fürtös' variety (Figure 1.) were the cyanidin-3-O-glucosyl-rutinoside, (2 mg/100 g), cyanidin-3-O-rutinoside, (183 mg/100 g) and cyanidin-3-O-monoglucoside (4.29 mg/100 g).

The antioxidant capacity of these components is determined by OH groups at positions C3' and C4' on the chalcone.

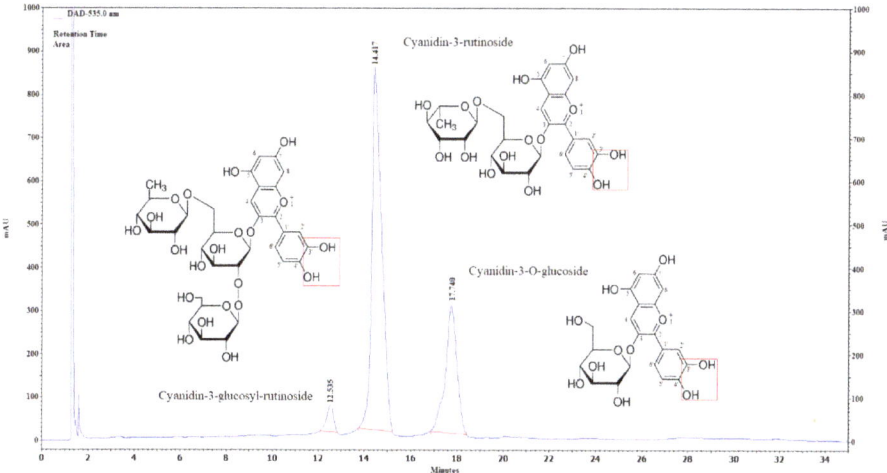

Figure 1. UHPLC chromatogram of sour cherry at 535 nm. Confirmed by standard.

2.3. Main Flavonoid and Phenolic Compounds of Sour Cherry

Quercetin, quercetin-3 rutinoside and apigenin (flavonoids) occur in abundant quantities in sour cherry (Figure 2.). These are precursor compounds in the biosynthesis of anthocyanins. There are other phenolic compounds like chlorogenic and caffeic acid in high concentrations in this fruit. The antioxidant activity of these compounds is also high.

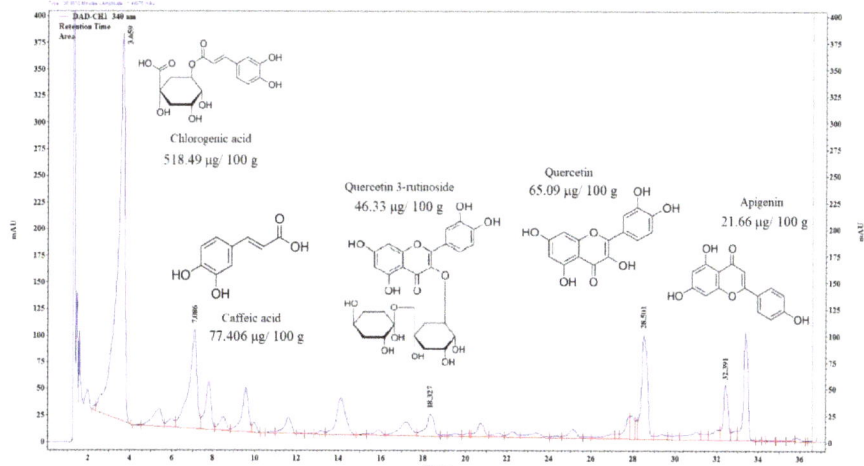

Figure 2. UHPLC chromatogram of sour cherry at 340 nm. Confirmed by standard.

2.4. Total Procyanidin Content (PAC) of Sour Cherry and Sour Cherry Residues

Several studies have been reported that procyanidins have strong protective properties regarding oxidative damage, microbial infection, prevention of colon cancer, and prevention of cardiovascular disease [37–40]. However, the degree of polymerization (DP) of procyanidins may be highly influential and determine these effects [41–43]. In the gastrointestinal tract, procyanidin monomers, dimers, and trimers are absorbed into the blood system to a much larger extent than larger oligomers and polymers [44,45]. The DP value of sour cherry procyanidins is lower than 4, indicating the relatively high levels of better absorbable short-chain procyanidin species [46], so sour cherry is an exceptional source of short-chain procyanidins, and a major food ingredient.

Measurably higher amounts of mono-, di-, and trimer procyanidins were extracted with the solvent combination 1, since fewer remained in the residue 1/R, however, the total amount of procyanidins could be not extracted (Figure 3.).

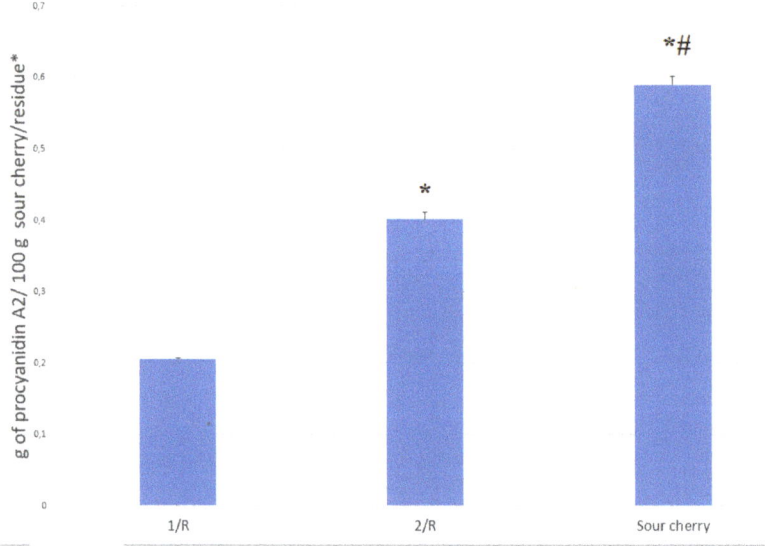

Figure 3. The total procyanidin content of sour cherry and sour cherry residues. * Units for different type of samples: sour cherry sample: g of procyanidin A2/100 g fresh weight sour cherry; residues: g of procyanidin A2/100 g dried residue. Abbreviations: 1/R: residue of 'solvent combination 1'; 2/R: residue of 'solvent combination 2'. * indicates significant difference ($p < 0.05$) from the 1/R. # indicates significant difference ($p < 0.05$) between the 2/R and the sour cherry.

2.5. Identification of Cinconain I

As you can see in the Table 1, the peaks for Cinchonain I isomers are 19.41, 21.81, 22.81, and 25.51 min. with $[M - H]^-$ ions at m/z 451.10291 were identified as distereomers of Cinchonain I on the bases of their exact molecular mass, isotopic pattern, and fragmentation. The characteristic fragment ions are 451.10400, 341.06747, and 217.0155 (Figure 4.).

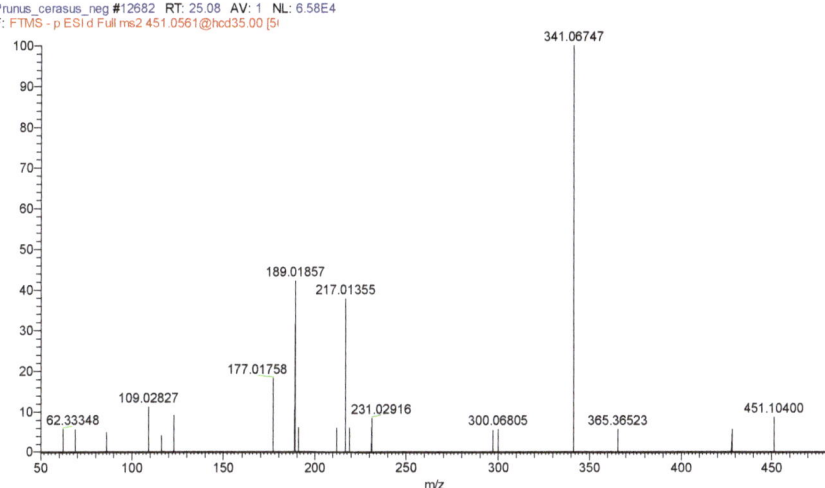

Figure 4. ESI-MS2 spectrum of Cinchonain I diastereoisomer at retention time 25.51.

2.6. Extractable Antioxidant Capacity of Sour Cherry Extracts

The antioxidant activites were compared in case of solvent combination 1 and 2, using the well-known measuring methods FRAP, DPPH, TEAC, ACL, ACW, and TPC (Figure 5A.).

Our results show that the amount of antioxidant compounds extracted by these two methods is not significantly different. The aqueous–alcoholic mixture is more advantageous for the processing industry and is sufficient to extract the most important compounds of the sour cherry (anthocyanins, procyanidines, phenolic components, and flavonoids). These compounds slightly soluble in water, but ethanol is a good solvent for them. Because of the polarity of 1/A mixture, it is also suitable for extraction of low molecular weight organic acids, which provides pH 3 in which glycolized anthocyanins maintain their chemical structure (more acid is not required.). All the other antioxidants can be extracted with ethanol (1/B).

UHPLC-MS measurements show (Table 1) that combinations of 1/A or 1/B and 2/A or 2/B are only partially applicable to the extraction of bioactive compounds, because all sour cherry extracts (1/AS, 1/BS, 2/AS, 2/BS) include 'anthocyanin and procyanidins', 'flavonoids', and 'other polyphenols'. The difference is only the amount of extracted compounds, that depends on solubility. It is therefore not surprising that methods based on the measurement of water-soluble polar components can measure a lower antioxidant concentration.

The used assays (except for ACL, ACW) are colorimetric methods based on complexometry, and have many disadvantages. The most significant drawback of the FRAP method is that it is only suitable for measuring water soluble components. In addition, not all antioxidants are able to reduce Fe^{3+}, antioxidants that act by H atom transfer are not detected [47–49]. During the application of the TEAC method, the problem is that the reaction of ABTS+• with the antioxidant compounds is strongly time-dependent, so components with 'slow kinetic' do not react with the radical in time [47]. DPPH is mainly used to measure the ability of polyphenols to transfer labile H atoms to radicals [50].

Obviously, the determination of antioxidant capacity of antioxidant compounds, that are extracted with solvent combination 1 and 2 by chemiluminescence technique seem to be the most appropriate. This method is suitable for selectively determining the concentration of water-soluble and lipid-soluble antioxidants. It can be used for antioxidants that act H atom transfer and electron transfer, because both groups react with the superoxide anion, which is one of the most important radicals in the living organisms [51,52].

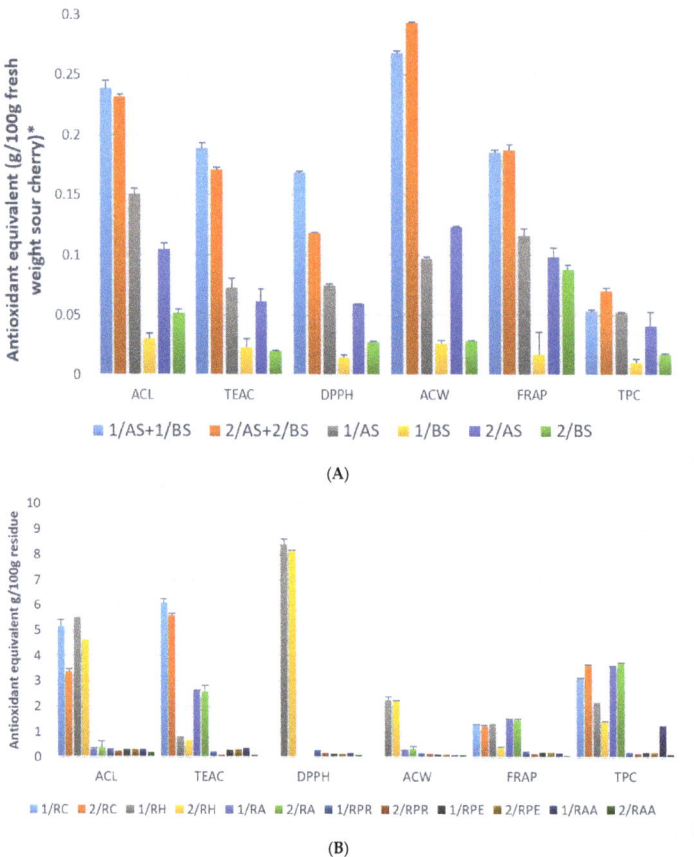

Figure 5. ESI-MS2 spectrum of procyanidin B. (**A**) Comparison of the extractable antioxidant capacity of sour cherry-extracts and the totalphenolic content. * Units for different measurement methods: ACL: Trolox equivalent g/100 g; TEAC: Trolox equivalent g/100 g; DPPH: Trolox equivalent g/100 g; ACW: Ascorbic acid g/100 g; FRAP: Ascorbic acid g/100 g; TPC: Gallic acid g/100 g. Abbreviations: 1/AS: evaporated ethanol:water extract; 1/BS: evaporated ethanol extract after ethanol:water extraction; 1/AS + 1/BS: 1/AS and 1/BS extracts evaporated together; 2/AS: evaporated acidic methanol:water extract; 2/BS: evaporated acetone:water extract after methanol:water extraction; 2/AS + 2/BS: 2/AS and 2/BS extracts evaporated together. The table form (Supplement 1) with the results of the statistical analysis can be found in the Supplemets secyion. (**B**) Comparison of the non-extractable antioxidant capacity of sour cherry residue extracts and the totalphenolic content. * Units for different measurement methods: ACL: Trolox equivalent g/100 g; TEAC: Trolox equivalent g/100 g; DPPH: Trolox equivalent g/100 g; ACW: Ascorbic acid g/100 g; FRAP: Ascorbic acid g/100 g; TPC: Gallic acid g/100 g. Abbreviations: 1/R: residue of 'solvent combination 1'; 1/RC: supernatant from the 'extraction of hydrolysable tannins' of 1/R; 1/RH: supernatant from the 'extraction of condensed tannins' of 1/R; 1/RA: supernatant from the 'alkaline hydrolysis' of 1/R; 1/RPR: supernatant from the 'protease hydrolysis' of 1/R; 1/RPE: supernatant from the 'pectinase hydrolysis' of 1/R; 1/RAA: supernatant from the 'α-amilase hydrolysis' of 1/R; 2/R: residue of 'solvent combination 2'; 2/RC: supernatant from the 'extraction of hydrolysable tannins' of 2/R; 2/RH: supernatant from the 'extraction of condensed tannins' of 2/R; 2/RA: supernatant from the 'alkaline hydrolysis' of 2/R; 2/RPR: supernatant from the 'protease hydrolysis' of 2/R; 2/RPE: supernatant from the 'pectinase hydrolysis' of 2/R; 2/RAA: supernatant from the 'α-amilase hydrolysis' of 2/R; The table form (Supplement 2) with the results of the statistical analysis can be found in the Supplemets chapter.

2.7. Capacity of Non-Extractable Antioxidants of Sour Cherry Extracts

The enzymatic digestion not resulted significant antioxidant activity (Figure 5B.). The explanation is that sour cherry does not contain large amounts of starch, so the α-amylase hydrolisis is not relevant. It does not contain large amounts of protein, so hydrolysis with protease is not important either. The use of pectinase is also more important for apple crops.

Significant amounts of antioxidant fragments were obtained in the case of the alkaline treatment, but mainly acidic hydrolysis. The results obtained using the HCl butanol extractant are not significantly different. Low molecular weight phenolic derivatives resulting from the degradation of polyphenols may be responsible for the apparently high antioxidant activity.

Proantocianines are considered as non-extractable components but some of them can be recovered with a solvent combination 1 and 2, as can be seen from the Table 1. However, non-extractable proantocianidines can not be identified in the hydrolysates.

The amount of antioxidants that extracted from the sour cherry and obtained from hydrolysis from the remaining residues were similar in case of the solvent combination (Figure 5A,B). Thus, the acidification (HCl) and the methanol–acetone–water solvent combination that was used by Saura-Calixto and Goñi [28] did not extract significantly higher amounts of antioxidant compounds. Consequently, it is not necessary to use HCl, and the methanol can be replaced by etanol in the first step, furthermore the acetone water combination can be replaced by 100% ethanol in the second step.

3. Experimental

3.1. Plant Material

Stoned, frozen sour cherry ('Újfehértói fürtös' variety) was bougth from Mirelite Mirsa Zrt (Albertirsa, Hungary) in 2017. Fruit samples were frozen ($-20\,^\circ$C) and stored in dark.

3.2. Chemicals and Reagents

Ethanol, acetic acid, and Folin–Ciocalteu's reagent were purchased from VWR (Randore, PA, USA). Hydrochloric acid and 1-Butanol were obtained from Merck (Damstadt, Germany). Methanol, acetone, sulfuric acid, 2, 4, 6-Tris(2-pyridyl)-s-triazine (TPTZ), 2,2-Diphenyl-1-picrylhydrazyl (DPPH), 2,2′-azino-bis(3-ethylbenzothiazoline-6-sulfonic acid) (ABTS), 4-(dimethylamino)cinnamaldehyde (DMAC), iron(III) chloride hexahydrate, sodium acetate trihydrate, potassium persulfate, procyanidin A2, sodium carbonate anhydrous, ascirbic acid, ($\pm$)-6-Hydroxy-2,5,7,8-tetramethylchromane-2-carboxylic acid (Trolox), gallic acid, sodium hydroxide, antioxidant standards, and the enzymes (protease, α-amylase) were purchased from Sigma-Aldrich (St. Louis, MO, USA). Pectinex XXL enzyme was obtained from Novozymes (Bagsværd, Denmark). Dulbecco's phosphate-buffered saline (DPBS) were obtained from iBioTech (Szigetszentmiklós, Hungary). ACL and ACW kits were obtained from Greenlab (Budapest, Hungary). In our experiments, all the reagents were analytical grade. HPLC-grade methanol and formic acid were purchased from Fisher Scientific (Hampton, NH, USA).

3.3. Extraction of Extractable Antioxidants

The sour cherry was defrosted and homogenized. Then two different solvents were used to extract antioxidant compounds. Each extraction was performed parallel three times.

3.3.1. Extraction with the Mixture of Ethanol and Water (Solvent Combination 1)

200 g of sample was extracted with 150 mL ethanol (96%) and 150 mL distilled water for 2 h (1/A). The samples were centrifuged (Eppendorf Cetrifuge 5810R)) for 15 min at 4000 rpm and the supernatant was recovered.

150 mL ethanol (96%) was added to the residue, and the mixture was mixed for 2 h (1/B). After centrifugation (15 min, 4000 rpm), the supernatant was recovered.

For the first time, supernatants from 1/A and 1/B were evaporated together (1/AS + 1/BS), but in the second case separately (1/AS and 1/BS). Evaporation was performed at 40 °C, 10 mbar (Figure 6).

The residue (1/R) was lyophilised (ScanVac CoolSafe 55-4 Pro lyophilizer), homogenized (Gorenje SMK 150 B coffee grinder), and stored in freezer (−20 °C) before use.

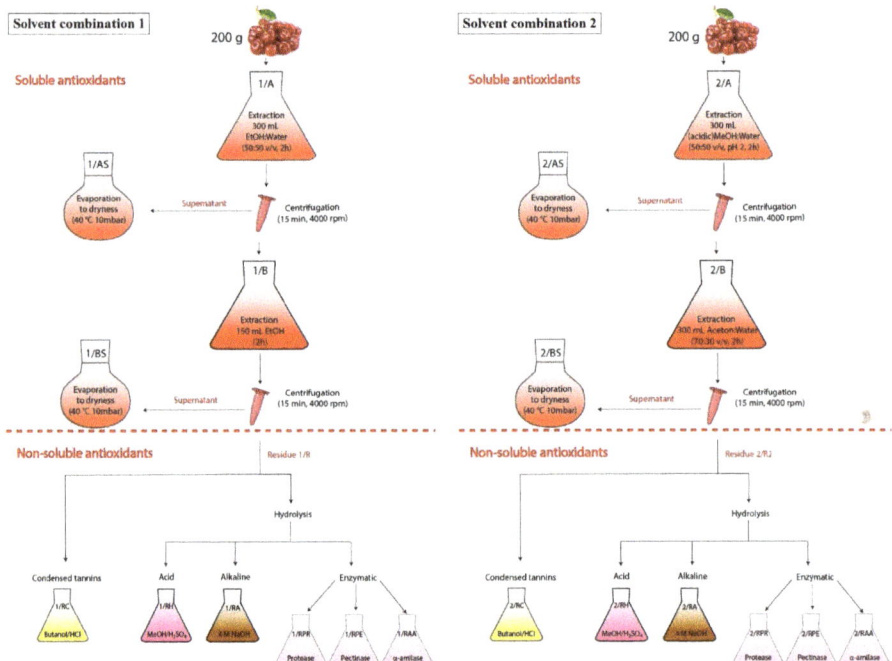

Figure 6. Scheme of the extraction of antioxidants from sour cherry. Abbreviations: 1/AS: evaporated ethanol:water extract; 1/BS: evaporated ethanol extract after ethanol:water extraction; 1/AS + 1/BS: 1/AS and 1/BS extracts evaporated together; 2/AS: evaporated acidic methanol:water extract; 2/BS: evaporated acetone:water extract after methanol:water extraction; 2/AS + 2/BS: 2/AS and 2/BS extracts evaporated together; 1/R: residue of 'solvent combination 1'; 1/RC: supernatant from the 'extraction of hydrolysable tannins' of 1/R; 1/RH: supernatant from the 'extraction of condensed tannins' of 1/R; 1/RA: supernatant from the 'alkaline hydrolysis' of 1/R; 1/RPR: supernatant from the 'protease hydrolysis' of 1/R; 1/RPE: supernatant from the 'pectinase hydrolysis' of 1/R; 1/RAA: supernatant from the 'α-amilase hydrolysis' of 1/R; 2/R: residue of 'solvent combination 2'; 2/RC: supernatant from the 'extraction of hydrolysable tannins' of 2/R; 2/RH: supernatant from the 'extraction of condensed tannins' of 2/R; 2/RA: supernatant from the 'alkaline hydrolysis' of 2/R; 2/RPR: supernatant from the 'protease hydrolysis' of 2/R; 2/RPE: supernatant from the 'pectinase hydrolysis' of 2/R; 2/RAA: supernatant from the 'α-amilase hydrolysis' of 2/R.

3.3.2. Extraction of Extractable Antioxidants According to Saura-Calixtoa and Goñi [28] (Solvent Combination 2)

200 g of sample was extracted with 300 mL acidic methanol/water/HCl (50:50; pH 2) were added (2/A) for 2 h, then centrifuged (15 min, 4000 rpm) and the supernatant was recovered.

300 mL acetone/water (70:30, v/v) was added to the residue, and the mixture was mixed for 2 h (2/B). After centrifugation (15 min, 4000 rpm), the supernatant was recovered [28].

The extraction was performed twice. For the first time, supernatants from 2/A and 2/B were evaporated together (2/AS + 2/BS), but in the second case separately (2/AS and 2/BS). Evaporation was performed at 40 °C, 10 mbar (Figure 6).

The residue (2/R) was lyophilised, homogenized, and stored in freezer (−20 °C) before use.

3.3.3. Preparation of Extracts from UHPLC

The purification of anthocyanins, a simple fractionation of sour cherry extracts (1/A + 1/B and 2/A + 2/B) was performed using preconditioned Supelclean ENVI-18 SPE tubes [53]. The tubes were conditioned with 5 mL MeOH then with 5 mL H$_2$O and finally 1 mL of fruit sample was applied. The anthocyanins were eluted with methanol:water; 80:20. Solvent was evaporated at 40 °C with Heidolph Hei-VAP Value rotary evaporator (Schwabach, Germany).

3.4. Acid Hydrolysis

3.4.1. Extraction of Hydrolysable Tannins

10–10 mg dried sour cherry residue powder from the two extractions were subjected to hydrolysis with 2 mL methanol and 200 µL sulphuric acid for 20 h at 85 °C. Samples are then centrifuged (2500 g, 10 min) and supernatants recovered. The residues was washed with 2–2 mL distilled water two times [54]. The supernatant from 1/R residue is 1/RH, and the extract from 2/R residue is 2/RH.

3.4.2. Extraction of Condensed Tannins

10–10 mg dried sour cherry residue powder from the two extractions were treated with 3 mL HCl/butanol (5:95) and 100 µL FeCl$_3$ (2 wt %) at 100 °C for 3 h. After centrifugation (2500 g, 10 min), the supernatant was recovered. The residues was washed with 2–2 mL HCl/butanol (5:95) two times. The supernatant from 1/R residue is 1/RC, and the extract from 2/R residue is 2/RC [55,56].

3.5. Alkaline Hydrolysis

0.1 g dried sour cherry residue powder from the two extractions were treated with 5 mL NaOH (4 mM) at 25 °C for 1 h. After centrifugation (4000 rpm, 10 min), the supernatant was recovered. The supernatant from 1/R residue is 1/RA, and the hydrolysate from 2/R residue is 2/RA [23].

3.6. Enzymatic Hydrolysis

3.6.1. Enzymatic Hydrolysis with Protease

5 mL DPBS and 10 µL tyrosine (50 mg/mL; 3550 tyrosine units/mL) was added to 0.1 g dried sour cherry residue powder from the two extractions. The samples were incubated at 60 °C for 1 h. To stop the enzymatic hydrolisis, the hydrolysates were placed in a water bath at 100 °C for 10 min. After centrifugation (5 min, 4000 rpm), the supernatant was recovered. The hydrolysate from 1/R residue is 1/RPR, and the supernatant from 2/R residue is 2/RPR.

3.6.2. Enzymatic Hydrolysis with Pectinase

5 mL DPBS and 10 µL pectinase (Pectinex XXL) was added to 0.1 g dried sour cherry residue powder from the two extractions. The samples were incubated at room temperature for 1 h. To stop the enzymatic hydrolisis, the hydrolysates were placed in a water bath at 100 °C for 5 min. After centrifugation (5 min, 4000 rpm), the supernatant was recovered. The supernatant from 1/R residue is 1/RPE, and the hydrolysate from 2/R residue is 2/RPE [22].

3.6.3. Enzymatic Hydrolysis with α-amilase

5 mL DPBS and 10 µL α-amilase (3000 Units/mL) was added to 0.1 g dried sour cherry residue powder from the two extractions. The samples were incubated at 37 °C for 10 min. To stop the

enzymatic hydrolisis, the hydrolysates were placed in a water bath at 100 °C for 20 min. After centrifugation (5 min, 4000 rpm), the supernatant was recovered. The supernatant from 1/R residue is 1/RAA, and the hydrolysate from 2/R residue is 2/RAA [23].

3.7. Determination of Total Phenolic Content (TPC)

Total phenolics in all extracts were determined with the Folin–Ciocalteu assay [57] with minor modifications. 10 µL of appropriately diluted extracts, standard gallic acid solutions (50, 100, 200, 400, 800, and 1600 µg/mL) or water (blank) was mixed with 190 µL of distilled water in a well of a 96-well plate; 25 µL of Folin–Ciocalteu reagent solution was then added. After 6 min, 75 µL of 7% Na_2CO_3 was added. The mixture was shaken gently and incubated in the pre-heated chamber (50 °C) for 10 min, and its absorbance was measured at 765 nm, using the microplate reader (SPECTROstar®Nano, BMG Labtech, Ortenberg, Germany). TPC was expressed as milligrams of gallic acid equivalents (mg GAE/100 g fresh weight sour cherry/dried residue). In some cases, the extract was too dilute, so 100 µL of sample and 100 µL of H_2O were mixed in a well.

3.8. Determination of Total Procyanidin Content (PAC)

Total procyanidin content was measured using the method of Prior et al. [58].

Dried powder of residuals and sour cherry were weighed (500 mg) into a 50 mL conical tube. 20 mL extraction solution (acetone/deionized water/acetic acid 75:24.5:0.5) was added to the samples. The samples were vortexed for 30 s followed by sonication for 1 h at room temperature. After centrifugation (4000 rpm, 10 min), the supernatant was collected for analysis.

70 µL of 96% ethanol for blank; or 70 µL of control (100 µg mL^{-1} Procyanidin A2 in ethanol)/standard/samples were added to 210 µL DMAC solution (0.1 wt % in ethanol) in a well of 96-well plate. The mixture was shaken gently and incubated in the pre-heated chamber (25 °C). The microplate was read for 25 min.

The plate reader protocol was set to read the absorbance (640 nm) of each well in the plate every min for 30 min. The maximum absorbance readings were used for calculation.

3.9. Determination of Antioxidant Capacity

In this experiment, FRAP, DPPH, TEAC, and PCL (Photochemiluminescence assay) methods were used to measure, the antioxidant capacity.

3.9.1. FRAP

The ferric reducing antioxidant power assay was performed as previously described by Benzie and Strain [59]. It is based on the reduction of the Fe^{3+}-TPTZ complex to the ferrous form at low pH. This reduction is monitored by measuring the absorption change at 593 nm.

The reaction was carried out in a microtiter plate. 30 µL of distilled water and 10 µL properly diluted samples/standard were pipetted in a well of 96-well plate, then 200 µL FRAP reagent (10 volumes of 250 mM acetate buffer (pH 3.6), one volume of 20 mM ferric chloride solution and one volume of 10 mM tripyridyl-s-triazin (TPTZ) in 40 mM HCl) were added. The mixture was incubated at 37 °C and the absorbance was taken after 8 min at 593 nm.

The FRAP values was calculated and expressed as ascorbic acid equivalents per 100 g sample (fresh weight sour cherry/dried residue).

3.9.2. DPPH

The DPPH free radical scavenging activity was measured using the method of Brand-Williams with modified as follows: 10 µL of appropriately diluted sample or Trolox solution (31.25, 62.5, 125, 250, 500, 750, and 1000 µM) and 50 µL distilled water was added to 190 µL of DPPH solution (0.1 mM in methanol) in a well of a 96-well plate. The mixture was shaken gently, incubated at 25 °C and the absorbance was taken after 30 min. The absorbance was measured at 517 nm, using the microplate reader. DPPH was expressed as milligrams of trolox equivalents (mg TE/100 g fresh weight sour cherry/dried residue) [26,60].

3.9.3. TEAC

Determination of Trolox Equivalent Antioxidant Capacity (TEAC). This assay was performed as reported previously with slight modification. ABTS radical cations were prepared by mixing equal volumes of ABTS (7 mM in H_2O) and potassium persulfate (4.9 mM in H_2O), and the solution was left to stand in the dark for 12–16 h at room temperature; then the above solution was filtered and diluted with 80% ethanol to an absorbance of about 2 at 734 nm. 70 µL of 80% ethanol and 10 µL properly diluted samples/standard were pipetted in a well of 96-well plate, then 190 µL ABTS solution in a well of a 96-well plate, and the absorbance was recorded at 734 nm after 30 min of incubation at room temperature. Trolox was used as standard, and a standard calibration curve was obtained for Trolox at concentrations of 15.65, 31.25, 62.5, 125, 250, 500, and 1000 µM. The TEAC of samples was calculated from the standard curve of Trolox and expressed as gram of Trolox equivalents (TE) per 100 g of fresh weight sour cherry/dried residue (g TE/100 g) [61].

3.9.4. Photochemiluminescence Assay (PLC)

This assay was described by Popov and Lewin, and distributed as a complete system under the name Photochem® by Analytik Jena AG (Jena, Germany).

In the PCL assay, the photochemical generation of ($O_2^{\bullet-}$) free radicals is combined with the sensitive detection by using chemiluminescence. The assay is initiated by optical excitation of photosensitizer (S), resulting in the generation of the superoxide radical anion.

$$S + h\upsilon + O_2 \rightarrow [S^*O_2] \rightarrow S^{\bullet+} + O_2^{\bullet-} \tag{1}$$

There are two different protocols: ACW (water-soluble antioxidant capacity) and ACL (lipid-soluble antioxidant capacity) so both of the hydrophilic and the lipophilic antioxidants can be measured separately. These are standardized conditions, so the results are comparable to other assays. The antioxidant potential was assayed by means of the lag phase (ACW) or by means of the area under the curve (ACL) at different concentrations [51,52].

A. ACL

The lipophilic antioxidants were measured with the ACL kit. The reaction solutions were prepared by mixing 2.3 mL Reagent 1 (methanol), 200 µL Reagent 2 (buffer solution), 25 µL Reagent 3 (photosensitizer and detection reagent), and 0–30 µL of Reagent 4 (calibration standard for quantification of lipophilic antioxidants in Trolox equivalents) or 10 µL of sample (beverage diluted with Reagent 1) were mixed and measured. The detector measures the current proportion to the generated luminescence as a function of measurement time. The detector signal, monitored for 180 s. Results are expressed as mg equivalents of trolox per 100 g fresh weight sour cherry/dried residue [52].

B. ACW

The hydrophilic antioxidants were measured with the ACW kit. The reaction solutions were prepared by mixing 1.5 mL of Reagent 1 (buffer solution pH 10.5), 1 mL of Reagent 2 (reaction buffer), 25 µL Reagent 3 (photosensitizer and detection reagent) and 0–30 µL of Reagent 4 (calibration standard for quantification of water-soluble antioxidants in ascorbic acid equivalents) or 10 µL of sample (beverage diluted with Reagent 1). The detector measures the current proportion to the generated luminescence as a function of measurement time. The detector signal, monitored for 250 s, includes a lag phase in which no luminescence can be detected. When the antioxidants are exhausted, the amount of radicals in the sample increases until the detected signal reaches the maximum. The length of the lag phase increases in function of the amount of the antioxidants in the sample, and it is calculated by determining the first derivative and the maximum point of the detected curve. The interstion point of the slope of the straight line with the *x*-axis defines the lag time. Results are expressed as mg equivalents of ascorbic acid per 100 g fresh weight sour cherry/dried residue [51].

3.10. UHPLC Analysis

Measurements were carried out using CromasterUltraRs UHPLC, equipped with diode array detector, automatic sampler and Agillent OpenLAB software. The sample components were separated on a Phenomenex Kinetex column (2.6μ, XB.C18, 100A, 100 × 4.6 mm).

UHPLC running conditions consisted of the following linear gradient steps
0 min solvent A 15%,
0–25 min solvent A to 30%,
25–30 min solvent A to 40%,
30–40 min solvent A to 50%.
Solvent A: MeOH; Solvent B: 3% HCOOH (Formic acid) in water.

Flow rate was 0.7 mL min^{-1} and oven temperature was kept at 25 °C. The anthocyanin content was analyzed quantitatively by comparison with the corresponding authentic standards. UV–vis detection was used at 535 nm wavelength for anthocyanins and 340 nm for flavonoid and phenolic compounds. The appropriate amounts of sour cherry extracts were measured and dissolved in solvent A. Injection volume was 10 μL.

3.11. UHPLC-MS Analysis

The UHPLC system (Dionex Ultimate 3000RS) was coupled to a Thermo Q Exactive Orbitrap mass spectrometer (Thermo Fisher Scientific Inc., Waltham, USA) equipped with an electrospray ionization source (ESI). The HPLC separation was achieved on a Themo Accucore C18 column (100 mm × 2.1 mm × 2.6 μm). Sampler and oven temperature were maintained at 25 °C, flow rate was 200 μL min^{-1}. Eluent A was water containing 0.1% formic acid and eluent B was methanol containing 0.1% formic acid. The following gradient elution program was used: 0 min, 95% A; 0–3 min, 95% A; 3–43 min, →0% A; 43–61 min, 0% A; 61–62 min, →95% A; 62–70 min, 95% A. 2 μL of the samples were injected in every run. The Q Exactive hybrid quadrupole-orbitrap mass spectrometer was operated with the following parameters: capillary temperature 320 °C, spray voltage 4.0 kV in positive and 3.8 kV in negative ionization mode. The resolution was set to 35,000. The mass range scanned was 150–1500 *m/z*. The maximum injection time was 100 ms. The resolution was set to 17,500 in the cases of MS2 scans. The collision energy was 35 NCE. Sheath gas and aux gas flow rates were 32 and 7 arb, respectively. Xcalibur 4.0 (Thermo Fisher Scientific Inc., Waltham, USA) software was used to collect and analyze data.

3.12. Statistical Analysis

Data were expressed as means ± standard errors. Data were statistically analyzed using the SPSS statistical software, version 23. (SPSS Inc, Chicago, IL, USA). One-way analysis of variance (ANOVA) with Tukey's honestly sgnificant difference test (homogeneity of variances) and Games–Howell significant difference test (not equal variances) were used to compare means among groups. The level of significance was set at $p < 0.05$.

4. Conclusions

It is known that different types of extractants can extract a variety of bioactive compounds. Accordingly, just one solvent is not sufficient to extract the total antioxidant compounds of foods, solvent combination is necessary, and the choice of suitable solvents is essential. As a result of our investigation, we found that the amounts and antioxidant properties of the dissolved compounds are not significantly different in case of solvent combination 1 and 2. However, Solvent combination 2 (methanol–acetone–water) can not be used in the food technology, only alcohol–water extraction is suitable.

The choice of the appropriate solvent is just the first step, the next is the determination of the exact antioxidant capacity. To do this you will need to find the most appropriate measurement method for the food type, because they contain different antioxidant compounds. FRAP method is good for the determination of water soluble, low molecular weight components. However, anthocyanins and associated flavonoids are only slightly soluble in water, so this method can not be measured these well. Although the solvent of DPPH and TEAC methods is ethanol, there are certain limitations that block measurement of the anthocyanins rich in sour cherry. For instance, because of the steric accessibility of DPPH• radical, the DPPH method can not adequately measure anthocyanin compounds [47], and in case of TEAC, the degree and position of hydroxylation and methoxylation in the B ring of anthocyanins, affects the stability and reactivity and thereby the antioxidant capacity [62]. However, the ACL and ACW methods are suitable to determine the antioxidant activity of various chemical components in SC.

Supplementary Materials: The following are available.

Author Contributions: J.R. conceived and designed the experiments. A.N., E.S., L.S., A.B., J.R.H., M.M.S., and Z.C. performed the experiments. P.B., Z.C., and J.R. analyzed the data. A.N. and J.R. wrote the paper. All authors read and approved the final manuscript.

Funding: This research received no external funding.

Acknowledgments: The work is supported by the GINOP-2.3.2-15-2016-00042 project. This project is co-financed by the European Union and the European Social Fund. Furthermore, the research was financed by the Higher Education Institutional Excellence Programme (20428-3/2018/FEKUTSTRAT) of the Ministry of Human Capacities in Hungary, within the framework of the 4. thematic programme of the University of Debrecen.

Conflicts of Interest: The authors declare no conflict of interest.

Dedication: This study is dedicated to Professor Sándor Biró on the occasion of his 70th birthday, and we honor his undisputed merits in the field of the microbial genetics.

References

1. Olden, E.J.; Nybom, N. On the origin of the *Prunus cerasus* L. *Hereditas* **1968**, *59*, 327–345. [CrossRef]
2. Wang, H.; Nair, M.G.; Iezzoni, A.F.; Strasburg, G.M.; Booren, A.M.; Gray, J.I. Quantification and Characterization of Anthocyanins in Balaton Tart Cherries. *J. Agric. Food Chem.* **1997**, *45*, 2556–2560. [CrossRef]
3. Myhrstad, M.C.; Carlsen, H.; Nordstrom, O.; Blomhoff, R.; Moskaug, J.O. Flavonoids increase the cellular glutathione level by transactivation of the g-glutamylcysteine synthetase catalytical subunit promoter. *Free Radic. Biol. Med.* **2002**, *32*, 386–393. [CrossRef]
4. Moskaug, J.O.; Carlsen, H.; Myhrstad, M.C.W.; Blomhoff, R. Polyphenols and glutathione synthesis regulation. *Am. J. Clin. Nutr.* **2005**, *81*, 277–283. [CrossRef] [PubMed]
5. Gutierrez, R.M. Effect of the hexane extract of Piper auritum on insulin release from beta-cell and oxidative stress in streptozotocin-induced diabetic rat. *Pharmacogn. Mag.* **2012**, *8*, 308–313. [CrossRef] [PubMed]
6. Mane, C.; Loonis, M.; Juhel, C.; Dufour, C.; Malien-Aubert, C. Food grade lingonberry extract: Polyphenolic composition and in vivo protective effect against oxidative stress. *J. Agric. Food Chem.* **2011**, *59*, 3330–3339. [CrossRef] [PubMed]
7. Martin, M.A.; Fernández-Millán, E.; Ramos, S.; Bravo, L.; Goya, L. Cocoa flavonoid epicatechin protects pancreatic beta cell viability and function against oxidative stress. *Mol. Nutr. Food Res.* **2014**, *58*, 447–456. [CrossRef]
8. Youdim, K.A.; Martin, A.; Joseph, J.A. Incorporation of the elderberry anthocya- nins by EC increases protection against oxidative stress. *Free Radic. Biol. Med.* **2000**, *29*, 51–60. [CrossRef]
9. Ciz, M.; Denev, P.; Kratchanova, M.; Vasicek, O.; Ambrozova, G.; Lojek, A. Flavonoids Inhibit the Respiratory Burst of Neutrophils in Mammals. *Oxid. Med. Cell. Longev.* **2012**, *2012*, 181295. [CrossRef]
10. Cassidy, A.; O'Reilly, E.J.; Kay, C.; Sampson, L.; Franz, M.; Forman, J.P.; Curhan, G.; Rimm, E.B. Habitual intake of flavonoid subclasses and incident hypertension in adults. *Am. J. Clin. Nutr.* **2011**, *93*, 338–347. [CrossRef]

11. Xu, J.W.; Ikeda, K.; Yamori, Y. Cyanidin-3-glucoside regulates phosphorylation of endothelial nitric oxide synthase. *FEBS Lett.* **2004**, *574*, 176–180. [CrossRef] [PubMed]
12. Watson, R.R.; Preedy, V.R.; Zibadi, S. *Polyphenols in Human Health and Disease*, 1st ed.; Academic Press: Oxford, UK, 2014; pp. 86–90. ISBN 978-0-12-398456-2. [CrossRef]
13. Guo, H.; Ling, W.; Wang, Q.; Liu, C.; Hu, Y.; Xia, M. Cyanidin 3-glucoside protects 3T3-L1 adipocytes against H_2O_2- or TNF-α-induced insulin resistance by inhibiting c-Jun NH2-terminal kinase activation. *Biochem. Pharmacol.* **2008**, *75*, 1393–1401. [CrossRef] [PubMed]
14. Tang, Y.; Zhang, B.; Li, X.; Chen, P.X.; Zhang, H.; Liu, R.; Tsao, R. Bound Phenolics of Quinoa Seeds Released by Acid, Alkaline, and Enzymatic Treatments and Their Antioxidant and α-Glucosidase and Pancreatic Lipase Inhibitory Effects. *J. Agric. Food Chem.* **2016**, *64*, 1712–1719. [CrossRef] [PubMed]
15. Shahidi, F.; Yeo, J.D. Insoluble-Bound Phenolics in Food. *Molecules* **2016**, *21*, 1216. [CrossRef] [PubMed]
16. Pérez-Jiménez, J.; Arranz, S.; Tabernero, M.; Díaz-Rubio, M.E.; Serrano, J.; Goñi, I.; Saura-Calixto, F. Updated methodology to determine antioxidant capacity in plant foods, oils and beverages: Extraction, measurement and expression of results. *Food Res. Int.* **2008**, *41*, 274–285. [CrossRef]
17. Andreasen, M.F.; Kroon, P.A.; Williamson, G.; Garcia-Conesa, M.T. Esterase Activity Able to Hydrolyze Dietary Antioxidant Hydroxycinnamates Is Distributed along the Intestine of Mammals. *J. Agric. Food Chem.* **2001**, *49*, 5679–5684. [CrossRef] [PubMed]
18. Pérez-Jiménez, J.; Díaz-Rubio, M.E.; Saura-Calixto, F. Non-extractable polyphenols, a major dietary antioxidant: Occurrence, metabolic fate and health effects. *Nutr. Res. Rev.* **2013**, *26*, 118–129. [CrossRef]
19. Pérez-Jiménez, J.; Saura-Calixto, F. Macromolecular antioxidants or non-extractable polyphenols in fruit and vegetables: Intake in four European countries. *Food Res. Int.* **2015**, *74*, 315–323. [CrossRef]
20. Kristl, J.; Slekovec, M.; Tojnko, S.; Unuk, T. Extractable antioxidants and non-extractable phenolics in the total antioxidant activity of selected plum cultivars (*Prunus domestica* L.): Evolution during on-tree ripening. *Food Chem.* **2011**, *125*, 29–34. [CrossRef]
21. Gómez-García, R.; Martínez-Ávila, G.C.G.; Aguilar, C.N. Enzyme-assisted extraction of antioxidative phenolics from grape (*Vitis vinifera* L.) residues. *3 Biotech* **2012**, *2*, 297–300. [CrossRef]
22. Guo, L. Enzymatic hydrolysis of lotus rhizome starch using alpha-amylase and glucoamylase. *J. Food Nutr. Res.* **2017**, *56*, 372–380.
23. Anokwuru, C.; Sigidi, M.; Boukandou, M.; Tshisikhawe, P.; Traore, A.; Potgieter, N. Antioxidant Activity and Spectroscopic Characteristics of Extractable and Non-Extractable Phenolics from Terminalia sericea Burch. ex DC. *Molecules* **2018**, *23*, 1303. [CrossRef] [PubMed]
24. Wang, H.; Cao, G. Oxygen radicals absorbing capacity of anthocyanins. *J. Agric. Food Chem.* **1997**, *45*, 304–309. [CrossRef]
25. Frankel, E.N.; Meyer, A.S. The problems of using one-dimensional methods to evaluate multifunctional food and biological antioxidants. *J. Sci. Agric.* **2000**, *80*, 1925–1941. [CrossRef]
26. Brand-Williams, W.; Cuvelier, M.E.; Berset, C. Use of a free radical method to evaluate antioxidant activity. *Food Sci. Technol.* **1995**, *28*, 25–30. [CrossRef]
27. Sanchez-Moreno, C.; Larrauri, J.A.; Saura-Calixto, F. A procedure to measure the antiradical efficiency of polyphenols. *J. Sci. Food Agric.* **1998**, *76*, 270–276. [CrossRef]
28. Saura-Calixto, F.; Goñi, I. Antioxidant capacity of the Spanish Mediterranean diet. *Food Chem.* **2006**, *94*, 442–447. [CrossRef]
29. Homoki, J.R.; Nemes, A.; Fazekas, E.; Gyémánt, G.; Balogh, P.; Gál, F.; Al-Asri, J.; Mortier, J.; Wolber, G.; Babinszky, L.; et al. Anthocyanin composition, antioxidant efficiency, and a-amylase inhibitor activity of different Hungarian sour cherry varieties (*Prunus cerasus* L.). *Food Chem.* **2016**, *194*, 222–229. [CrossRef] [PubMed]
30. Chaovanalikit, A.; Wrolstad, R.E. Anthocyanin and polyphenolic composition of fresh and processed cherries. *J. Food Sci.* **2004**, *69*, 73–83. [CrossRef]
31. Levaj, B.; Dragović-Uzelac, V.; Delonga, K.; Ganić, K.K.; Banović, M.; Kovačević, D.B. Polyphenols and volatiles in fruits of two sour cherry cultivars, some berry fruits and their jams. *Food Technol. Biotechnol.* **2010**, *48*, 538–547.
32. Han, J.H.; Lee, H.J.; Cho, M.R.; Chang, N.; Kim, Y.; Oh, S.Y.; Kang, M.H. Total antioxidant capacity of the Korean diet. *Nutr. Res. Pract.* **2014**, *8*, 183–191. [CrossRef] [PubMed]

33. Bonerz, D.; Würth, K.; Dietrich, H.; Will, F. Analytical characterization and the impact of ageing on anthocyanin composition and degradation in juices from five sour cherry cultivars. *Eur. Food Res. Technol.* **2007**, *224*, 355–364. [CrossRef]
34. Wojdyło, A.; Nowicka, P.; Laskowski, P.; Oszmiański, J. Evaluation of sour cherry (*Prunus cerasus* L.) fruits for their polyphenol content, antioxidant properties, and nutritional components. *J. Agric. Food Chem.* **2014**, *51*, 12332–12345. [CrossRef] [PubMed]
35. Jakobek, L.; Seruga, M.; Seruga, B.; Novak, I.; Medvicovic-Kosanovic, M. Phenolic compound composition and antioxidant activity of fruits of Rubus and Prunus species from Croatia. *Int. J. Food Sci. Technol.* **2009**, *44*, 860–868. [CrossRef]
36. Toydemir, G.; Capanoglu, E.; Gomez-Roldan, M.V.; de Vos, R.C.H.; Boyacioglu, D.; Hall, R.D.; Beekwilder, M.J. Industrial processing effects on phenolic compounds in sour cherry (*Prunus cerasus* L.) fruit. *Food Res. Int.* **2013**, *53*, 218–225. [CrossRef]
37. Arteel, G.E.; Sies, H. Protection against peroxinitrite by cocoa polyphenol oligomers. *FEBS Lett.* **1999**, *462*, 167–170. [CrossRef]
38. Lunder, T.L. Catechins of green tea: Antioxidant activity. In *Phenolic Compounds in Food and Their Effects on Health II*, 1st ed.; Huang, M.T., Ho, C.T., Lee, C.Y., Eds.; American Chemical Society Inc.: Washington, DC, USA, 1992; Volume 507, pp. 114–120. ISBN 9780841224766.
39. Pannala, A.S.; Chan, T.S.; O'Brien, P.J.; Rice-Evans, C.A. Flavonoid B-ring chemistry and antioxidant activity: Fast reaction kinetics. Biochem. *Biophys. Res. Commun.* **2001**, *282*, 1161–1168. [CrossRef]
40. Rice-Evans, C.A.; Packer, L. *Flavonoids in Health and Disease*; Dekker: New York, NY, USA, 1997.
41. Gonzales-Manzano, S.; Santos-Buelga, C.; Perez-Alonso, J.J.; Rivas-Gonzalo, J.C.; Escribano-Bailon, M.T. Characterization of the mean degree of polymerization of proanthocyanidins in red wines using Liquid Chromatography-Mass Spectrometry (LC-MS). *J. Agric. Food Chem.* **2006**, *54*, 4326–4332. [CrossRef]
42. Hagerman, A.E.; Riedl, K.M.; Jones, G.A.; Sovik, K.N.; Ritchard, N.T.; Hartzfeld, P.W.; Riechel, T.L. High molecular weight plant polyphenolics (tannins) as biological antioxidants. *J. Agric. Food Chem.* **1998**, *46*, 1887–1892. [CrossRef]
43. Shi, J.; Yu, J.; Pohorly, J.E.; Kakuda, Y. Polyphenolics in grape seeds-biochemistry and functionality. *J. Med. Food* **2003**, *6*, 291–299. [CrossRef]
44. Khanal, R.C.; Howard, L.R.; Prior, R.L. Procyanidin content of grape seed and pomace, and total anthocyanin content of grape pomace as affected by extrusion processing. *J. Food Sci.* **2009**, *74*, 174–182. [CrossRef] [PubMed]
45. Manach, C.; Williamson, G.; Morand, C.; Scalbert, A.; Remesy, C. Bioavailability and bioefficacy of polyphenols in humans. I. Review of 97 bioavailability studies. *Am. J. Clin. Nutr.* **2005**, *81*, 230–242. [CrossRef] [PubMed]
46. Capanoglu, E.; Boyacioglu, D.; de Vos, R.C.H.; Hall, R.D.; Beekwilder, J. Procyanidins in fruit from Sour cherry (*Prunus cerasus*) differ strongly in chainlength from those in Laurel cherry (*Prunus lauracerasus*) and Cornelian cherry (*Cornus mas*). *J. Berry Res.* **2011**, *1*, 137–146. [CrossRef]
47. Boligon, A.A.; Machado, M.M.; Athayde, M.L. Technical evaluation of antioxidant activity. *Med. Chem.* **2014**, *4*, 517–522. [CrossRef]
48. Prior, R.L.; Cao, G. Analysis of botanicals and dietary supplements for antioxidant capacity: A review. *J. AOAC Int.* **2000**, *83*, 950–955. [PubMed]
49. Huang, D.; Ou, B.; Prior, R.L. The chemistry behind antioxidants capacity assays. *J. Agric. Food Chem.* **2005**, *53*, 1841–1856. [CrossRef] [PubMed]
50. Litwinienko, G.; Ingold, K.U. Abnormal solvent effects on hydrogen atom abstractions. 1. The reactions of phenols with 2,2-diphenyl-1-picrylhydrazyl (dpph•) in alcohols. *J. Org. Chem.* **2003**, *68*, 3433–3438. [CrossRef] [PubMed]
51. Popov, I.N.; Lewin, G. Photochemiluminescent detection of antiradical activity. 2. Testing nonenzymic water-soluble antioxidants. *Free Radic. Biol. Med.* **1994**, *17*, 267–271. [CrossRef]
52. Popov, I.N.; Lewin, G. Photochemiluminescent detection of antiradical activity; IV: Testing of lipid-soluble antioxidants. *J. Biochem. Biophys. Methods* **1996**, *31*, 1–8. [CrossRef]
53. Kim, D.; Heo, H.J.; Yang, H.S.; Lee, C.Y. Sweet and sour cherry phenolics and their protective effects on neuronal cells. *J. Agric. Food Chem.* **2005**, *53*, 9921–9927. [CrossRef]

54. Hartzfeld, P.W.; Forkner, R.; Hunter, D.M.; Hagerman, A.E. Determination of hydrolysable tannins (gallotannins and ellagitannins) after reaction with potassium iodate. *J. Agric. Food Chem.* **2002**, *50*, 1785–1790. [CrossRef] [PubMed]
55. Porter, L.; Hrstich, L.; Chan, B. The conversion of procyanidins and prodelphinidins to cyaniding and delphinidin. *Phytochemistry* **1985**, *25*, 223–230. [CrossRef]
56. Reed, J.; McDowell, R.E.; Van Soest, P.J.; Horvarth, P.J. Condensed tannins: A factor limiting the use of cassava forage. *J. Sci. Food Agric.* **1982**, *33*, 213–220. [CrossRef]
57. Singleton, V.L.; Orthofer, R.; Lamuela-Raventós, R.M. Analysis of total phenols and other oxidation substrates and antioxidants by means of folin-ciocalteu reagent. *Methods Enzymol.* **1999**, *299*, 152–178. [CrossRef]
58. Prior, R.L.; Fan, E.; Ji, H.; Howell, A.; Nio, C.; Payne, M.J.; Reed, J. Multi-laboratory validation of a standard method for quantifying proanthocyanidins in cranberry powders. *J. Sci. Food Agric.* **2010**, *90*, 1473–1478. [CrossRef] [PubMed]
59. Benzie, I.F.; Strain, J.J. The ferric reducing ability of plasma (FRAP) as a measure of "antioxidant power": The FRAP assay. *Anal. Biochem.* **1996**, *239*, 70–76. [CrossRef] [PubMed]
60. Blois, M.S. Antioxidant determinations by the use of a stable free radical. *Nature* **1958**, *181*, 1199–1200. [CrossRef]
61. Miller, N.J.; Rice-Evans, C.A.; Davies, M.J.; Gopinathan, V.; Milner, A. A novel method for measuring antioxidant capacity and its application to monitoring the antioxidant status in premature neonates. *Clin. Sci.* **1993**, *84*, 407–412. [CrossRef]
62. Montoro, P.; Tuberoso, C.I.; Piacente, S.; Perrone, A.; De Feo, V.; Cabras, P.; Pizza, C. Stability and antioxidant activity of polyphenols in extracts of Myrtus communis L. berries used for the preparation of myrtle liqueur. *J. Pharm. Biomed. Anal.* **2006**, *41*, 1614–1619. [CrossRef]

Sample Availability: Samples of the compounds are not available from the authors.

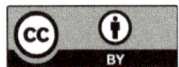

© 2018 by the authors. Licensee MDPI, Basel, Switzerland. This article is an open access article distributed under the terms and conditions of the Creative Commons Attribution (CC BY) license (http://creativecommons.org/licenses/by/4.0/).

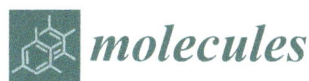

Article

A Novel HPLC Method for Direct Detection of Nitric Oxide Scavengers from Complex Plant Matrices and Its Application to *Aloysia triphylla* Leaves

Didier Fraisse [1], Alexandra Degerine-Roussel [1], Alexis Bred [1], Samba Fama Ndoye [2], Magali Vivier [3], Catherine Felgines [1] and François Senejoux [1,*]

1. Université Clermont Auvergne, INRA, UNH, F-63000 Clermont-Ferrand, France; didier.fraisse@uca.fr (D.F.); alexandra.degerine@uca.fr (A.D.-R.); alexis.bred@uca.fr (A.B.); catherine.felgines@uca.fr (C.F.)
2. Laboratory of Organic and Therapeutic Chemistry, Faculty of Medicine, Pharmacy and Odontology (F.M.P.O.), Cheikh Anta Diop University (U.C.A.D.), Dakar-Fann PB 5005, Senegal; sambabathie0806@yahoo.fr
3. UMR IMoST 1240 Inserm, Université Clermont Auvergne, 63005 Clermont-Ferrand, France; magali.vivier@uca.fr
* Correspondence: francois.senejoux@uca.fr; Tel.: +334-731-780-33, Fax: +334-731-780-37

Academic Editor: Alessandra Durazzo
Received: 4 June 2018; Accepted: 26 June 2018; Published: 28 June 2018

Abstract: The present study aimed at developing an original pre-column HPLC assay allowing rapid characterization of nitric oxide (NO) scavengers from complex plant extracts. Sodium nitroprusside (SNP) was employed as a NO donor and spiked with an aqueous extract from *Aloysia triphylla* leaves prior to HPLC analysis. Relying on the ability of radical scavenging constituents to be oxidized upon reaction with radicals, this assay successfully allowed direct identification of three potential NO scavengers, including verbascoside, isoverbascoside, and luteolin-7-*O*-diglucuronide. These three phenolics were also individually assessed for their NO scavenging activities by using a Griess colorimetric assay. With respective IC_{50} values of 56 ± 4, 51 ± 3, and 69 ± 5 µg/mL, verbascoside, isoverbascoside, and luteolin-7-*O*-diglucuronide were all reported as potent NO scavenging compounds, confirming the efficiency of the SNP spiking HPLC assay. The present method can, thus, be considered as a valuable and effective approach for speeding up the discovery of NO scavenging constituents.

Keywords: nitric oxide scavengers; pre-column HPLC method; *Aloysia triphylla*; phenolics; antioxidants

1. Introduction

Nitric oxide (NO) is an important signaling molecule with dual effects. Generated by nitric oxide synthases through the conversion of L-arginine to L-citrulline, NO plays a key role in regulating vasodilation, neurotransmission, and the immune system, as well as cardiovascular and renal functions [1–3]. Low concentrations are, in most cases, sufficient to exert these beneficial effects. However, overproduction of this free radical may induce several undesired deleterious effects, including inflammatory and autoimmune diseases [4,5]. The search for substances capable of preventing overproduction of NO has, therefore, received increasing attention, and numerous extracts of edible and/or medicinal plants have been shown to exert potent NO scavenging activities [6,7]. Nevertheless, the main pitfall to drug discovery or plant extract standardization remains the characterization of bioactive principles. Traditional bioassay-guided fractionation has been successfully conducted in some investigations [8], but several major limitations arise from this time-consuming, labor intensive, and expensive strategy. Thus, there is a need to develop new approaches capable of speeding up the discovery of NO scavenging natural compounds. Of interest, several pre-column HPLC spiking methods have been recently reported to directly detect radical scavenging compounds from complex matrices, such as plant extracts [9,10]. These experiments consist of spiking extracts with a radical solution prior to HPLC analysis, and rely on the ability of antioxidant constituents to be oxidized upon reaction with radicals. On this basis, peak areas of radical scavenging compounds are reduced in HPLC chromatograms of spiked extracts whereas peak areas of inactive constituents are not affected. Of note, such a kind of approach has already been successfully adapted to identify DPPH [11] and ABTS [12], as well as peroxynitrite scavengers [13]. However, a method capable of detecting NO scavengers has yet to be devised. By using sodium nitroprusside (SNP) as an NO source, the present study aimed at developing a novel spiking HPLC assay that allows direct detection of NO scavenging constituents from herbal products. Lemon verbena (*Aloysia triphylla* (L'Hér.) Britt., Verbenaceae), a widely consumed herbal tea known to exert significant anti-oxidant and anti-inflammatory effects [14,15], was chosen as the case study plant material.

2. Results and Discussion

2.1. NO Scavenging Activity and Total Phenolic Content of an Aqueous Extract from A. triphylla *Leaves*

Native to western South America, *A. triphylla* is a widely consumed edible plant whose leaves are mostly employed as herbal tea. To be relevant to this mode of consumption, an aqueous infusion was prepared. *A. triphylla* aqueous extract (ATAE) was first assessed for its NO scavenging activity by using common colorimetric evaluation. This method relies on the principle that, in aqueous solution and at physiological pH, SNP spontaneously generate NO radicals, which subsequently react with oxygen to produce nitrite ions that can be estimated with Griess reagent. Scavengers of NO compete with oxygen, thus, leading to a lower production of nitrite ions. The present study demonstrates, for the first time, that ATAE exerts potent NO scavenging effects, as attested by its low IC_{50} value of 231 ± 17 µg/mL. These results tend to suggest that *A. triphylla* leaves can be regarded as a suitable herbal product to counteract NO overproduction. Considering that polyphenols are regarded as the most prevalent radical scavenging phytochemicals in the plant kingdom [16], total phenolic content of the extract was also evaluated. Of interest, a substantial value of 148 ± 1 mg gallic acid equivalent per g of dried extract was determined for ATAE. Taken together, these preliminary results indicated that ATAE was a suitable candidate for the development of a straightforward HPLC method, aiming at directly detecting NO scavenging compounds from a complex plant extract.

2.2. Separating Constituents from ATAE by HPLC

Ensuring the separation of all compounds in a plant extract is a crucial first step in analytical HPLC. Different modes of elution and mobile phase compositions were screened to obtain chromatograms with a sufficient resolution and within an acceptable time of analysis. Under the chosen conditions, a satisfying resolution was achieved and all the major compounds reached base-line separation. As illustrated in Figure 1, six main constituents were observed on the ATAE chromatogram.

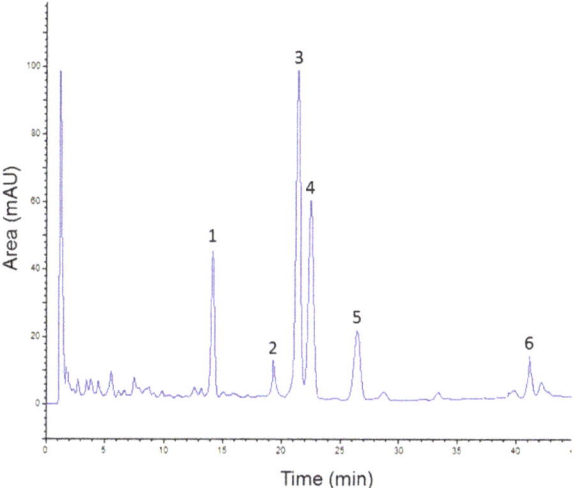

Figure 1. HPLC-UV profile of aqueous extract from *Aloysia triphylla* leaves with detection at 280 nm. Peaks: 1, luteolin-7-O-diglucuronide; 2, apigenin-7-O-diglucuronide; 3, verbascoside; 4, diosmetin-7-O-diglucuronide; 5, isoverbascoside; and 6, apigenin-7-O-glucoside.

2.3. SNP Spiking HPLC Analysis for Screening of Main Scavengers in ATAE

Unlike commonly employed synthetic radicals, such as DPPH and ABTS [10,12], NO is not stable enough to be prepared prior to spiking experiments. Thus, the present method had to be developed with a reagent able to extemporaneously generate NO during pretreatment of the extract. As for colorimetric evaluation, SNP was chosen as the NO donor. Spiking experiments were performed with three different concentrations of SNP (1, 2.5, and 5 mM). It was hypothesized that pretreatment of ATAE with a low concentrated solution of SNP would only oxidize the most reactive scavengers, while solutions containing higher concentrations of SNP would affect additional antioxidant constituents. As shown in Figure 2, the chromatogram of ATAE spiked with a 1 mM solution of SNP indicated that peak areas of compounds **3** and **5** were significantly reduced ($p < 0.05$) whereas other constituents were not affected. As expected, peak area diminutions were more pronounced when higher concentrations of SNP were employed (2.5 and 5 mM). Indeed, compound **1** was significantly affected by the SNP pretreatment at these two concentrations ($p < 0.05$). In addition, compounds **3** and **5** almost disappeared from the corresponding chromatograms. Conversely, the peak areas of compounds **2**, **4**, and **6** were not significantly modified over all the SNP concentrations. According to these spiking experiments, it was possible to assume that three constituents (**1**, **3**, and **5**) are mainly contributing to ATAE scavenging effect, while compounds **2**, **4**, and **6** only play a negligible role. To confirm this hypothesis and to validate the proposed method, all major constituents of the extract were identified and assessed for their individual NO scavenging activities.

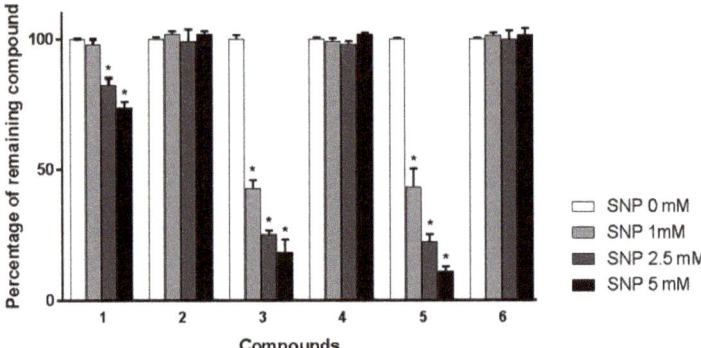

Figure 2. Percentage of remaining compounds (1–6) after incubation of aqueous extract from *Aloysia triphylla* leaves with various concentrations of SNP (0, 1, 2.5, and 5 mM). Data are presented as means ± SEM (n = 3). * $p < 0.05$ vs. control (SNP = 0 mM).

2.4. Characterization and Identification of the Main Constituents of ATAE

Analysis of the UV data of the six major components of ATAE revealed the presence of two different classes of metabolites (Table 1). Indeed, compounds **3** and **5** showed highly similar profiles with two maximum absorption bands at 217 nm and 325–330 nm, which were consistent with caffeoyl derivatives [17]. On the other hand, with maximum absorption bands at 250–270 nm and 330–350 nm, the UV profiles of constituents **1**, **2**, **4**, and **6** were typical of flavonoid derivatives [18]. These assumptions were further confirmed by examining previous chemical investigations of *A. triphylla* [19] and by comparing retention times and UV spectra of ATAE components with that of authentic commercial standards. Compounds **2** and **6** were corresponding to flavonoid derivatives, and were identified as apigenin-7-*O*-diglucuronide and apigenin-7-*O*-glucoside, respectively. In addition, compounds **3** and **5** were characterized as two caffeoyl phenylethanoid glycosides, respectively known as verbascoside and isoverbascoside. However, compounds **1** and **4** did not match with any available standards and purification of these two constituents was achieved to unambiguously determine their structures. ATAE was first fractionated using gel filtration chromatography and two fractions containing important amounts of the targeted compounds were subsequently submitted to semi-preparative HPLC purification. ^{1}H and ^{13}C NMR analyses were then performed on the two purified compounds and confirmed their assumed flavonoid nature. Indeed, compound **1** exhibited characteristic signals of a luteolin glycoside, while the NMR data of compound **4** matched with a diosmetin derivative. In both cases, typical signals attributable to two β-glucuronide units were observed. Deeper investigations of NMR analyses allowed the unequivocal identification of compounds **1** and **4**, which were, respectively, characterized as luteolin-7-*O*-diglucuronide and diosmetin-7-*O*-diglucuronide. All spectral data of these compounds agreed with respective published data [20,21]. Of note, the occurrence of compounds **1**, **2**, **3**, **5**, and **6** is consistent with previous phytochemical investigations of *A. triphylla* leaves [19,20]. By contrast, diosmetin-7-*O*-diglucuronide (**4**) is unambiguously identified for the first time in this species. Also known as fargenin C, this compound is very scarcely distributed in the plant kingdom and had only been isolated once in *Meehania fargesii*, an Asian species belonging to the Lamiaceae family [21].

Table 1. Retention time and UV maximum absorption of major constituents from *Aloysia triphylla* leaves.

Peak Number	Compound	Retention Time (min)	UV, λ_{max} (nm)
1	Luteolin-7-O-diglucuronide	14.3	255, 347
2	Apigenin-7-O-diglucuronide	19.3	265, 333
3	Verbascoside	21.6	217, 330
4	Diosmetin-7-O-diglucuronide	22.9	253, 346
5	Isoverbascoside	26.8	217, 326
6	Apigenin-7-O-glucoside	41.4	266, 332

2.5. NO Radical Scavenging Activity of Isolated Components

To ascertain the efficiency of the present HPLC spiking assay, all the compounds affected by SNP pretreatment (**1**, **3**, and **5**) were individually assessed for their NO scavenging properties by using a common colorimetric method. In addition, two assumed inactive constituents (**4** and **6**) were also evaluated to be employed as negative controls. As indicated in Table 2, very low IC_{50} values were determined for compounds **1**, **3**, and **5**, confirming that a decrease in peak area during spiking experiments is indicative of NO scavenging properties. Of note, constituents **3** and **5** were both shown to exert higher NO scavenging activity than the positive control, ascorbic acid. The presumed weak effect of compounds **4** and **6** was also confirmed, as attested by their IC_{50} being superior to 200 µg/mL.

Table 2. Nitric oxide scavenging activity of major constituents from *Aloysia triphylla* leaves.

Compound	Nitric oxide Scavenging Activity (IC_{50}, µg/mL)
Luteolin-7-O-diglucuronide	69 ± 5 [b]
Verbascoside	56 ± 4 [a]
Diosmetin-7-O-diglucuronide	>200 [c,*]
Isoverbascoside	51 ± 3 [a]
Apigenin-7-O-glucoside	>200 [c,*]
Ascorbic acid (positive control)	71 ± 2 [b]

Values with different superscripts are significantly different ($p < 0.05$). * For statistical analysis, IC_{50} values of diosmetin-7-O-diglucuronide and apigenin-7-O-glucoside was assumed to be 200 µg/mL.

All these results are consistent with SNP spiking HPLC experiments, establishing that the method has successfully led to the detection of bioactive constituents of the studied extract. Additionally, compounds **3** and **5** were confirmed to be significantly more effective than compound **1** ($p < 0.05$), signifying that pretreatment with a low concentrated solution of SNP had only oxidized the most reactive scavengers. Of interest, the present study reports, for the first time, the potent NO scavenging properties of **1**, thus, highlighting the efficacy of the spiking method in the search of new NO scavengers. It can also be regarded as an effective experiment to quickly determine bioactive markers from plant extracts, and may be of major interest to support the standardization process of herbal products. Besides, it must be noted that this assay can be considered as more physiologically relevant than a DPPH spiking experiment. Indeed, in addition to using an endogenous radical, SNP spiking experiments are performed in aqueous solutions buffered at pH 7.4 while DPPH cannot be solved in water solution. It is well known that the pH value, as well as the solvent composition, strongly influences the reactivity of radical scavenging compounds [22].

3. Materials and Methods

3.1. Plant Material and Reagents

Dried leaves of *A. triphylla* were obtained from Biosphère 99 (Saint Bonnet de Rochefort, France). Acetonitrile was of chromatographic grade Carlo Erba Reagents SAS (Val de Reuil, France). Phosphoric acid (purity 85%) was purchased from VWR prolabo (Fontenay-sous-Bois, France). Sodium nitroprusside (SNP), N-(1Naphthyl) ethylenediamine dihydrochloride (NED), and sulfanilamide were bought from Sigma–Aldrich Chemical (Saint Quentin Fallavier, France). SNP solutions were freshly prepared in distilled water every half-day and kept protected from light.

3.2. Preparation of Aqueous Extract from A. triphylla Leaves

An infusion of *A. triphylla* leaves was prepared by adding 500 mL of boiling distilled water to powdered plant material (10 g) and was left at room temperature for 30 min. The extract was then filtered and concentrated under reduced pressure using a rotary evaporator. The obtained dried residue (2.57 g) was kept at 4 °C until further analyses.

3.3. Colorimetric NO Scavenging Assay and Total Phenolic Content Evaluation

Nitric oxide scavenging colorimetric assay was performed using Griess reagent as previously described by Silva and Soysa [23]. Briefly, SNP (10 mM in PBS) was mingled with different concentrations of ATAE (50–300 µg/mL in PBS) or pure compounds (5–200 µg/mL in PBS). A reaction mixture without extract or pure compound was also prepared on the same basis to be employed as the negative control. After 2 h incubation at 37 °C, Griess reagent (1% sulfanilamide, 5% phosphoric acid, and 0.1% NED) was added to the reaction mixtures. Absorbance was recorded at 540 nm after 10 min incubation. NO scavenging activities were expressed as IC_{50} values, which correspond to the concentration required to reduce 50% of the NO formation. Ascorbic acid was employed as the positive control.

Total phenolic content (TPC) was estimated by the Folin–Ciocalteu method as previously reported by Meda et al. [11]. The amount of TPC was indicated as a milligram of gallic acid equivalent per gram of dried extract.

3.4. HPLC Analysis of ATAE

Analytical HPLC consisted of two L7100 pumps, an L7200 autosampler, an L2450 LaChrom Elite diode array detector, a D7000 interface system controller, and an EZ Chrom Elite software (VWR-Hitachi, Radnor, Pennsylvania, PA, USA). ATAE samples (2 mg/mL) were analyzed using a LiChrospher® RP8 column (125 × 4 mm, 5 µm particle size). A gradient elution was employed with a mobile phase consisting of water containing 1% of phosphoric acid (A) and acetonitrile (B). The program was set as follows: 0–15 min, 10–15% B; 15–25 min, 15% B; 25–40 min, 15–20% B; 40–50 min, 20–40% B; 50–60 min, 40–60% B. The flow rate was 1.0 mL/min and the injection volume was 30 µL. All analyses were performed at a detection wavelength of 280 nm and the column was maintained at ambient temperature.

3.5. Pre-Column SNP–HPLC Analysis for Screening of Main NO Scavengers in ATAE

Briefly, ATAE was dissolved in PBS at a concentration of 10 mg/mL and was subsequently mixed with SNP solutions of different concentrations (1, 2.5, and 5 mM, final concentrations) at the ratio of 1:5 (*v/v*). The resulting mixtures were incubated for 30 min at 37 °C prior to HPLC analyses in previously reported conditions (Section 3.4). As a control, ATAE was identically treated except that PBS was substituted for the SNP solution. All solutions were prepared and analyzed in triplicate. The percentage of the remaining compound was calculated as the ratio between the compound peak area after the reaction with SNP divided by the compound peak area of the control sample.

3.6. Isolation and Identification of Compounds 1 and 4

A portion of ATAE (500 mg) was subjected to exclusion chromatography (Sephadex® LH-20, 75 g) eluted with H_2O/MeOH (40:60) to yield a total of 8 combined fractions. Fractions 6 (30 mg) and 7 (40 mg) were then submitted to semi-preparative HPLC (Nucleosil® RP-18, 250 mm × 100 mm, 5 µm particle size) eluted with a mobile phase consisting of water containing 0.1% trifluoroacetic acid and acetonitrile to obtain compounds **1** (7 mg) and **4** (11 mg). Proton and carbon nuclear magnetic resonance spectra were recorded in DMSO-d_6 on a Bruker DRX 500 spectrometer (11.7 T:^{1}H:500 MHz, ^{13}C:125 MHz) (Bruker Biospin SAS, Wissembourg, France).

3.7. Statistical Analyses

The statistical significance of difference was analyzed by one-way ANOVA, followed by a Fisher's LSD test, and values $p < 0.05$ were considered significant. All data are indicated as mean ± standard error of mean (SEM, $n = 3$).

4. Conclusions

In the present study, a novel SNP spiking HPLC assay has been successfully devised to quickly and directly detect NO scavengers from *A. triphylla* leaves. Three compounds, including luteolin-7-*O*-diglucuronide, as well as verbascoside and isoverbascoside, were shown to be the main contributors to the activity of the studied extract. It must be noted that the potent NO scavenging activities of luteolin-7-*O*-diglucuronide is reported for the first time, thus, highlighting the usefulness of this novel approach in the search of new bioactive chemical entities. Of interest, this method can be applied in all laboratories with common HPLC-UV equipment and can, thus, be widely adopted for the analysis of other NO scavenging plant extracts.

Author Contributions: Conceptualization, F.S.; Investigation, D.F., A.D.-R. and M.V.; Project administration, C.F.; Resources, A.B.; Supervision, F.S.; Validation, D.F. and S.F.N.; Writing—original draft, F.S.; Writing—review & editing, C.F.

Funding: This research received no external funding.

Conflicts of Interest: The authors declare that there is no conflict of interest.

References

1. Knott, A.B.; Bossy-Wetzel, E. Nitric Oxide in Health and Disease of the Nervous System. *Antioxid. Redox Signal.* **2009**, *11*, 541–553. [CrossRef] [PubMed]
2. Kone, B.C. Nitric oxide in renal health and disease. *Am. J. Kidney Dis.* **1997**, *30*, 311–333. [CrossRef]
3. Rastaldo, R.; Pagliaro, P.; Cappello, S.; Penna, C.; Mancardi, D.; Westerhof, N.; Losano, G. Nitric oxide and cardiac function. *Life Sci.* **2007**, *81*, 779–793. [CrossRef] [PubMed]
4. Blantz, R.C.; Munger, K. Role of Nitric Oxide in Inflammatory Conditions. *Nephron* **2002**, *90*, 373–378. [CrossRef] [PubMed]
5. Singh, V.K.; Mehrotra, S.; Narayan, P.; Pandey, C.M.; Agarwal, S.S. Modulation of autoimmune diseases by nitric oxide. *Immunol. Res.* **2000**, *22*, 1–19. [CrossRef]
6. Jagetia, G.C.; Baliga, M.S. The evaluation of nitric oxide scavenging activity of certain Indian medicinal plants in vitro: A preliminary study. *J. Med. Food* **2004**, *7*, 343–348. [CrossRef] [PubMed]
7. Yokozawa, T.; Chen, C.P.; Tanaka, T. Direct scavenging of nitric oxide by traditional crude drugs. *Phytomedicine* **2000**, *6*, 453–463. [CrossRef]
8. Dirsch, V.M.; Stuppner, H.; Vollmar, A.M. The Griess assay: Suitable for a bio-guided fractionation of anti-inflammatory plant extracts? *Planta Med.* **1998**, *64*, 423–426. [CrossRef] [PubMed]
9. Li, Y.-J.; Chen, J.; Li, Y.; Li, Q.; Zheng, Y.-F.; Fu, Y.; Li, P. Screening and characterization of natural antioxidants in four *Glycyrrhiza* species by liquid chromatography coupled with electrospray ionization quadrupole time-of-flight tandem mass spectrometry. *J. Chromatogr. A* **2011**, *1218*, 8181–8191. [CrossRef] [PubMed]
10. Zhang, Y.-P.; Shi, S.-Y.; Xiong, X.; Chen, X.-Q.; Peng, M.-J. Comparative evaluation of three methods based on high-performance liquid chromatography analysis combined with a 2,2′-diphenyl-1-picrylhydrazyl assay for the rapid screening of antioxidants from *Pueraria lobata* flowers. *Anal. Bioanal. Chem.* **2012**, *402*, 2965–2976. [CrossRef] [PubMed]
11. Meda, N.R.; Fraisse, D.; Gnoula, C.; Vivier, M.; Felgines, C.; Senejoux, F. Characterization of antioxidants from *Detarium microcarpum* Guill. et Perr. leaves using HPLC-DAD coupled with pre-column DPPH assay. *Eur. Food Res. Technol.* **2017**, *243*, 1659–1666. [CrossRef]

12. Shui, G.; Peng, L.L. An improved method for the analysis of major antioxidants of *Hibiscus esculentus* Linn. *J. Chromatogr. A* **2004**, *1048*, 17–24. [CrossRef]
13. Könczöl, Á.; Kéry, Á.; Keserű, G.M.; Balogh, G.T. LC Determination of Peroxynitrite Scavenging Activity of Phenols from *Salvia* spp. *Chromatographia* **2010**, *71*, 51–59. [CrossRef]
14. Abderrahim, F.; Estrella, S.; Susín, C.; Arribas, S.M.; González, M.C.; Condezo-Hoyos, L. The antioxidant activity and thermal stability of lemon verbena (*Aloysia triphylla*) infusion. *J. Med. Food* **2011**, *14*, 517–527. [CrossRef] [PubMed]
15. Lenoir, L.; Joubert-Zakeyh, J.; Texier, O.; Lamaison, J.-L.; Vasson, M.-P.; Felgines, C. *Aloysia triphylla* infusion protects rats against dextran sulfate sodium-induced colonic damage. *J. Sci. Food Agric.* **2012**, *92*, 1570–1572. [CrossRef] [PubMed]
16. Tabart, J.; Kevers, C.; Pincemail, J.; Defraigne, J.-O.; Dommes, J. Comparative antioxidant capacities of phenolic compounds measured by various tests. *Food Chem.* **2009**, *113*, 1226–1233. [CrossRef]
17. Matsumoto, T. *Phytochemistry Research Progress*; Nova Science Publishers: New York, NY, USA, 2008; ISBN 978-1-60456-232-3.
18. Mabry, T.J.; Markham, K.R.; Thomas, M.B. *The Systematic Identification of Flavonoids*; Springer: Berlin, Germany, 1970; ISBN 978-3-64288-460-3.
19. Felgines, C.; Fraisse, D.; Besson, C.; Vasson, M.-P.; Texier, O. Bioavailability of lemon verbena (*Aloysia triphylla*) polyphenols in rats: Impact of colonic inflammation. *Br. J. Nutr.* **2014**, *111*, 1773–1781. [CrossRef] [PubMed]
20. Carnat, A.; Carnat, A.P.; Chavignon, O.; Heitz, A.; Wylde, R.; Lamaison, J.L. Luteolin 7-diglucuronide, the major flavonoid compound from *Aloysia triphylla* and *Verbena officinalis*. *Planta Med.* **1995**, *61*, 490. [CrossRef] [PubMed]
21. Murata, T.; Miyase, T.; Yoshizaki, F. Cyclic spermidine alkaloids and flavone glycosides from *Meehania fargesii*. *Chem. Pharm. Bull.* **2010**, *58*, 696–702. [CrossRef] [PubMed]
22. Amorati, R.; Pedulli, G.F.; Cabrini, L.; Zambonin, L.; Landi, L. Solvent and pH Effects on the Antioxidant Activity of Caffeic and Other Phenolic Acids. *J. Agric. Food Chem.* **2006**, *54*, 2932–2937. [CrossRef] [PubMed]
23. Silva, I.K.; Soysa, P. Evaluation of phytochemical composition and antioxidant capacity of a decoction containing *Adenanthera pavonina* L. and *Thespesia populnea* L. *Pharmacogn. Mag.* **2011**, *7*, 193–199. [CrossRef] [PubMed]

Sample Availability: Samples of the compounds are not available from the authors.

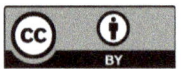

© 2018 by the authors. Licensee MDPI, Basel, Switzerland. This article is an open access article distributed under the terms and conditions of the Creative Commons Attribution (CC BY) license (http://creativecommons.org/licenses/by/4.0/).

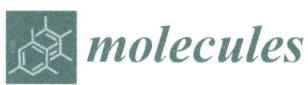

Article

Physicochemical, Functional, and Nutraceutical Properties of Eggplant Flours Obtained by Different Drying Methods

Jenny R. Rodriguez-Jimenez [1], Carlos A. Amaya-Guerra [1,*], Juan G. Baez-Gonzalez [1], Carlos Aguilera-Gonzalez [1], Vania Urias-Orona [2] and Guillermo Nino-Medina [3,*]

[1] Facultad de Ciencias Biologicas, Universidad Autonoma de Nuevo Leon, Ave. Universidad S/N, Cd. Universitaria, 66450 San Nicolas de los Garza, Mexico; ing.rodriguezjimenez@hotmail.com (J.R.R.-J.); baezjuan@yahoo.com.mx (J.G.B.-G.); carlos.aguileragn@uanl.edu.mx (C.A.-G.)
[2] Laboratorio de Quimica y de Alimentos, Facultad de Salud Publica y Nutricion, Universidad Autonoma de Nuevo Leon, Col. Mitras Centro, C.P. 64460 Monterrey, Nuevo Leon, Mexico; vania.uriaso@uanl.mx
[3] Laboratorio de Quimica y Bioquimica, Facultad de Agronomia, Universidad Autonoma de Nuevo Leon, Francisco Villa S/N, Col. Ex-Hacienda El Canada, C.P. 66050 General Escobedo, Nuevo Leon, Mexico
* Correspondence: numisamaya@hotmail.com (C.A.A.-G.); guillermo.ninomd@uanl.edu.mx (G.N.-M.)

Academic Editors: Alessandra Durazzo and Massimo Lucarini
Received: 29 October 2018; Accepted: 2 December 2018; Published: 5 December 2018

Abstract: The importance of consuming functional foods has led the food industry to look for alternative sources of ingredients of natural origin. Eggplants are a type of vegetable that is valued for its content in phytochemical compounds and it is due to the fact that this research is conducted towards the development of eggplant flour as a proposal to be used as a functional ingredient in the food industry. In this study, the eggplant fruits were divided into four groups, based on the drying method and the equipment used: Minced, drying oven (T1); sliced, drying oven (T2); sliced and frozen, drying tunnel (T3); and sliced, drying tunnel (T4). All the eggplant flours showed the same trend regarding their antioxidant capacity and phenolic content in the order T2 > T4 > T1 > T3. The freezing of eggplant was found to have a negative effect on functional and antioxidant properties. With respect to their nutritional composition, the flours did not change in their crude fiber, protein, and fat contents. In general terms, the T2 flour is a potential ingredient for the preparation of foods with functional properties since it is rich in phenolic compounds and antioxidants.

Keywords: eggplant; flour; phenolics; antioxidant activity; functional ingredient

---

1. Introduction

In recent years, the food industry has focused its efforts in the development of new products with properties that not only provide the necessary nutrients for human food, but also help prevent diseases related to nutrition such as diabetes, obesity, hypertension, and cardiovascular complications. It has been found that there is a significant correlation between the regular intake of phytochemicals and the prevention of these lifestyle-related diseases [1]. Antioxidants have attracted great attention as possible agents to prevent and treat diseases related to oxidative stress [2]. The antioxidants used by the food industry can be either from natural sources or from a synthetic origin (such as butylated hydroxytoluene and butylated hydroxyanisole). The latter has been found to be potentially carcinogenic and toxic [3]. Consequently, a niche in the food industry is opened to replace the existing synthetic antioxidants with those of natural origin found in fruits and vegetables, which are mainly vitamins and polyphenols [2].

Eggplant is an economically important vegetable crop from the tropical and subtropical zones of the world [4]. This crop produces fruit of different colors, sizes, and shapes [5]. Eggplant is a valued vegetable for its composition in phytochemicals considered as nutraceuticals [6], in particular, polyphenols and dietary fiber [4].

In Mexico, eggplant production was 172,112 tons in 2016. It is mostly exported to the United States as this vegetable is not commonly consumed domestically [7] due to a lack of information regarding its preparation and characteristics. Eggplant has a non-climacteric pattern of respiration, which leads to a short shelf life despite being harvested in immature stages of development [8]. Therefore, the use of eggplant is suggested as a flour with high nutritional value, which can also be used as an antioxidant of natural origin. Therefore, the objective of this work is to evaluate the physicochemical, functional, and nutraceutical properties of eggplant flour as a proposed functional ingredient.

2. Results and Discussion

2.1. Eggplant Flour Samples

The eggplant flour produced was labelled as T1 (eggplant minced and dried at 45 °C–50 °C in a drying oven), T2 (sliced eggplant dried at 45 °C–50 °C in a drying oven), T3 (sliced eggplant was frozen and dried at 40 °C–45 °C in a tunnel dryer), and T4 (sliced eggplant dried at 40 °C–45 °C in a tunnel dryer). Eggplant is a vegetable with a high percentage of water (approximately 90%), which allows microorganisms and biochemical reactions to deteriorate, thus reducing its shelf life. In general, eggplant is a difficult vegetable to dehydrate due to its high percentage of water, which implies long drying times. With the use of the drying tunnel, the drying time was reduced from 48 h (drying oven) to 16 h (70% reduction in efficiency), showing that dehydration is faster when the air speed increases [9] and the speed of drying at high temperature decreases due to the hardening phenomenon [10–12].

2.2. Proximal Chemical Analysis

The results of the nutritional composition of the eggplant flours are shown in Table 1. Eggplant flour has low values for moisture content (1.5% to 8.5%), below the Mexican standard (NOM-247-SSA1-2008) of 15% [13]. The T2 sample had the highest moisture content, while the T4 sample had the lowest moisture content. The moisture content obtained in this study was lower than other results (7.7% to 9.45%) reported from different types of *Solanum melongena*, dried in the same range (45 °C to 50 °C) of temperature [4,14].

Table 1. Nutritional components of different obtained flours.

Component (%)	T1	T2	T3	T4
Moisture	5.26 ± 0.4 [b]	8.57 ± 0.26 [a]	4.55 ± 0.32 [c]	1.57 ± 0.09 [d]
Ash	6.47 ± 0.38 [b]	7.31 ± 0.03 [a]	7.31 ± 0.08 [a]	6.53 ± 0.25 [b]
Fat	1.79 ± 0.07 [a]	1.75 ± 0.03 [a]	1.73 ± 0.0 [a]	1.73 ± 0.02 [a]
Protein	12.57 ± 0.39 [a]	12.5 ± 0.45 [a]	12.68 ± 0.29 [a]	12.77 ± 0.24 [a]
Crude Fiber	12.74 ± 0.37 [a]	12.32 ± 0.43 [a]	11.8 ± 0.59 [a]	12.17 ± 0.92 [a]
Carbohydrates [+]	61.17 ± 0.7 [b]	57.54 ± 0.52 [c]	61.92 ± 0.18 [b]	65.22 ± 1.22 [a]

Eggplant minced and dried in a drying oven (T1), sliced eggplant dried in a drying oven (T2), sliced eggplant frozen and dried in a tunnel dryer (T3), and sliced eggplant dried in a tunnel dryer (T4). Average values with three replicates ± standard deviations, of three different lots. Mean values labeled with a different letter in the same file are significantly different ($p < 0.05$). [+] Carbohydrates (%) = 100 − (% moisture + % ash + % fat + % protein + % crude fiber).

Flour having a moisture content of 9% to 10% is suitable for extended shelf life [15] since a lower moisture content in flour shows a better storage stability. The range of the average ash content determined among the four eggplant flours was 6.47%–7.31%, and it was similar to the eggplant ash content of other investigations treated under the same drying temperature conditions [4,14], compared to the ash content obtained from different types of eggplants (0.48%–1%), and 4.93%–13.7% (dry base) [16]; the drying treatment allows the concentration of the eggplant nutrients. Regarding the determination of proteins, the results obtained fell in a small range of 12.55%–12.77%. The results of this study are in accordance with the USDA database [17]. They have reported that protein content for fresh eggplant was 0.98% (12.73% in dry basic). Various types (Indian, Thai, Chinese, and white) of eggplants dried at the same temperature produced similar protein contents (12%–15%) [4] to the results obtained in this study.

The average fat content (1.75%) of the flour in this study was higher than that reported by Nino-Medina et al. [16] in fresh eggplant (Chinese, Philippine, Thai, Hindu and American types), with obtained values between 0.3% and 0.4% (dry base). Uthumporn et al. [4] found levels of 0.88% to 5.18% in different types (Indian, Thai, Chinese, and white) of eggplant flour; the lowest values were for flour samples made at 50 °C. Carbohydrates contents for the samples were between 57% and 65%. The result of the present investigation is similar in the amount of carbohydrates contained in the eggplant flour mentioned before, which were in the range of 62%–68%. The main soluble sugars were glucose and fructose [18]. They reported starch content between 1.43% and 2.38% in fresh eggplant. Eggplant flour contained a lower amount of carbohydrates and moisture compared with wheat flour, yet it had more fiber.

2.3. Physicochemical Parameters

The pH and titratable acidity are analytically determined in separate ways, and each has its own particular impact on food quality [19]. The pH is a good predictor of the ability of a microorganism to grow in a specific food, while the titratable acidity is a good predictor of the impact of acid content on the flavor of food [20]. On the other hand, color is the first notable characteristic of a food and often predetermines our expectations. Natural and synthetic colors play several roles in foods and consumers use the color as a way to identify a food and also as a way to judge the quality of a food [21].

With the exception of the titratable acidity and b^* chromatic property, in which statistical differences were not observed ($p > 0.05$), other physicochemical parameters showed statistical differences ($p < 0.05$) between eggplant flour samples (Table 2). The values of pH of eggplant flours were slightly acidic and ranged from 3.89 to 4.14, while titratable acidity values were low ranging from 0.46% to 0.47%. In addition, chromatic values were from 52.50 to 64.60, 4.55 to 9.65, 20.15 to 21.65, 21.09 to 23.60, and 65.98 to 77.54 in L^*, a^*, b^*, C^*, and h, respectively. All the eggplant flours had a "mostly desaturated dark orange" color. However, the color of the treatments 1 and 2 can be classified as a "pale brown", while the treatments the color of the treatments 3 and 4 can be classified as "clear brown"; the main difference among these two colors tonalities is due mainly to the L^* value.

Table 2. Physicochemical parameters of different eggplant flours.

Flour	pH	TA (%)	Chromatic Properties					View
			L^*	a^*	b^*	C^*	h	
T1	3.89 ± 0.04 [b]	0.47 ± 0.004 [a]	52.50 ± 0.14 [c]	9.65 ± 0.49 [a]	21.65 ± 0.49 [a]	23.60 ± 0.65 [a]	65.98 ± 0.60 [b]	
T2	3.97 ± 0.02 [b]	0.47 ± 0.004 [a]	52.55 ± 0.49 [c]	9.25 ± 0.63 [ab]	21.05 ± 0.49 [a]	22.99 ± 0.71 [ab]	66.29 ± 0.95 [b]	
T3	4.19 ± 0.01 [a]	0.46 ± 0.009 [a]	57.40 ± 0.42 [b]	6.90 ± 0.56 [b]	20.15 ± 0.21 [a]	21.30 ± 0.01 [b]	71.10 ± 1.62 [b]	
T4	4.14 ± 0.03 [a]	0.46 ± 0.004 [a]	64.60 ± 0.42 [a]	4.55 ± 0.07 [c]	20.60 ± 0.14 [a]	21.09 ± 0.16 [b]	77.54 ± 0.10 [a]	

Potential of hydrogen (pH), titratable acidity (TA) and chromatic properties (L^*, a^*, b^*, C^*, h) of eggplant flours. Values are the average of three replicates ± standard deviations, of three different lots. Mean values labeled with a different letter in the same column are significantly different ($p < 0.05$).

The cause of this color difference is attributed to the enzymatic browning of vegetable tissue, which is one of the main causes of loss of quality in food drying. The color values corresponding to the T1 and T2 samples show the effect caused by the Maillard reaction in eggplant during the drying process due to the formation of brown complex polymers (melanins) [22]. The T1 and T2 samples are more affected by this phenomenon due to the long drying times in the drying oven. The sample T3 shows a color similar to the aforementioned samples due to the damage by the low temperatures to which it was subjected before drying.

There is no literature available for comparison with the current report as there are no studies on the evaluation of chromatic properties of eggplant flour; however, flours obtained from other vegetables through similar methods to the ones used in this study have been previously reported. In this regard, Noor and Komathi [23] obtained flour from peeled pumpkin pulp and unpeeled pumpkin pulp. Their process for production of flour consisted in soaking the pumpkin pulps in a 0.1% sodium methabisulphite for 30 min; after that, the pulps were washed, sliced, and dried overnight at 60 °C. The chromatic properties of the obtained flours were 63.45, 15.68, 53.83, 56.07, and 73.76 for peeled pumpkin pulp flour and 64.93, 13.53, 49.45, 51.27, and 74.70 for unpeeled pumpkin pulp flour in L^*, a^*, b^*, C^* and h chromatic parameters. On the other hand, Que et al. [24] (2007) also obtained flour from pumpkin through hot air-drying procedures. In this study, the pumpkin flesh was cut into slices and hot air-dried at 70 °C for 54 h. Both products were ground and sieved using a 60 mesh screen (250 μm). The chromatic properties of the obtained flours were 80.15, 13.43, 48.63, 50.45, and 74.56 for freeze-dried flour, and 61.83, 11.12, 41.87, 43.32, and 75.13 for hot air-dried flour in L^*, a^*, b^*, C^* and h chromatic parameters.

All the chromatic parameters obtained in the studies mentioned above were higher than the chromatic properties of our eggplant flours; this could be mainly attributed to the fact that pumpkin has different chemical and physical characteristics from eggplant. Another important fact that produces a lower L^* value in eggplant in contrast to pumpkin is the high concentration of phenolics in the eggplant skin (anthocyanins) and pulp (phenolic acids), which are oxidized by an enzymatic mechanism once they are sliced, and also to the non-enzymatic browning due to the heat treatment used in the production of the flour.

2.4. Functional Properties

The water holding capacity (WHC) of the samples was between 1.2 to 2 g water/g flour (Table 3). Sample T4 (2.08 g water/g flour) had the highest amount of WHC and T1 (1.28 g water/g flour) had the lowest values. Similar values were found in frozen-dried flour from soy beans (1.8 g water/g flour) and pumpkin flour (1.5–2.5 g water/g flour) dried at 60 °C [23,25]. The capacity to absorb water is considered a functional property of proteins, fundamental in viscous foods such as sauces, soups, baked goods, and doughs, products where a good protein-water interaction is required [26]. Different protein structure and different hydrophilic carbohydrates contribute to the variation in WHC of flours [27,28]. This agrees with the result of Chen and et al. [29], study which reported that high WHC of fruit fibers is linked to the high pectin content of the fruits. The WHC aids modification of texture and viscosity in formulated food.

Table 3. Functional properties of eggplant flours.

Flour	WHC (g Water/g Flour DW)	OHC (g Oil/ g Flour DW)	EC (%)
T1	1.28 ± 0.1 [b]	2.13 ± 0.26 [d]	25.00 ± 0.10 [c]
T2	1.61 ± 0.16 [b]	4.49 ± 0.59 [b]	37.33 ± 0.57 [a]
T3	1.40 ± 0.25 [b]	3.79 ± 0.16 [c]	34.50 ± 0.50 [b]
T4	2.08 ± 0.13 [a]	5.22 ± 0.11 [a]	37.83 ± 0.28 [a]

Water holding capacity (WHC), oil holding capacity (OHC) and emulsion capacity (EC) of eggplant flours. DW = dried weight. Values are the average of three replicates ± standard deviations, of three different lots. Mean values labeled with a different letter in the same column are significantly different ($p < 0.05$).

The oil holding capacity (OHC) differed significantly ($p \leq 0.05$) among T1, T2, T3, and T4 (Table 3). *Treculia africana* seed flour, prepared at 100 °C, parboiled and dried (55 °C, 24 h) had an OHC in the range of 1.14–1.3 g oil/g for flour [30,31] and the flour from soy beans (1.93 g oil/g flour) [25] had lower values than the eggplant samples. However, the *Canavalia ensiformis* flour (3.15 g oil/g flour) [32] had similar values to these results. This high oil holding capacity can be attributed to the high levels of nonpolar residues protein molecules [32]. On the other hand, the heat treatment increases the absorption of oil [31]. This is an increase attributed to the dissociation and denaturation of proteins by heat. The T4 and T2 treatments have a greater water/oil retention capacity than the T1 and T3 samples; these changes in the retention capacity can be attributed to the modification of the physical structure of the food. Methods of food processing such as freezing and mincing can affect protein conformation and hydrophobicity [33,34].

For the emulsification capacity (EC), T1 (25%) had the lowest value with respect to the T2, T3, and T4 (Table 3), as Yu et al. [34] suggests, food processing methods affect protein conformation and hydrophobicity. The mincing process was the most probable reason for the lower EC of the T1 sample. Emulsification capacity is considered as an index of the ability of proteins or peptides to adsorb on the new created surface, delaying coalescence [35]. According to Kinsella et al. and Sathe et al. [36,37], the emulsifying capacity of proteins tend to decrease as protein concentration is increased; nevertheless, it was the opposite in this study.

In short, these functional properties verify the application of this flour as an ingredient in the formulation of a food, as the physical-chemical characteristics define the behavior of proteins, carbohydrates, and fibers in the processed food.

2.5. Total Phenols Content (TPC)

Polyphenols are a large group of phytochemicals that are considered responsible for the health benefits associated with fruits and vegetables [38]. Plant polyphenols can scavenge free radicals due to their chemical structure. The total phenols content (TPC) was markedly higher in samples T2 and T4 (Table 4), while it was lower for samples T3 and T1 (4183 and 8211 mg chlorogenic acid/kg flour, respectively). Similar data were reported [39] in the juice from 31 eggplant varieties (commercial varieties, landraces, and hybrids between the landraces) that were in the range of 5450 to 10,480 (mg chlorogenic acid/kg of sample). It was found that eggplant displays an important intraspecific variation for the composition traits studied, and in some cases, there are considerable differences among the varietal types.

Table 4. Phenolic compounds of eggplant flours.

Flour	TPC (mgCAE/kg Flour DW)	TFC (mgCatE/kg Flour DW)	TCC (mgCatE/kg Flour DW)	TAC (mgC3GE/kg Flour DW)
T1	8211 ± 452 [c]	2060 ± 396 [c]	3022 ± 330 [a]	1612 ± 44 [a]
T2	18,227 ± 442 [a]	15,753 ± 1027 [a]	1461 ± 176 [c]	679 ± 12 [b]
T3	4183 ± 123 [d]	1473 ± 188 [c]	1240 ± 206 [c]	230 ± 13 [d]
T4	10,866 ± 673 [b]	10,300 ± 467 [b]	2307 ± 145 [b]	519 ± 10 [c]

Total phenols content (TPC), total flavonoid content (TFC) and condensed tannin content (CTC). mgCAE = milligrams of chlorogenic acid equivalents, mgCatE = milligrams of catechin equivalents, mgC3G = milligrams of cyanidin-3-glucoside, DW = dried weight. Values are the average of three replicates ± standard deviations, of three different lots. Mean values labeled with a different letter in the same column are significantly different ($p < 0.05$).

Nino-Medina et al. [16] report similar results in their report based on a study in frozen, dried eggplant from different varieties (Chinese, Philippine, American, Hindu, and Thai); the total phenols content ranged from 15,120 to 20,490 (mg chlorogenic acid/kg of sample). The results obtained in this study were higher than the results of fresh eggplant by Nisha et al. [38] on different eggplant varieties that reported to contain between 490 to 1070 (mg gallic acid equivalents/kg of sample) and 570 to 650 (mg chlorogenic acid/kg of sample) for Black Beauty and Violetta Lunga varieties [40]. The low value of the T3 sample is due to the freezing before the dehydration; freezing reduces the original value of the food up to 80% due to the increase in water activity [41]. This has a greater effect than the mincing the sample, as it was in the case of the T1 sample.

2.6. Total Flavonoids Content (TFC)

The total flavonoids content of different eggplant flours is shown in Table 4. TFC content follows the order T2 > T4 > T1 > T3. According to these results, a significant difference was found between the pre-drying treatments (mincing, slicing, and slicing/freezing), where the T3 sample was the most affected by the freezing treatment of eggplant slices before drying, showing the same behavior as the TPC. The decrease in TFC level in the flour subjected to pre-drying treatments (mincing and slicing/freezing) could occur because part of the anthocyanin was degraded during these treatments. Ninfali et al. [40] report a total flavonoid content between 257 and 284 mg caffeic acid equivalents/kg of the sample in fresh Black Beauty and Violetta Lunga eggplant varieties. Uthumporn et al. [4] found a range between 9090 and 29,180 mg catechin equivalent/kg, but their report was based on a study of eggplant flour dried at same temperature range as the one used in this study.

2.7. Total Catechins Content (TCC)

The content of total catechins was maintained in the range of 1240 to 3022 (mg catechins/kg flour), which reveals a significant difference between tannin contents of the four eggplant flour extracts ($p < 0.05$). Indeed, the T1 extract presented the highest level among the four flour samples. Alkurd et al. [42] obtained 4137 mg tannic acid equivalents/kg from eggplant extract whole fruit, while Boulekbache et al. [43] obtained 42.6 mg tannic acid equivalents/kg from eggplant peels extract. The mincing of the eggplants before the drying process had a significant effect on the TCC in comparison with the other treatments after drying the eggplant.

2.8. Total Anthocyanins

The total anthocyanins content of different eggplant flours is shown in Table 4. The results were in the range of 230 a 1612 (mgC3GE/kg Flour DW) and follows the order T1 > T2 > T4 > T3. Anthocyanins results obtained in this study were similar to those reported by Nino et al. [16] in different eggplant types of Chinese (1287 mgC3GE/kg of eggplant), Philippine (1610 mgC3GE/kg of eggplant), American (1234 mgC3GE/kg of eggplant), Hindu 828 mgC3GE/kg of eggplant), Thai (39 mgC3GE/kg of eggplant), and higher than those reported in the Black Bell eggplant type [6], Tunisina, Buia, and L305 [44] raw, grill and boiled (50 to 90, 15 to 41, 31 to 155, and 17 to 96 mg D3R/ 100 g of dry matter, respectively).

2.9. Antioxidant Capacity

Currently, there are numerous methods to measure the antioxidant capacity of a food. In this study, the antioxidant capacity of the flours was measured by using three methods (DPPH, ABTS, and FRAP), using vitamin E analogue as reference (Trolox).

Determination of scavenging stable DPPH free radical is a quick way to evaluate the antioxidant activity of the extracts [45]. Table 5 shows the DPPH activity results of all four different samples. The range was between 9111 to 54,815 (μM Trolox equivalents/kg flour). Nino-Medina et al. [16] found higher results than the results of this study, which were 78,500 μM Trolox equivalents/kg on frozen, dried American eggplant type.

The ABTS (2,2'-azinobis-(3-ethylbenzothiazoline-6-sulfonic acid) assay is generated by the oxidation of the ABTS with potassium persulfate [46]. The results for ABTS assay ranged from 14,272 to 63,583 (μM Trolox equivalents/g flour). These results can be seen in Table 5. The results of this study were higher than those reported by Okmen et al. [47]. Their report was based on a study of total water soluble antioxidant activity of 26 eggplant (*Solanum melongena* L.) cultivars from Turkish with an antioxidant activity range from 2664 μM Trolox equivalents/kg to 8247 μM Trolox equivalents/kg.

Table 5. Antioxidant activity of eggplant flours.

Flour	ABTS (μMTE/kg Flour DW)	DPPH (μMTE/kg Flour DW)	FRAP (μMTE/kg Flour DW)
T1	25,484 ± 1166 [c]	15,160 ± 142 [c]	29,534 ± 315 [c]
T2	63,583 ± 1689 [a]	54,815 ± 2447 [a]	105,617 ± 3917 [a]
T3	14,272 ± 433 [d]	9111 ± 160 [d]	17,820 ± 587 [d]
T4	43,205 ± 673 [b]	43,167 ± 3611 [b]	75,361 ± 773 [b]

μMTE = micromoles Trolox equivalents. DW = dried weight. Values are the average of three replicates ± standard deviations of three different lots. Mean values labeled with a different letter in the same column are significantly different ($p < 0.05$).

The ferric reducing antioxidant power (FRAP) assay measures the ability of eggplant flour to reduce Fe^{3+}/tripyridyltriazine complex to its ferrous form [48]. The results shown in Table 5 reveal a significant difference between μM Trolox equivalents/kg flour; the results ranged from 17,820 to 105,617 μM Trolox equivalents/kg flour. Results reported for eggplant extract [43] with different solvents (acetone, methanolic, and ethanolic) were in the range of 21,000 to 27,000 mg of quercetin equivalent/kg of extract.

In general terms, the results of antioxidant activity, such as the content of total phenols content and total flavonoids content, follow the following order T1 > T4 > T1 > T3. A highly significant difference was found between the samples; the sample treated with a pre-treatment of slicing/freezing before drying was the most affected sample, followed by the sample crushed before drying, as explained above in Sections 2.5 and 2.6. Concellon et al. Reference [49] found that eggplant (American type) stored at 0 °C had a rapid degradation of antioxidant compounds. This behavior was described by other authors [49,50] as related to the antioxidant and phenolic content with the degree of browning of the eggplant. Eggplants generate a cellular disruption when being cut, with a loss of compartmentalization that allows contact between enzymes responsible for browning, such as polyphenoloxidase (PPO) and phenolic substrates [49,51–53]. Treatments such as mincing and freezing, and the time of exposure to air and light contribute to the generation of the browning of the eggplant, thus affecting both its content and antioxidant capacity.

3. Materials and Methods

3.1. Flour Preparation

The eggplants fruits used in this study did not had the quality requirements for exportation market (American type) and were purchased from local market in San Nicolas de los Garza County (Nuevo Leon, Mexico). The chemical composition of the eggplant was: Moisture 90%, ash 0.55%, protein 1.07%, fat 0.15%, 1.03% crude fiber, and carbohydrate 5.69%. The fruits (60 units, 25 kg) were washed and separated into four treatments. The fruits of treatment one (T1) were minced (Cyclone Sample mill-model 3010-030, UDY Corporation, Fort Collins, CO, USA) and dried in the drying oven (Model 630, Napco, Oregon, OR, USA) at 45 °C to 50 °C for 2 days. The fruits of treatment two (T2) were sliced and dried using the same condition of the first group. The fruits of treatment 3 (T3) were sliced, frozen, and dried in a tunnel dryer (Procmex Model LQ001, Procomm, Mexico) at 40 °C to 45 °C for 16 h. In the treatment four (T4) the fruits were sliced and dried with the same condition of the third group. The drying temperature range were based on the experience of Uthumporn et al. and Vega-Galvez et al. [4,9] in order to keep the content of phenolic compounds. To determine the drying time, the humidity content was measured as a preliminary result until a percentage below 15% (Mexican Standard NOM-247-SSA1-2008) [13] was obtained. Two drying methods were used, a drying oven (no air circulation and in total darkness, 15.5% humidity,) and a drying tunnel (air circulation, which passes through a set of resistance becomes dry air, 2.5% humidity). The tunnel design allows for the entrance of light, yet it was controlled. The flour was stored in a refrigerator at 4 °C prior to use. Table 6 describes the conditions of the treatments.

Table 6. Pre-treatments and drying method for obtaining of eggplant flours.

Flour	Pre-Treatments	Equipment
T1	Mincing	Drying oven
T2	Cutting in slices	Drying oven
T3	Cutting in slices and freezing	Tunnel dryer
T4	Cutting in slices	Tunnel dryer

3.2. Proximate Composition

Analyses were performed according to the Association of Official Analytical Chemistry [54]. Ash, moisture, and crude fiber content were evaluated gravimetrically (method AOAC 14.006, AOAC 925.15, and AOAC 962.09, respectively). The Goldfisch method (AOAC 920.36C) was used to determine the fat content. The protein content was measured using the Kjeldahl method (AOAC 930.29), and total carbohydrates were determined by difference.

3.3. Physicochemical Properties

In order to measure the potential of hydrogen (pH) and titratable acidity (TA), 10 mL of sample were diluted with 40 mL of distilled water; then, the pH was read. After that, samples were titrated with 0.1 M NaOH to a pH 8.2 (citric acid as predominant) using a Corning, 440 pH meter (Woburn, MA, USA) according to the Association of Official Analytical Chemist methods [55].

For color determination, a 1.5 mL spectrophotometric cuvette was filled with sample and color and was measured using a CR-20 Konica Minolta Color Reader (Tokyo, Japan). Chromatic parameters were obtained using CIELAB (L^*, a^*, b^*) and CIELCH (L^*, C^*, h) color systems according to Commission Internationale De L'ecleirage [56]. L^* defines Lightness (0 = black, 100 = white), a^* indicates red (positive a^*) or green value (negative a^*) and b^* indicates yellow (positive b^*) or blue value (negative b^*), C^* (Chroma; saturation level of h), and h (hue angle: 0° = red, 90° = yellow, 180° = green, 270° = blue). Color view was obtained by using the online software ColorHexa, color converter using L^*, a^*, and b^* values [57].

3.4. Functional Properties

Water and oil holding capacity were determined according to the method described by Beuchat [58] with some modifications; 0.5 g of the sample were taken in 5 mL of distilled water (pH was adjusted to 7) or vegetable oil and mixed by vortexing (model V2H, Boeco, Hamburg, Germany) for 1 min. Then, it was centrifuged at 3000 rpm/30 min. The results were expressed in grams of water-oil retained per gram of sample. The measurements were carried out at room temperature.

For the emulsifying activity, the methods described by Yasumatsu et al. [59] and Zhao et al. [60] were used; 0.5 g of sample with 20 mL of distilled water were mixed in a vortex for 15 min and the pH was adjusted to 7. Vegetable oil was mixed in a relation 1:1 (20 mL) and homogenized (OMNI GLH model glh-01, OMNI International, Georgia, GE, USA) for 3 min at medium speed, and it was then centrifuged at 1300 rpm. The results were expressed as a percentage of the height of the emulsification layer with respect to the total liquid.

3.5. Preparation of the Eggplant Flour Extracts (EFE)

Dried powder (90 mg) was extracted with 5 mL of 80% methanol. The extraction was carried out at room temperature, using a magnetic stirrer. After 40 min, the solution was centrifuged for 5 min at 9500× g (10 °C). The supernatant was collected and stored under refrigerated conditions until it was used.

3.6. Total Phenols Content (TPC)

The total phenols content was determined by using the Folin-Ciocalteu method [61]. This was carried out by mixing 200 µL of the samples extract with 2.6 mL of distilled water, 200 µL of Folin-Ciocalteu reagent, and 2 mL of sodium carbonate solution (7%). After 120 min in the dark (incubation was at room temperature, 23 °C–25 °C), absorbance was measured at 730 nm. The total phenolic content was expressed as mg of chlorogenic acid equivalent (CAE) per 100 g of eggplant flour.

3.7. Total Flavonoids Content (TFC)

The total flavonoids content was measured using the Xiong et al. [62] method, with slight modifications. Briefly, 200 µL of the samples extract were mixed with 3.5 mL of distilled water and 150 µL of 5% $NaNO_2$ solution. After 5 min, 150 µL of 10% $AlCl_3$ solution were dissolved in distilled water, which was added. The mixture was incubated at room temperature for 5 min; then, 1 mL of 1 M NaOH was added and vortexed well for 5 s and left for 15 min. TFC was expressed as mg of catechins equivalent (CAE) per 100 g of eggplant flour.

3.8. Total Catechins Content (TCC)

The total catechins content of the extract was determined by using the vanillin method [63] with some modifications. The sample extract (250 µL) was mixed with a solution of 1% vanillin (650 µL) and a solution of 25% H_2SO_4 (650 µL). After 15 min, the solution was incubated at 30 °C; absorbance was measured at 500 nm. TCC was expressed as mg of catechins equivalent (CAE) per gram of eggplant flour.

3.9. Total Anthocyanins (TAC)

The total anthocyanins content was evaluated according to Abdel-Aal and Hucl [64]. For the extraction of anthocyanins, 200 mg of maize flour was mixed with 10 mL of ethanol-HCl 1N (85:15 v/v, pH 1, 4 °C), purged for 30 s with argon and stirred for 30 min at 200 rpm. Afterwards, the sample was centrifuged at $7759 \times g$ (4 °C, 15 min) and finally, 3.5 mL of sample was measured at 535 nm. The content of was reported as milligrams of cyanidin-3-glucoside (C3G) per kilogram of flour (mgC3GE/kg) as follows: $C = (A/\varepsilon) \times (V/1000) \times MW \times (1/\text{weight of sample}) \times 10^6$, where: C = concentration in mgC3GE/L, A = absorbance of sample, ε = molar absortivity (mgC3GE = 26,965 $cm^{-1}mol^{-1}$), V = volume of sample, and MW = molecular weight of C3G (449.2 g/mol).

3.10. Determination of Antioxidant Capacity

The electron-hydrogen donation ability of eggplant flour extract was measured by using DPPH, ABTS, and FRAP methods. The DPPH method was performed according to the method described by Tai et al. [65] with slight modifications. For this, 1.5 mL of 2 mg/L DPPH solution in methanol 80% and 50 µL of sample were mixed, and incubated at room temperature (23 °C–25 °C) in darkness for 30 min. The absorbance was measured at 517 nm against a blank. Results were expressed in micromoles of Trolox equivalents (µMTE)/g eggplant flour.

For the ABTS assay, the procedure followed the method used in previous assays [66,67] with a few modifications. The stock solutions included 2.6 mM potassium persulfate solution and 7.7 mM ABTS·+ solution; these solutions were mixed in equal quantities. After 12 h at room temperature in the darkness, the ABTS·+ solution was diluted with methanol 80% to obtain an absorbance of 1.000 units at 734 nm using the spectrophotometer. The eggplant flour extract (50 µL) was allowed to react with 1500 µL of ABTS·+ solution for 30 min in the dark; then, the absorbance was measured at 734 nm. Results are expressed in micromoles of Trolox equivalents (µMTE)/g eggplant flour.

The ferric reducing-antioxidant capacity was measured according to the method described by Suárez et al. [68] with slight modifications. The working FRAP reagent was prepared with 5 mL of TPTZ (10 mM), 5 ml of $FeCl_3$ (20 mM), and 50 mL of sodium acetate buffer (300 mM, pH = 3.6). Then,

50 µL of the sample extract were mixed with 1.5 mL of freshly working FRAP reagent. The FRAP assay was carried out at 37 °C in an incubator. The absorbance was measured at 595 nm and the results were expressed in micromoles of Trolox equivalents (µMTE)/g eggplant flour.

3.11. Statistical Analysis

Data from the three replicated experiments were analyzed to determine whether the variances were statistically homogeneous, and the results were expressed as means ± SD. Statistical comparisons were made by one-way analysis of variance (ANOVA) followed by a Tukey's test using SPSS 17 Software. Difference between means were considered significant at $p < 0.05$.

4. Conclusions

All the eggplant flours showed the same trend regarding their antioxidant capacity and phenolic content in the order T2 > T4 > T1 > T3. The freezing of eggplant was found to have a negative effect on functional and antioxidant properties. With respect to their nutritional composition, the flours did not change in their crude fiber, protein, and fat contents. In general terms, the T2 flour is a potential ingredient for the preparation of foods with functional properties since it is rich in phenolic compounds and antioxidants.

Author Contributions: J.R.R.-J., C.A.A.-G. and G.N.-M. conceived and designed the experiments; J.R.R.-J. performed the experiments; J.R.R.-J, C.A.A.-G and G.N.-M. analyzed data; C.A.A.-G., G.N.-M., J.G.B.-G., V.U.-O. and C.A.-G. contributed with reagents, materials, and analysis tools; J.R.R.-J., C.A.A.-G. and G.N.-M. wrote and edited the original draft. Carlos A. Amaya-Guerra and Guillermo Niño-Medina contributed equally to this work.

Funding: This research received no external funding.

Acknowledgments: We would like to thank Consejo Nacional de Ciencia y Tecnologia (CONACyT) for financially supporting J.R.R.-J. to obtain her Ph.D. (scholarship 331700).

Conflicts of Interest: The authors reported no potential conflict of interest.

References

1. Gresele, P.; Cerletti, C.; Guglielmini, G.; Pignatelli, P.; de Gaetano, G.; Violi, F. Effects of resveratrol and other wine polyphenols on vascular function: An update. *J. Nutr. Biochem.* **2011**, *22*, 201–211. [CrossRef] [PubMed]
2. Fu, L.; Xu, B.-T.; Xu, X.-R.; Qin, X.-S.; Gan, R.-Y.; Li, H.-B. Antioxidant capacities and total phenolic contents of 56 wild Fruits from South China. *Molecules* **2010**, *15*, 8602–8617. [CrossRef] [PubMed]
3. Botterweck, A.; Verhagen, H.; Goldbohm, R.A.; Kleinjans, J.; Van den Brandt, P.A. Intake of butylated hydroxyanisole and butylated hydroxytoluene and stomach cancer risk: Results from analyses in the Netherlands cohort study. *Food Chem. Toxicol.* **2000**, *38*, 599–605. [CrossRef]
4. Uthumporn, U.; Fazilah, A.; Tajul, A.; Maizura, M.; Ruri, A. Physico-chemical and antioxidant properties of eggplant flour as a functional ingredient. *Adv. J. Food Sci. Technol.* **2016**, *12*, 235–243. [CrossRef]
5. Nino-Medina, G.; Urias-Orona, V.; Muy-Rangel, M.; Heredia, J. Structure and content of phenolics in eggplant (*Solanum melongena*)—A review. *S. Afr. J. Bot.* **2017**, *111*, 161–169. [CrossRef]
6. Lo Scalzo, R.; Fibiani, M.; Francese, G.; D'Alessandro, A.; Rotino, G.L.; Conte, P.; Mennella, G. Cooking influence on physico-chemical fruit characteristics of eggplant (*Solanum melongena* L.). *Food Chem.* **2016**, *194*, 835–842. [CrossRef] [PubMed]
7. Atlas Agroalimentario. 2017. Available online: http://online.pubhtml5.com/clsi/ibhs/#p=1 (accessed on 26 March 2018).
8. Muy-Rangel, D.; Siller-Cepeda, J.; Garcia-Estrada, R.; Baez-Sanudo, M. Caracterizacion poscosecha de berenjenas producidas en Sinaloa, Mexico. *Rev. Chapingo Serie Hortic.* **2002**, *8*, 171–181. [CrossRef]
9. Vega-Galvez, A.; Ah-Hen, K.; Chacana, M.; Vergara, J.; Martinez-Monzo, J.; Garcia-Segovia, P.; Lemus-Mondaca, R.; Di Scala, K. Effect of temperature and air velocity on drying kinetics, antioxidant capacity, total phenolic content, color, texture and microstructure of apple (var. Granny Smith) slices. *Food Chem.* **2012**, *132*, 51–59. [CrossRef] [PubMed]

10. Hincapie, G.; Omana, M.; Hincapie, C.; Arias, Z.; Velez, L. Efecto de la temperatura de secado sobre las propiedades funcionales de la fibra dietaria presente en la citropulpa. *Rev. Lasallista Investig.* **2010**, *7*, 85–93.
11. Femenia, A.; García-Pascual, P.; Simala, S.; Rossello, C. Effects of heat treatment and dehydration on bioactive polysaccharide acemannan and cell wall polymers from *Aloe barbadensis* Miller. *Carbohyd. Polym.* **2003**, *51*, 397–405. [CrossRef]
12. Demirel, D.; Turhan, M. Air-drying behavior of Dwarf Cavendish and Gros Michel banana slices. *J. Food Eng.* **2003**, *59*, 1–11. [CrossRef]
13. Norma Oficial Mexicana, NOM-247-SSA1-2008. Productos y Servicios. Cereales y sus Productos. Cereales, Harinas de Cereales, Sémolas o Semolinas. Alimentos a base de: Cereales, Semillas Comestibles, de Harinas, Sémolas o Semolinas o sus Mezclas. Productos de Panificación. Disposiciones y Especificaciones Sanitarias y Nutrimentales. Métodos de Prueba. 2008. Available online: http://depa.fquim.unam.mx/amyd/archivero/NOMcereales_12434.pdf (accessed on 1 February 2018).
14. Hussain, J.; Rehman, N.; Khan, A.; Hussain, H.; Al-Harrasi, A.; Ali, L.; Sami, F.; Shinwari, Z. Determination of macro and micronutrients and nutritional prospects of six vegetable species of Mardan, Pakistan. *Pak. J. Bot.* **2011**, *43*, 2829–2833.
15. Nasir, M.; Butt, M.; Anjum, F.; Sharif, K.; Minhas, R. Effect of moisture on the shelf life of wheat flour. *Int. J. Agric. Biol.* **2003**, *5*, 458–459.
16. Niño-Medina, G.; Muy-Rangel, D.; Gardea-Béjar, A.; González-Aguilar, G.; Heredia, B.; Báez-Sañudo, M.; Siller-Cepeda, J.; Vélez-de la Rocha, R. Nutritional and nutraceutical components of commercial eggplant types grown in Sinaloa, Mexico. *Not. Bot. Horti Agrobot.* **2014**, *42*, 538–544. [CrossRef]
17. United States Drug Administration (USDA). Agricultural Research Service; National Nutrient Database for Standard Reference. 2018. Available online: https://ndb.nal.usda.gov/ndb/search/list (accessed on 1 March 2018).
18. San José, R.; Sánchez, M.; Cámara, M.; Prohens, J. Composition of eggplant cultivars of the Occidental type and implications for the improvement of nutritional and functional quality. *Int. J. Food Sci. Technol.* **2013**, *48*, 2490–2499. [CrossRef]
19. Sadler, S.; Murphy, P. Chapter 13. pH and titratable acidity. In *Food Analysis*, 1st ed.; Nielsen, S.S., Ed.; Springer Science: Cham, Switzerland, 2010; p. 219.
20. Tyl, C.; Sadler, G. Chapter 22. pH and titratable acidity. In *Food Analysis*, 5th ed.; Nielsen, S.S., Ed.; Springer Science: Cham, Switzerland, 2017; p. 389.
21. Griffiths, J. Coloring food and beverages. *Food Technol. (Chic.)* **2005**, *59*, 38–44.
22. Tomás-Barberán, F.; Ferreres, F.; Gil, M. Antioxidant phenolic metabolites from fruit and vegetables and changes during postharvest storage and processing. *Stud. Nat. Prod. Chem.* **2000**, *23*, 739–795. [CrossRef]
23. Noor, A.; Komathi, C. Physicochemical and functional properties of peeled and unpeeled pumpkin flour. *J. Food Sci.* **2009**, *74*, S328–S333. [CrossRef]
24. Que, F.; Mao, L.; Fang, X.; Wu, T. Comparison of hot air-drying and freeze-drying on the physicochemical properties and antioxidant activities of pumpkin (*Cucurbita moschata* Duch.) flours. *Int. J. Food Sci. Technol.* **2008**, *43*, 1195–1201. [CrossRef]
25. Chau, C.F.; Cheung, P.C.K. Functional properties of flours prepared from three Chinese indigenous legume seeds. *Food Chem.* **1998**, *61*, 429–433. [CrossRef]
26. Granito, M.; Guerra, M.; Torres, A.; Guinand, J. Efecto del procesamiento sobre las propiedades funcionales de vigna sinensis. *Interciencia* **2004**, *29*, 521–526.
27. Kaur, M.; Sandhu, K.; Singh, N. Comparative study of the functional, thermal and pasting properties of flours from different field pea (*Pisum sativum* L.) and pigeon pea (*Cajanus cajan* L.) cultivars. *Food Chem.* **2007**, *104*, 259–267. [CrossRef]
28. Hodge, J.; Osman, E. Carbohydrates, principles of food science. Part I. In *Food Chemistry*; Fennema, R.O., Ed.; Marcel Dekker Inc.: New York, NY, USA, 1976; pp. 97–200.
29. Chen, J.; Piva, M.; Labuza, T. Evaluation of water binding capacity (WBC) of food fiber sources. *J. Food Sci.* **1984**, *49*, 59–63. [CrossRef]
30. Akubor, P.; Badifu, G. Chemical composition, functional properties and baking potential of African breadfruit kernel and wheat flour blends. *J. Food Sci. Technol.* **2004**, *39*, 223–229. [CrossRef]
31. Fasasi, O.; Eleyinmi, A.; Fasasi, A.; Karim, O. Chemical properties of raw and processed breadfruit (*Treculia africana*) seed flour. *J. Food Agric. Environ.* **2004**, *2*, 65–68.

32. Chel-Guerrero, L.; Perez, V.; Betancur, D.; Dávila, G. Functional properties of flours and protein isolate from *Phaseolus lunatus* and *Canavalia ensiformis* seeds. *J. Agric. Food Chem.* **2002**, *50*, 584–591. [CrossRef] [PubMed]
33. Sangnark, A.; Noomhorm, A. Chemical, physical and baking properties of dietary fiber prepared from rice straw. *Food Res. Int.* **2004**, *37*, 66–74. [CrossRef]
34. Yu, J.; Ahmedna, M.; Goktepe, I. Peanut protein concentrate: Production and functional properties as affected by processing. *Food Chem.* **2007**, *103*, 121–129. [CrossRef]
35. Mahmoud, M. Physicochemical and functional properties of protein hydrolysates in nutritional products. *Food Technol.* **1994**, *48*, 89–95.
36. Kinsella, J.E.; Damodaran, S.; German, B. Physicochemical and functional properties of oil seed proteins with emphasis on soy proteins. *New Protein Foods* **1985**, *5*, 107–179.
37. Sathe, S.; Desphande, S.; Salunhkhe, D. Functional properties of lupin seed (*Lupinus mutabilis*) proteins and protein concentrates. *J. Food Sci.* **1982**, *47*, 491–497. [CrossRef]
38. Nisha, P.; Nazar, N.; Jayamurthy, P. A comparative study on antioxidant activities of different varieties of *Solanum melongena*. *Food Chem. Toxicol.* **2009**, *47*, 2640–2644. [CrossRef] [PubMed]
39. Raigón, M.; Prohens, J.; Muñoz-Falcón, J.; Nuez, F. Comparison of eggplant landraces and commercial varieties for fruit content of phenolics, minerals, dry matter and protein. *J. Food Compos. Anal.* **2008**, *21*, 370–376. [CrossRef]
40. Ninfalli, V.; Mea, G.; Giorgini, S.; Rocchi, M.; Bacchiocca, M. Antioxidant capacity of vegetables, spices and dressings relevant to nutrition. *Brit. J. Nutr.* **2005**, *93*, 257–266. [CrossRef]
41. Molina, Y.; Caez-Ramirez, G.; Rodríguez, M.; Cerón, M.; Garnica, A. Contenido de antioxidantes en papas criollas nativas (*Solanum tuberosum* L. grupo phureja) en proceso de precocción y congelación. *Aliment. Hoy* **2015**, *23*, 31–41. Available online: http://www.alimentoshoy.acta.org.co/index.php/hoy/article/view/341 (accessed on 10 February 2018).
42. Alkurd, A.; Takruri, H.; Al-Sayyed, H. Tannin contents of selected plants used in Jordan. *Jordan J. Agric. Sci.* **2008**, *4*, 265–274. Available online: https://www.uop.edu.jo/download/research/members/1046_2725_Refa.pdf (accessed on 30 February 2018).
43. Boulekbache-Makhlouf, L.; Medouni, L.; Medouni-Adrar, S.; Arkoub, L.; Madani, K. Effect of solvents extraction on phenolic content and antioxidant activity of the byproduct of eggplant. *Ind. Crop. Prod.* **2013**, *49*, 668–674. [CrossRef]
44. Lo Scalzo, R.; Fibiani, M.; Mennella, G.; Rotino, G.; Dal Sasso, M.; Culici, M.; Spallino, A.; Braga, P. Thermal Treatment of Eggplant (*Solanum melongena* L.) Increases the Antioxidant Content and the Inhibitory Effect on Human Neutrophil Burst. *J. Agric. Food Chem.* **2010**, *58*, 3371–3379. [CrossRef]
45. Mokrani, A.; Madani, K. Effect of solvent, time and temperature on the extraction of phenolic compounds and antioxidant capacity of peach (*Prunus persica* L.) fruit. *Sep. Purif. Technol.* **2016**, *162*, 68–76. [CrossRef]
46. Re, R.; Pellegrini, N.; Protteggente, A.; Pannala, A.; Yang, M.; Rice-Evans, C. Antioxidant activity applying an improved ABTS radical cation decolorization assay. *Free Radic. Biol. Med.* **1999**, *26*, 1231–1237. [CrossRef]
47. Okmen, B.; Sigva, H.; Mutlu, S.; Doganlar, S.; Yemenicioglu, A.; Frary, A. Total antioxidant activity and total phenolic contents in different Turkish eggplant (*Solanum melongena* L.) Cultivars. *Int. J. Food Prop.* **2009**, *12*, 616–624. [CrossRef]
48. Moon, J.; Shibamoto, T. Antioxidant assays for plant and food components. *J. Agric. Food Chem.* **2009**, *57*, 1655–1666. [CrossRef] [PubMed]
49. Concellón, A.; Añón, M.; Chaves, A. Effect of low temperature storage on physical and physiological characteristics of eggplant fruit (*Solanum melongena* L.). *LWT-Food Sci. Technol.* **2007**, *40*, 389–396. [CrossRef]
50. Oms-Oliu, G.; Rojas-Graü, M.; González, L.; Varela, P.; Soliva-Fortuny, R.; Hernando, M.; Martín-Belloso, O. Recent approaches using chemical treatments to preserve quality of fresh-cut fruit: A review. *Postharvest Biol. Technol.* **2010**, *57*, 139–148. [CrossRef]
51. Prohens, J.; Rodríguez-Burruezo, A.; Raigón, M.; Nuez, F. Total phenolic concentration and browning susceptibility in a collection of different varietal types and hybrids of eggplant: Implications for breeding for higher nutritional quality and reduced browning. *J. Am. Soc. Hortic. Sci.* **2007**, *132*, 638–646. Available online: http://journal.ashspublications.org/content/132/5/638.short (accessed on 15 February 2018).
52. Mishra, B.; Gautam, S.; Sharma, A. Free phenolics and polyphenol oxidase (PPO): The factors affecting post-cut browning in eggplant (*Solanum melongena*). *Food Chem.* **2013**, *139*, 105–114. [CrossRef]

53. José Zaro, M. Análisis de Factores que Afectan la Acumulación, Distribución y Estabilidad de Antioxidantes de Naturaleza Fenólica en Berenjena (*Solanum melongena* L.). 2014. Available online: http://sedici.unlp.edu.ar/handle/10915/35592 (accessed on 25 February 2018).
54. Association of Official Analytical Chemist (AOAC). *Official Methods of Analysis of International*, 16th ed.; AOAC: Maryland, MD, USA, 1998.
55. Association of Official Analytical Chemist (AOAC). *Official Methods of Analysis of International*, 17th ed.; AOAC: Gaithersburg, MD, USA, 2006; ISBN 0935584773-9780935584776.
56. Commission Internationale De L'ecleirage. *Cie 15: Technical Report: Colorimetry*, 3rd ed.; CIE Publications: Vienna, Austria, 2004; p. 7.
57. Colorhexa. Color Encyclopedia: Information and Conversion. Computer Software. 2018. Available online: http://www.colorhexa.com/ (accessed on 28 August 2018).
58. Beuchat, L. Functional and electrophoretic characteristics of succinylated peanut flour proteins. *J. Agric. Food Chem.* **1977**, *25*, 258–263. [CrossRef]
59. Yasumatsu, K.; Sawada, K.; Moritaka, S.; Misaki, M.; Toda, J.; Wada, T.; Ishii, K. Studies on the functional properties of food grade soybean products: Whipping and emulsifying properties of soybean products. *Agric. Biol. Chem.* **1992**, *36*, 719–727. [CrossRef]
60. Zhao, X.; Zhang, X.; Liu, H.; Zhang, G.; Ao, Q. Functional, nutritional and flavor characteristic of soybean proteins obtained through reverse micelles. *Food Hydrocolloids* **2018**, *74*, 358–366. [CrossRef]
61. Singleton, V.L.; Orthofer, R.; Lamuela-raventos, R.M. Analysis of total phenols and other oxidation substrates and antioxidants by means of Folin-Ciocalteu reagent. *Methods Enzymol.* **1999**, *299*, 152–178. [CrossRef]
62. Xiong, L.; Yang, J.; Jiang, Y.; Lu, B.; Hu, Y.; Zhou, F.; Mao, S.; Shen, C. Phenolic compounds and antioxidant capacities of 10 common edible flowers from China. *J. Food Sci.* **2014**, *79*, C517–C525. [CrossRef] [PubMed]
63. Sun, B.; Ricardo-da-Silva, J.M.; Spranger, I. Critical factors of vanillin assay for catechins and proanthocyanidins. *J. Agric. Food Chem.* **1998**, *46*, 4267–4274. [CrossRef]
64. Abdel-Aal, E.S.; Hucl, P. A rapid method for quantifying total anthocyanins in blue aleurone and purple pericarp wheats. *Cereal Chem.* **1999**, *76*, 350–354. [CrossRef]
65. Tai, Z.; Cai, L.; Dai, L.; Dong, L.; Wang, M.; Yang, Y.; Cao, Q.; Ding, Z. Antioxidant activity and chemical constituents of edible flower of *Sophora viciifolia*. *Food Chem.* **2011**, *126*, 1648–1654. [CrossRef] [PubMed]
66. Arnao, M.B.; Cano, A.; Acosta, M. The hydrophilic and lipophilic contribution to total antioxidant activity. *Food Chem.* **2001**, *73*, 239–244. [CrossRef]
67. Thaipong, K.; Boonprakob, U.; Crosby, K.; Cisneros-Zevallos, L.; Hawkins Byrne, D. Comparison of ABTS, DPPH, FRAP and ORAC assays for estimating antioxidant activity from guava fruit extracts. *J. Food Compos. Anal.* **2006**, *19*, 669–675. [CrossRef]
68. Suárez, B.; Álvarez, Á.L.; García, Y.D.; Barrio, G.; Lobo, A.P.; Parra, F. Phenolic profiles, antioxidant activity and in vitro antiviral properties of apple pomace. *Food Chem.* **2010**, *120*, 339–342. [CrossRef]

Sample Availability: Samples of the compounds are not available from the authors.

© 2018 by the authors. Licensee MDPI, Basel, Switzerland. This article is an open access article distributed under the terms and conditions of the Creative Commons Attribution (CC BY) license (http://creativecommons.org/licenses/by/4.0/).

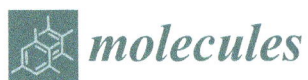

Article

Increasing Antioxidant Activity and Protein Digestibility in *Phaseolus vulgaris* and *Avena sativa* by Fermentation with the *Pleurotus ostreatus* Fungus

Edith Espinosa-Páez [1], Ma. Guadalupe Alanis-Guzmán [1], Carlos E. Hernández-Luna [1], Juan G. Báez-González [1,*], Carlos A. Amaya-Guerra [1] and Ana M. Andrés-Grau [2]

1 Facultad de Ciencias Biológicas, Universidad Autónoma de Nuevo León, Ave. Universidad s/n, Cd. Universitaria, 66450 San Nicolás de los Garza, Mexico; edith.espinosapz@uanl.edu.mx (E.E.-P.); maria.alanisgm@uanl.edu.mx (M.G.A.-G.); carlosehlmx@yahoo.com (C.E.H.-L); numisamaya@hotmail.com (C.A.A.-G.)
2 Instituto Universitario de Ingeniería de Alimentos para el Desarrollo, Universitat Politècnica de València, Camino de Vera s/n, 46022 Valencia, Spain; aandres@tal.upv.es
* Correspondence: juan.baezgn@uanl.edu.mx or baezjuan@yahoo.com.mx; Tel.: +52-(81)-83294000 (ext. 3654)

Received: 7 November 2017; Accepted: 16 December 2017; Published: 20 December 2017

Abstract: The aim of the research was to determine the impact of fermentation with *Pleurotus ostreatus* on kidney beans, black beans, and oats. The results indicate that the fungus has a positive effect on the substrates when compared to the controls. The antioxidant activity (39.5% on kidney beans and 225% on oats in relation to the controls) and content of total polyphenols (kidney beans three times higher regarding the controls) increased significantly by the presence of the fungus mycelium, even after simulated digestion. There was a significant increase in protein digestibility (from 39.99 to 48.13% in black beans, 44.06 to 69.01% in kidney beans, and 63.25 to 70.01% in oats) and a decrease of antinutrient tannins (from 65.21 to 22.07 mg in black beans, 35.54 to 23.37 in kidney beans, and 55.67 to 28.11 in oats) as well as an increase in the contents of some essential amino acids. Overall, this fermentation treatment with *Pleurotus ostreatus* improved the nutritional quality of cereals and legumes, making them potential ingredients for the elaboration and/or fortification of foods for human nutrition.

Keywords: *Pleurotus ostreatus*; antioxidant activity; polyphenols; digestibility; fermentation; cereals; legumes

1. Introduction

Foods today are intended not only to satisfy hunger and provide the necessary nutrients for humans but also to prevent nutrition-related diseases that impact physical and mental wellness [1]. Functional foods have been introduced in markets, and they are usually defined as "modified foods which contain ingredients that have demonstrated actions that increase the welfare of the individual or decrease disease risk beyond the traditional role" [2]. The legume, a particularly common bean (*Phaseolus vulgaris*), is one of the main sources of vegetable protein available in developing countries [2]. The high lysine content protein of *Phaseolus vulgaris* makes it an ideal cereal protein; it supplements the deficiency in this essential amino acid and is also a staple ingredient in developing countries, where the availability of animal protein is low. Also, it provides adequate nutrition due to its contribution of carbohydrates [3] and high-quality protein. *Phaseolus vulgaris* has also been associated with various health benefits, including the reduced risk of diabetes and cardiovascular disease attributed to the presence of polyphenols [4,5]. *Phaseolus vulgaris*, however, contains antinutritional factors such as protein inhibitors (inhibitors of trypsin, chymotrypsin, and amylase), lectins, phytates, and tannins [6].

The common oat (*Avena sativa*) is among the major cereals used for human food [7]; it is the cereal with the highest percentage of vegetable fat and has a variety of minerals, trace elements and vitamins such as calcium, copper, iron, magnesium, potassium, selenium, zinc and vitamins: B1, B2, B3, B6 and E, and trace amounts of vitamin D [8].

The disadvantage of using legumes in food fortification is the presence of antinutrients such as phytates, tannins, and trypsin inhibitors, which decrease the digestibility of the protein [7].

Fungi are considered a source of food with incalculable value for their nutritional quality, being low in calories and rich in carbohydrates, essential amino acids, fiber, vitamins, and minerals [9,10]. Studies indicate that *Pleurotus* species are potent biological agents that convert non-food organic products into palatable human food [11]. They are able to synthesize a greater proportion of essential amino acids, which promotes a positive balance of amino acids, as well as improving the taste. They can grow on a variety of substrates, such as straw (wheat, oats, and rice), sawdust, cotton waste, banana leaves, corn stalks, and other agricultural wastes [12].

Pleurotus ostreatus is the second most cultivated edible mushroom worldwide after *Agaricus bisporus*; it has a high nutritional value as it contains minerals, vitamins, and proteins. While it has a low content of fat and sodium, it is high in potassium [10]. This fungus also has antioxidant properties [13,14].

The production of fermented foods is one of the oldest food processing technologies, [15] and it is an economic and simple process that causes chemical changes and modifies the functionality of foods [16]. Many of these foods are manufactured for their unique flavor, aroma, and texture attributes that are highly appreciated by the consumer. Furthermore, filamentous fungi simultaneously decrease anti-nutrients components and partially hydrolyzed biopolymers substrates. The byproduct of the fermentation can be used as an inexpensive food and as a supplement to support marketing demands [15]. Considering the above and the growing industry of ingredients and functional foods, the aim of this research was to evaluate the effect of fermentation with *Pleurotus ostreatus* on protein digestibility, antioxidant activity, and nutritional quality of cereals (oats) and legumes (black and kidney beans).

2. Results and Discussion

The obtained amount of flour, including mycelium produced during fermentation with *Pleurotus ostreatus*, is equivalent to the grams of substrate used in dry weight (BB, KB, OG), so there is only one bioconversion of the substrate to mycelium.

2.1. Proximal Chemical Analysis

The results of the chemical composition of dry matter corresponding to the non-fermented varieties of black beans, kidney beans and oats (BB, KB, OG) and fermented ones with *Pleurotus ostreatus* (FBB, FKB, FOG) are shown in Table 1. The effect of fermentation with a significant increase of 13% and 6% in kidney beans and oats protein, respectively, can be observed. This is attributed to the increase of amino acid synthesis as a consequence of the fermentation with *Pleurotus ostreatus* [12]. With respect to the dietary fiber content, values obtained for the legumes were as follows: 45.09 g (BB), 27.80 g (KB) and 13.48 g (OG), which are greater than those reported by the USDA, which are 5.5 g for raw black beans, 8.7 g for cooked black beans, 4.9 g for raw kidney beans, 9.3 g for cooked kidney beans, and 10.6 g for raw oats and 2.6 g for cooked oats [17]. In the fermented black beans and oats, the dietary fiber contents significantly decreased by 59% and 22% respectively, attributable to the action of the enzymes from *Pleurotus ostreatus* such as cellulase, hemicellulase, xynalases and laccases [18], which selectively use the lignin and cellulose for their growth; lignin and cellulose form the major composite of the dietary fiber in legumes and cereals. The decrease in these structural carbohydrates allows the transformation of resistant starch into available starch, which in the case of black beans is a cause of the high observed value of dietary fiber (48.73%). In contrast to FKB, the fiber significantly increased 16%. These differences could be explained, as the action of the fungus depends on the substrate, species, or the variety of substrate being used; the fungus adjusts its enzymatic systems (hydrolase enzymes, oxide reductases, etc.) in relation to the conditions of the substrate, mainly the presence of carbon and nitrogen, selective delignification, crude protein content, dry matter and the threshold availability of the substrate in the grain for the growth of the fungus after inoculation [19]. The way in which enzymes of the fungus act to obtain the nutrients necessary for growth depends on the substrate; in the case of FB, it has a higher hardness index [20], having less permeability so the fungus could not act the same way as in the black beans, which could explain the differences in the composition [21]. This hypothesis is confirmed by data shown in Table 2; in the case of unfermented and fermented kidney beans, they do not show an increase in the total polyphenol content and antioxidant activity. The fat content highlights a significant increase of 97% in the FOG regarding OG treatment, which may have been provided by the fungus fat, since a 4.8% value of this component in *Pleurotus ostreatus* was reported [22]; this also happened to the legumes, assuming that the fungus is found in a greater proportion in oats, due to the fact that cereals such as grains of beer, wheat, rice, oats, and corn are more accessible substrates for the fungus, thus growing easier on them [23], as observed with other species of this fungus such as *Pleurotus pulmonaris*, which report a 3% value of this component [18]. It is important to consider that increases in some nutrients may be a response to the percentage decrease in others.

Table 1. Nutritional components of different obtained flours.

Parameter (%)	BB	FBB	KB	FKB	OG	FOG
Protein	23.62 ± 1.12^c	22.80 ± 2.85^c	22.81 ± 1.3^c	25.78 ± 2.35^d	11.78 ± 1.28^a	12.56 ± 0.63^b
Fat	2.08 ± 0.32^{bc}	1.67 ± 0.34^{abc}	1.86 ± 0.66^{ab}	1.68 ± 0.17^a	2.44 ± 0.45^c	4.80 ± 0.60^d
Minerals	4.90 ± 0.15^c	4.58 ± 0.31^c	4.63 ± 0.24^c	4.02 ± 0.01^c	1.61 ± 0.09^b	0.83 ± 0.52^a
Fiber	48.73 ± 0.56^f	20.0 ± 0.51^c	29.18 ± 0.15^d	33.88 ± 0.28^e	14.00 ± 0.07^b	10.92 ± 0.70^a
Carbohydrates	20.69 ± 0.79^a	50.95 ± 0.96^d	41.52 ± 0.59^c	34.64 ± 1.5^b	70.17 ± 0.44^e	70.89 ± 0.66^f

Black beans (BB); Black beans with *Pleurotus ostreatus* (FBB); kidney beans (KB); kidney bean with *Pleurotus ostreatus* (FKB); oats (OG) and oats with *Pleurotus ostreatus* (FOG). Average values with three replicates ± standard deviations, of three different lots. Mean values labeled with a different letter in the same file are significantly different ($p < 0.05$).

Table 2. Effect of *Pleurotus ostreatus* on antioxidant activity and total phenol content in different flours.

Flour	FOLIN (mg Acid Gallic/g Flour)			DPPH (mg Trolox/g Flour)		
	Initial	G.D. *	I.D. **	Initial	G.D.	I.D.
BB	1.48 ± 0.01^b	1.94 ± 0.05^c	3.30 ± 0.06^a	1.24 ± 0.04^b	2.89 ± 0.53^b	8.97 ± 0.73^d
FBB	1.87 ± 0.24^b	2.10 ± 0.00^d	6.85 ± 0.03^c	1.73 ± 0.09^c	3.90 ± 2.21^d	13.31 ± 1.63^f
KB	1.59 ± 0.10^b	1.82 ± 0.02^{ab}	4.23 ± 0.09^a	1.2 ± 0.01^b	2.42 ± 0.51^a	7.2 ± 0.29^c
FKB	1.59 ± 0.01^b	1.77 ± 0.06^a	4.78 ± 0.20^b	1.2 ± 0.08^b	3.24 ± 0.04^c	9.39 ± 0.01^e
OG	0.85 ± 0.76^a	1.88 ± 0.02^b	2.72 ± 0.49^a	0.40 ± 0.03^a	2.27 ± 0.77^a	3.04 ± 0.31^a
FOG	2.89 ± 0.34^c	2.12 ± 0.08^d	4.91 ± 0.06^b	1.30 ± 0.08^b	2.85 ± 0.37^b	5.04 ± 0.25^b

* Gastric digestion; ** Intestinal digestion. Black bean (BB); black bean with *Pleurotus ostreatus* (FBB); kidney beans (KB); kidney bean with *Pleurotus ostreatus* (FKB); oats (OG) and oats with *Pleurotus ostreatus* (FOG). Values are the average of three replicates ± standard deviations, of three different lots. Mean values labeled with a different letter in the same column are significantly different ($p < 0.05$).

2.2. Antioxidant Activity and Total Phenols

The content of total phenolic and antioxidant activity in flours was assessed before and after simulated gastric and intestinal digestion. The presence of total phenols in legumes and cereals has been documented in previous studies [5]. The initial content of phenols for the different treatments (Table 2) was 0.85 to 2.89 mg of gallic acid/g of flour, while Zielin´ski and Kozłowska [24] obtained 2.89 mg/g for FOG as the highest. Treatments of black beans and oats with *Pleurotus ostreatus* had a significant increase in the total phenol contents, i.e., 26.35% on BB and 240% in relation to the OG. This fungus is basidiomycete, which excreted at least three different oxidases of phenol; these are used to degrade lignin and obtain carbon and other nutrients. These laccases (phenol oxidases) are independent agents that catalyze reactions, including the oxidation of Mn^{+2} and Fe^{+2}, that can polymerize, depolymerize or transform a wide range of phenolic compounds [25].

This increase may be due not only to the synthesis of phenols in the mycelium or hydrolysis of conjugated phenolics [26], but also to the deamination of aromatic amino acids phenylalanine and tyrosine precursor of phenolic acids [27]; in addition, the phenol oxidases of the fungus also produced interesting industrial bioconversions of many aromatic xenobiotic compounds from lignin [28]. The antioxidant activity in the treatments was 1.2 to 1.73 mg Trolox equivalent/g in legume flours—higher than the values obtained for oats 0.40 mg/g OG and 1.30 mg/g FOG; this variation between oat and bean flours may be due simply to the different types of antioxidant compounds that they contain, as well as to their concentration [29,30]. In relation to the effect of the fungus in the flour, the fermented black bean and oat treatments significantly increased antioxidant activity; FBB presented an increase of 39.5% on BB and FOG 225% in relation to the OG, attributing it to the fungus in these treatments. There was a significant increase of polyphenols due to depolymerization or hydrolysis of conjugated polyphenols, not occurring in FKB, in which there was no antioxidant activity increase; assuming that the threshold availability of the compounds is not the same due the fact that the kidney bean hull is harder [20] because it has a higher cellulose content than the black bean hull [31]. The fungus degrades lignin molecules by the action of ligninolytic enzymes (lignin peroxidase, manganese peroxidase and laccase) and can then access energy-rich polysaccharides for growth and metabolism [32]. In this case, the phenol oxidase enzymes could not act in the same way, degrading conjugated phenolic compounds by not having enough access to them [33]. The varieties of beans have different characteristics. Depending on the natural adaptation to the environment and the harder seed coat (hull), the permeability and the possibility of access of microorganisms decrease, so the hull protects the endosperm from microbial attacks, assuming greater resistance to the action of the fungus [21]. After digestion, the antioxidant activity increased both in non-fermented flour and fermented flour, reaching values of Trolox 3.04 to 8.97 mg/g and 5.04 to 13.31 mg/g, respectively. This presented a seven-fold increase in FBB.

Concerning the activities of the total phenolic content in simulated digestion, it was observed that at the end of the digestion, values ranged from 2.72 to 4.23 mg/g in non-fermented and from 4.91 to 6.85 mg/g in fermented flours with the fungus, increasing three-fold in FBB. This increase was the tendency in all treatments. This is contrary to the results published by other authors [34], reporting that the content of total phenolic and antioxidant activity tended to decrease after digestion, due to the low pH fluids during gastric digestion and the interaction with other compounds such as minerals, fiber, and protein in foods, affecting the solubility and availability of polyphenols. However, it is well known that anthocyanins (antioxidant compounds present in many legumes), resist low pH and protect themselves; this probably explains the tendency observed in our results. In addition, we attribute it to the action of the enzymes of the fungus in the fiber, leaving it more available or accessible to antioxidants. This is very important since antioxidants play a protective role in the gastrointestinal tract while keeping the redox balance against harmful antioxidant agents, helping the prevention of gastrointestinal diseases during the process of digestion [34].

2.3. In Vitro Digestibility, Soluble Nitrogen and Tannins

In vitro digestibility values obtained for non-fermented bean flours shown in Table 3, were BB 39.99% and KB 44.06%. These were higher than those reported previously [35], which reported values below 35% in *Phaseolus vulgaris* in raw and pre-cooked flours. Fermented black beans with the fungus (FBB) presented a digestibility of 48.13%, which is similar to values reported for black beans fermented with *Bacillus* sp. [36]. The kidney bean with *Pleurotus ostreatus* (FKB) had a higher digestibility with 69%, and is higher than other reports [35], which have values below 50% for raw and cooked carica beans. Similarly, both treatments of fermented beans (FBB and FKB) had a higher digestibility than those reported for beans fermented with other microorganisms, such as *Rhizopus microsporus* var., *Chinensis* and *Lactobacillus plantarum* 33.87 and 35.09%, respectively [37]. The digestibility values for OG and FOG flours were 63.25% and 70% respectively, being similar to those reported by other authors [38]. The protein digestibility increased significantly in all fermented with *Pleurotus ostreatus* because this fungus has a great selectivity of delignification, which degrades the substrate and makes proteins more digestible [39].

Table 3. Protein digestibility, soluble nitrogen and tannin content.

Flour	Protein Digestibility (%)	Soluble Nitrogen (%)	Tannin Content (mg/100 g)
BB	39.99 ± 1.71 [a]	0.60 ± 0.80 [b]	65.21 ± 0.027 [f]
FBB	48.13 ± 0.78 [c]	1.34 ± 2.3 [d]	22.07 ± 0.016 [a]
KB	44.06 ± 1.71 [b]	0.30 ± 1.0 [a]	35.54 ± 0.086 [d]
FKB	69.01 ± 1.14 [de]	0.60 ± 1.5 [b]	23.37 ± 0.017 [b]
OG	63.25 ± 1.65 [d]	0.61 ± 0.4 [b]	55.67 ± 0.057 [e]
FOG	70.01 ± 0.30 [e]	0.91 ± 0.22 [c]	28.11 ± 0.030 [c]

Black bean (BB); black bean with *Pleurotus ostreatus* (FBB); kidney beans (KB); kidney bean with *Pleurotus ostreatus* (FKB); oats (OG) and oats with *Pleurotus ostreatus* (FOG). Values are the average of three replicates ± standard deviations, of three different lots. Mean values labeled with a different letter in the same column are significantly different ($p < 0.05$).

Soluble nitrogen values presented a significant difference between fermented and non-fermented treatments with *Pleurotus ostreatus*, confirming the effect of *Pleurotus ostreatus* on the availability of the protein (Table 3). In addition, the ability of the fungus to reduce tannins favored the increase in protein digestibility [40]. Tannin contents presented in Table 3 show a significant decrease in all fermented products with 66% for FBB, 34% for FKB and 49% for FOG. Fan et al. [41] reported that the fungus is able to reduce or eliminate tannin antinutrients mainly by the action of a tannase present in the fungus, which ultimately destroys the tannins [42]. The tannin values of non-fermented beans samples were similar to those previously reported [43]. The decrease in the concentration of tannins has been reported in the lactic fermentation of *Phaseolusvulgaris* [27].

2.4. Amino Acid Profile

The results of the amino acid profiles are shown in Table 4. It is observed that in oats, as well as in fermented legumes, a significant increase of most of the essential amino acids (isoleucine, leucine, phenylalanine, valine, threonine, and methionine) is present, confirming the effect of *Pleurotus ostreatus* in the synthesis of essential amino acids [12]. This also highlights a significant increase in sulfur amino acids such as methionine and cysteine with values of 22.4 mg/g of protein and 49.19 mg/g of protein in fermented treatments of kidney beans and oats respectively; this is considered relevant to improve the quality of the protein in the flour. Basic amino acids such as lysine and arginine decreased in all treatments in the fermentation process with the fungus. These amino acids were probably destabilized by the acidic conditions associated with the fermentation since the process was maintained at pH < 4 [44,45]. The values of these amino acids in the fermented products are similar to those reported for *Pleurotus ostreatus* [12].

Table 4. Effect of *Pleurotus ostreatus* on the amino acid profile.

	Flours					
Amino Acid (mg/g Protein)	BB	FBB	KB	FKB	OG	FOG
Asparagine	125.29 [e]	124.22 [c]	125.40 [e]	124.88 [d]	87.30 [a]	88.33 [b]
Threonine	46.11 [c]	47.30 [d]	49.51 [e]	49.56 [e]	37.04 [a]	39.17 [b]
Serine	53.10 [d]	51.60 [c]	53.68 [e]	52.96 [d]	46.74 [b]	45.00 [a]
Glutamine	157.89 [c]	154.80 [b]	153.63 [a]	154.52 [b]	217.81 [e]	212.50 [d]
Proline	46.58 [b]	48.73 [c]	34.71 [a]	49.08 [d]	60.85 [e]	61.67 [f]
Glycine	41.92 [a]	43.00 [b]	44.89 [c]	43.25 [b]	54.67 [d]	56.67 [e]
Alanine	42.85 [a]	45.87 [d]	44.89 [b]	45.19 [c]	50.26 [e]	53.33 [f]
Valine	59.62 [b]	64.50 [f]	60.62 [c]	63.65 [e]	57.32 [a]	61.67 [d]
Methionine + Cysteine	20.44 [a]	22.45 [c]	21.29 [a]	21.87 [b]	47.62 [d]	49.19 [d]
Isoleucine	49.84 [c]	53.03 [d]	49.98 [c]	52.96 [d]	41.45 [a]	45.83 [b]

Table 4. Cont.

Amino Acid (mg/g Protein)	Flours					
	BB	FBB	KB	FKB	OG	FOG
Leucine	87.10 [d]	88.87 [e]	86.07 [c]	89.89 [f]	82.01 [a]	84.17 [b]
Tyrosine	30.74 [c]	32.97 [e]	32.39 [d]	33.04 [e]	27.34 [a]	28.33 [b]
Phenylalanine	61.95 [d]	63.07 [e]	60.62 [c]	63.65 [f]	56.44 [a]	57.50 [b]
Hydroxylysine	1.40 [a]	3.34 [d]	1.39 [a]	1.94 [b]	2.65 [c]	3.33 [d]
Ornithine	0.47 [a]	0.96 [d]	0.93 [c]	0.97 [d]	0.88 [b]	1.67 [e]
Lysine	68.93 [d]	52.56 [b]	68.49 [d]	56.37 [c]	47.62 [b]	34.17 [a]
Histidine	28.88 [f]	25.80 [d]	28.69 [e]	25.27 [c]	22.93 [b]	20.83 [a]
Arginine	57.29 [c]	49.21 [a]	60.62 [d]	51.02 [b]	67.02 [e]	60.83 [d]
Tryptophan	10.71 [c]	10.51 [b]	11.11 [d]	11.18 [d]	14.99 [e]	10.00 [a]

Black bean (BB); black bean with *Pleurotus ostreatus* (FBB); kidney beans (KB); kidney bean with *Pleurotus ostreatus* (FKB); oats (OG) and oats with *Pleurotus ostreatus* (FOG). Mean values labeled with a different letter in the same file are significantly different ($p < 0.05$).

3. Materials and Methods

3.1. Seeds, Microorganism and Maintenance

The black beans (BB), kidney beans (KB) and oats grain (OG) were obtained from the local food market in Gpe, N. L. Mexico. *Pleurotus ostreatus* CS155 strain was obtained from Laboratorio de Enzimología, Facultad de Ciencias Biológicas, Universidad Autónoma de Nuevo León, San Nicolas de los Garza, N.L., Mexico. This strain was maintained by periodic transfers (2–3 months) in Petri dishes with growth medium prepared with 0.4% yeast extract, 0.1% malt extract, 0.4% glucose and 1.5% agar (YMGA) [46].

3.2. Inoculum Production

Seeds of fresh black beans, kidney beans and oats were obtained from local suppliers; they were washed and sterilized in mason jars with autoclave 121 °C for 45 min and water rational of 1:1, 1:1.10, and 1:1.35 (w:v), respectively. The strain fungus was inoculated in a YMG medium (0.44% yeast extract, 0.1% malt extract and 0.4% glucose) and incubated under agitation (150 rpm) for two weeks at room temperature, based on the studies by Hernandez, et al., 2008 and Gan, et al., 2017 [46,47]. The culture was homogenized during four periods of 15 s and used as inoculum. Then, 8 mL of the homogenized culture that contains 2.64 mg of biomass [d.w.] per gram of the homogenized culture [48] was added to each pre-treated jar for solid fermentation, looking for the inoculum to cover the whole sample while affecting the ratio of nutrients as little as possible. Afterwards, looking for sufficient biomass, the jars with the inoculated substrates were incubated for 2 weeks at room temperature under agitated anaerobic conditions. Subsequently, at the beginning of the idiophase, the highest ratio of biomass to the volume of medium nutrient-limited liquid was obtained, according to preliminary tests performed in our laboratory, where we observed that in a period of two weeks, the seeds were 100% colonized. The grains with mycelium were ground (Moulinex, Écully, France) and dehydrated in a convection furnace at 70 °C. Flours obtained with fermented and unfermented grains were labeled as black bean (BB); black bean with *Pleurotus ostreatus* (FBB); kidney beans (KB); kidney bean with *Pleurotus ostreatus* (FKB); oats (OG) and oats with *Pleurotus ostreatus* (FOG) [46].

3.3. Proximal Chemical Analysis

All proximal analyses were performed using standard methods of Association of Official Analytical Chemistry [49]. Protein content was determined with the Kjeldahl method (AOAC 930.29). Fat content was measured using the Goldfish method (AOAC 920.36C). Ash content was evaluated gravimetrically (AOAC 14.006), and dietary fiber and available carbohydrates were measured with the gravimetric-enzymatic (AOAC 985.29) and chemical (AOAC 962.09) methods, respectively.

3.4. Simulated In Vitro Digestion

A protocol based on the use of digestive enzymes was followed [50] and simulated fluids were prepared according to the protocol proposed by Minekus et al. (2014) [51]. Portions of 5 g of each sample were placed into a 50-mL tube. For the oral phase, 5 mL of FOS (simulated oral fluid) was added, incubated for 5 min at 37 °C in agitation. Then, 12 mL of FGS (simulated gastric fluid) with pepsin at pH 2.3 was added following incubation for 2 h at 37 °C in 55 rpm orbital agitation for the gastric phase. Finally, 20 mL FIS (simulated intestinal fluid) with 1.98 mg of pancreatin and bile extract at pH 8 was added and incubated for 2 h at 37 °C on orbital agitation for the intestinal phase.

3.5. Antioxidant Activity

Antioxidant activity was measured in samples before and after in vitro digestion. For undigested samples, the determination was made with extractions, using methanol 80% 1:5 ($p:v$) for each sample. The determinations of the extractions after gastric and intestinal digestion were performed with methanol 80% 1:20 ($v:v$) from 4 mL of the product of the gastric phase and 8 mL of the product of the intestinal phase. Of each extraction, 0.1 mL was mixed with 3.9 mL of DPPH (1 N), incubated for 30 min in darkness and measured at 515 nm absorbance. The results were expressed in the mg equivalent of Trolox [52].

3.6. Total Phenol Content

Total phenol content was determined in all samples before and after in vitro digestion. All the sample extractions were made with methanol 80% 1:5 ($w:v$) for undigested samples. For determination after gastric and intestinal digestion, extractions were performed with methanol 80% 1:20 ($v:v$) from 4 mL of the product of the gastric phase and 8 mL of the product of the intestinal phase. A 1 mL of extract was mixed with 0.025 mL of Folin–Ciocalteu (1 N), 2.5 mL of sodium carbonate (20%), incubated for 40 min in darkness, and then measured at 725 nm absorbance. The results were expressed as equivalents of gallic acid [52].

3.7. Protein Digestibility

A simulated digestion was performed and 37 mL of intestinal phase product was obtained; protein not digested was precipitated with trichloroacetic acid (TCA) and was prepared to a final concentration of 12% (w/w). It was centrifuged at 3500 rpm for 15 min and was then decanted. The precipitate was washed and centrifuged twice, and its nitrogen content was determined by the Kjeldahl [51,53].

3.8. Soluble Nitrogen

For soluble nitrogen, a 0.15-g sample was placed into a 50-mL tube, to which 49.5 mL of NaOH 0.02 N was added; it was then stirred for 1 h and centrifuged for 5 min at 3000 rpm. The content of nitrogen in the supernatant was determined by micro-Kjeldahl [54].

3.9. Tannins Content

Tannin content was measured using the AOAC 952.03 method (AOAC 1990). The standard curve was prepared with 100, 200, 400, 600 and 800 aliquots in 1000 µL of a tannic acid stock solution of 0.1 mg/mL. Each 10 mg sample was dissolved in 10 mL of water and 1 mL was taken to make the determinations. We then added 7.5 mL of water, 500 µL of Folin–Deniss and 1 mL of Na_2CO_3 at 35%; 10 mL was taken and stirred. After 30 min, a spectrophotometer at 760 nm absorbance was used to measure results. The results are expressed as equivalents of tannic acid [49].

3.10. Amino Acids Profile

The amino acid profile was determined using high-performance liquid chromatography (HPLC), gas-liquid chromatography (GLC) and mass spectrometry (MS), according to the method AOAC 982.30 E (a,b,c) [49].

3.11. Statistical Analysis

Data from the three replicated experiments were analyzed to determine whether the variances were statistically homogeneous, and the results expressed as means ± SD. Statistical comparisons were made by one-way analysis of variance (ANOVA) followed by a Duncan´s test using SPSS 17 Software. Difference between means were considered significant at $p < 0.05$.

4. Conclusions

Pleurotus ostreatus has a positive effect on the two varieties of beans and oats, increasing the content of polyphenols and their antioxidant activity even during digestion, thus improving the digestibility of the protein and decreasing tannins. The impact on the content of amino acids shows an increase of sulfur amino acids promoted by the fermentation of legumes and cereal, increasing the potential of these flours as functional ingredients in the production of food for human nutrition.

Acknowledgments: We would like to thank Consejo Nacional de Ciencia y Tecnología (CONACyT) for financially supporting E.E.-P to obtain her Ph.D. (scholarship 446871). We would also like to thank David Lazcano for the revision of this manuscript.

Author Contributions: E.E.-P. conceived the experiments; M.G.A.-G., C.E.H-L., J.G.B.-G, C.A.A.-G. and A.M.A.-G. performed the experiments, analyzed the data and contributed to reagents/materials/analysis tools; E.E.-P. wrote the paper. All authors read and approved the final version of this document.

Conflicts of Interest: No potential conflict of interest was reported by the authors.

References

1. Betoret, E.; Betoret, N.; Vidaland, D.; Fito, P. Functional foods development: Trends and technologies. *Trends Food Sci. Technol.* **2011**, *22*, 498–508. [CrossRef]
2. Caballero, B.; Allen, L.; Prentice, A. *Encyclopedia of Human Nutrition*, 3rd ed.; Academic Press: Cambridge, MA, USA, 2013; pp. 366–371, ISBN 9780123848857.
3. Sathe, S.K.; Deshpande, S.S. *Encyclopedia of Food Science and Nutrition*, 2nd ed.; Academic Press: Cambridge, MA, USA, 2003; pp. 403–412, ISBN 9780080917917.
4. Herrera, F.; Betancur, D.; Segura, M.R. Compuestos bioactivos de la dieta con potencial en la prevención de patologías relacionadas con sobrepeso y obesidad; péptidos biológicamente activos. *Nutr. Hosp.* **2014**, *29*, 10–20.
5. Xu, B.J.; Yuan, S.H.; Chang, S.K. Comparative analyses of phenolic composition, antioxidant capacity, and color of cool season legumes and other selected food legumes. *J. Food Sci.* **2007**, S167–S177. [CrossRef] [PubMed]
6. Luo, Y.W.; Xie, W.H. Effect of different processing methods on certain antinutritional factors and protein digestibility in green and white faba bean (*Vicia. faba* L.). *CyTA J. Food* **2012**, *11*, 43–49. [CrossRef]
7. Astiasarán, I.; Martínez, J.A. *Alimentos Composición y Propiedades*, 2nd ed.; McGraw Hill—Interamericana: Madrid, Spain, 2000; pp. 135–168, ISBN 84-486-0305-2.
8. López, A.L.; Divo, D.; Pizzorno, M.; Villela, F.; Stella, A.M. Utilización de extractos de *Avena sativa* L. en dermatitis. *Rev. Argent. Dermatol.* **2006**, *87*, 100–105.
9. Sharma, S.P.; Yadav, R.K.; Pokhrel, C.P. Growth and Yield of Oyster mushroom (*Pleurotus. ostreatus*) on different substrates. *JNBR* **2013**, *2*, 3–8.
10. Sánchez, C. Cultivation of *Pleurotus. ostreatus* and other edible mushrooms. *Appl. Microbiol. Biotechnol.* **2010**, *85*, 1321–1337. [CrossRef] [PubMed]

11. Bermúdez, R.C.; Morris, Q.H.; Danoso, F.C.; Martínez, M.C.; Ramos, S.E. Influencia de la luz en la calidad proteica de *Pleurotus ostreatus* var. Florida. *Rev. Cubana. Investig. Biomed.* **2003**, *22*, 226–231.
12. Bautista, M.; Alanís, M.; González, E.; García, C. Composición química de tres cepas mexicanas de setas (*Pleurotus ostreatus*). *Archiv. Latinoam. Nutr.* **1998**, *48*, 359–363.
13. Taofi, O.; Heleno, S.; Calhelha, R.; Alves, M.; Barros, L.; Barreiro, M.; González, A.; Ferreira, I. Development of Mushroom-Based Cosmeceutical Formulations with Anti-Inflammatory, Anti-Tyrosinase, Antioxidant, and Antibacterial Properties. *Molecules* **2016**, *21*, 1372. [CrossRef] [PubMed]
14. Jayakumar, T.; Thomas, P.; Geraldine, P. In-vitro antioxidant activities of an ethanolic extract of the oyster mushroom, *Pleurotus. ostreatus*. *Innov. Food Sci. Emerg. Technol.* **2009**, *10*, 228–234. [CrossRef]
15. Certík, M.; Sláviková, L.; Masrnová, S.; Sjbidor, J. Enhancement of Nutritional Value of Cereals with g-Linolenic Acid by Fungal Solid-State Fermentations. *Food Technol. Biotechnol.* **2006**, *44*, 75–82.
16. Davila, M.A.; Sangronis, E.; Granito, M. Leguminosas germinadas o fermentadas: Alimentos o ingredientes de alimentos funcionales. *Archiv. Latinoam. Nutr.* **2003**, *53*, 348–354.
17. USDA. *Agricultural Research Service*; National Nutrient Database for Standard Reference. Available online: https://ndb.nal.usda.gov/ndb/search/list (accessed on 17 October 2017).
18. Vega, A.; Franco, H. Productividad y calidad de los cuerpos fructíferos de los hongos comestibles *Pleurotus pulmonarius* RN2 y *P. djamor* RN81 y RN82 cultivados sobre sustratos lignocelulósicos. *Inf. Tecnol.* **2012**, *24*, 69–78. [CrossRef]
19. Raya, J.; Gutiérrez, G.; Ramírez, J.; Prieto, J.; Aguirre, C. Caracterización de proteínas y contenido mineral de dos variedades nativas de frijol de México. *Agron. Mesoam.* **2014**, *25*, 1–11. [CrossRef]
20. Deshpande, S.; Sathe, S.; Salunkhe, D. Interrelationships between certain physical and chemical properties of dry bean (*Phaseolus vulgaris* L.). *Qual. Plant. Plant. Foods Hum. Nutr.* **1984**, *34*, 53–65. [CrossRef]
21. Morales, M.; Peña, C.; García, A.; Aguilar, G.; Kohashi, J. Características físicas y de germinación en semillas y plántulas de frijol (*Phaseolus. Vulgaris L.*) silvestre, domesticado y su progenie. *Agrociencia* **2017**, *51*, 43–62.
22. Papaspyridi, L.; Aligiannis, N.; Topakas, E.; Christakopoulos, P.; Skaltsounis, A.; Fokialakis, N. Submerged Fermentation of the Edible Mushroom *Pleurotus ostreatus* in a Batch Stirred Tank Bioreactor as a Promising Alternative for the Effective Production of Bioactive Metabolites. *Molecules* **2012**, *17*, 2714–2724. [CrossRef] [PubMed]
23. Wang, D.; Sakoda, A.; Suzuki, M. Biological efficiency and nutritional value of *Pleurotus. ostreatus* cultived on spent beer grain. *Bioresour. Technol.* **2001**, *78*, 293–300. [CrossRef]
24. Zieliński, H.; Kozłowska, H. Antioxidant Activity and Total Phenolics in Selected Cereal Grains and Their Different Morphological Fractions. *J. Agric. Food Chem.* **2000**, *48*, 2008–2016. [CrossRef] [PubMed]
25. Sinsabaugh, R.L. Phenol oxidase, peroxidase and organic matter dynamics of soil. *Soil Biol. Biochem.* **2010**, *42*, 391–404. [CrossRef]
26. Vergara, H.; Gandul, B.; Roca, M. Formation of oxidised chlorophyll catabolites in olives. *J. Food Comp. Anal.* **2011**, *24*, 851–857. [CrossRef]
27. Granito, M.; Paolini, M.; Pérez, S. Polyphenols and antioxidant capacity of *Phaseolus. vulgaris* extreme conditions and processed. *LWT Food Sci. Technol.* **2008**, *41*, 994–999. [CrossRef]
28. Giardina, P.; Palmieri, G.; Fontanella, B.; Rivieccio, V.; Sannia, G. Manganese Peroxidase Isoenzymes Produced by *Pleurotus. ostreatus* Grown on Wood Sawdust. *Arch. Biochem. Bioph.* **2000**, *376*, 171–179. [CrossRef] [PubMed]
29. Cardador, M.A.; Loarca, P.G.; Dave, O.B. Antioxidant Activity in Common Beans (*Phaseolus. vulgaris*). *J. Agric. Food Chem.* **2002**, *50*, 6975–6980. [CrossRef]
30. Peterson, M. Oats Antioxidants. *J. Cereal Sci.* **2001**, *33*, 115–129. [CrossRef]
31. Labaneiah, M.; Luh, B. Changes of starch, crude fiber, and oligosaccharides in germinating dry beans. *Cereal Chem.* **1981**, *58*, 135–138.
32. Sharma, R.; Aora, D. Fungal degradation of lignocellulosic residues: An aspect of improved nutritive quality. *Crit. Rev. Microbiol.* **2015**, 1–9. [CrossRef] [PubMed]

33. Xu, B.J.; Chang, S.K. Total phenolic ceontent and antioxidant properties of eclipse black beans (*Phaseolus. vulgaris* L.) as affected by processing methods. *J. Food Sci.* **2008**, *73*, H19–H27. [CrossRef] [PubMed]
34. Bouayed, J.; Hoffmann, L.; Bhon, T. Total phenolics, flavonoids, anthocyanins and antioxidant activity following simulated gastro-intestinal digestion and dialysis of apple varieties: Bioaccessibility and potential uptake. *Food Chem.* **2011**, *128*, 14–21. [CrossRef] [PubMed]
35. Mojica, L.; Chen, K.; González, E. Impact of Commercial Precooking of Common Bean (*Phaseolus. vulgaris*) on the Generation of Peptides, After Pepsin–Pancreatin Hydrolysis, Capable to Inhibit Dipeptidyl Peptidasa-IV. *J. Food Sci.* **2014**, *80*, H188–H198. [CrossRef] [PubMed]
36. Ribero, D.; Patto, C.M.; Pinto, M. In vitro protein digestibility of enzymatically pre-treated bean (*Phaseolus. vulgaris* L.) flour using commercial protease and Bacillus sp. protease. *Food Sci. Technol.* **2010**, *30*, 94–99.
37. Starzynska-Janiszewska, A.; Stodolak, B.; Mickowska, B. Effect of controlled lactic acid fermentation on selected bioactive and nutritional parameters of tempeh obtained from unhulled common bean (*Phaseolus. vulgaris*) seeds. *J. Sci. Food Agric.* **2014**, *94*, 359–366. [CrossRef] [PubMed]
38. Mkandawire, N.L.; Weier, S.A.; Weller, C.L.; Jackson, D.S.; Rose, D.J. Composition, in vitro digestibility, and sensory evaluation of extruded whole grain sorghum breakfast cereals. *LWT Food Sci. Technol.* **2015**, *62*, 662–667. [CrossRef]
39. Tripathi, J.P.; Yadav, J.S. Optimisation of solid substrate fermentation of wheat straw into animal feed by *Pleurotus. ostreatus*: A pilot effort. *Anim. Feed Sci. Technol.* **2015**, 662–667. [CrossRef]
40. Aw, T.L.; Swanson, B.G. Influence of Tannin on *Phaseolus. vulgaris* Protein Digestibility and QualityAuthorsT-L. *J. Food Sci.* **1985**, *50*, 67–71. [CrossRef]
41. Fan, L.; Pandey, A.; Mohan, R.; Soccol, C.R. Use of Various Coffee Industry Residues for the Cultivation of *Pleurotus. ostreatus* in Solid State Fermentation. *Eng. Life Sci.* **2000**, *20*, 41–52.
42. Rodrigues, J.M.; Albino, S.; Pereira, D.; Dias, M.; Soares, J.; Cuquetto, H.; Megumi, M.C. Production of edible mushroom and degradation of antinutritional factors in jatropha biodiesel residues. *Food Sci. Technol.* **2013**, *50*, 575–580.
43. Díaz, A.M.; Caldas, G.V.; Blair, M.W. Concentrations of condensed tannins and anthocyanins in common bean seed coats. *Food Res. Int.* **2010**, *43*, 595–601. [CrossRef]
44. Martínez, D.A.; Buglione, M.B.; Filippi, M.V.; Reynoso, L.D.; Rodríguez, G.E.; Agüero, M.S. Evaluación del crecimiento micelial de *Pleurotus ostreatus* y *Agrocybe aegerita* sobre orujos de pera. *An. Biol.* **2005**, *37*, 1–10. [CrossRef]
45. Badui, D.S. *Quimica de los Alimentos*, 4th ed.; Pearson Educación: Ciudad de México, Mexico, 2006; pp. 121–130, ISBN 970-26-0670-5.
46. Hernández, C.; Gutiérrez, G.; Salcedo, S. Screening for decolorizing basidiomycetes in Mexico. Screening and Selectión of Ligninolytic basidiomycetes with decolorizing ability in Northeast Mexico. *World J. Microbiol. Biotechnol.* **2008**, *24*, 465–473. [CrossRef]
47. Gan, R.; Li, H.; Gunaratne, A.; Sui, Z.; Corke, H. Effects of fermented edible seeds and their products on human health: Bioactive components and bioactivities. *Comp. Rev. Food Sci. Food Saf.* **2017**, *16*, 489–531. [CrossRef]
48. Hu, J.; Duvnjak, Z. The production of a laccase and the decrease of the phenolic content in canola meal during the growth of the fungus *Pleurotus. ostreatus* in solid state fermentation processes. *Eng. Life Sci.* **2004**, *4*, 50–55. [CrossRef]
49. Association of Analytical Communities (AOAC). *Official Methods of Analysis of the Association of Official Analytical Chemists*, 17th ed.; AOAC: Gaithersburg, MD, USA, 2006; ISBN 0935584773-9780935584776.
50. Lamothe, S.; Corbeil, M.M.; Turgeon, S.L.; Britten, M. Influence of cheese matrix on lipid digestion in a simulated gastro-intestinal environment. *Food Funct.* **2012**, *3*, 681–774. [CrossRef] [PubMed]
51. Minekus, M.; Alminger, M.; Alvito, P.; Ballance, S.; Bohn, T.; Bourlieu, C.; Carriere, F.; Boutrou, R.; Corredig, M.; Dupont, D.; et al. A standardised static in vitro digestion method suitable for food—An international consensus. *Food Funct.* **2014**, *5*, 1113–1124. [CrossRef] [PubMed]

52. Aruguman, S.; Perumal, S. Effect of indigenous processing methods on phenolics and antioxidant potential of Underutilized legumes *Acacia auriculiformis* and *Parkia. roxburghii*. *J. Food Qual.* **2012**, *36*, 99–112. [CrossRef]
53. Reyes, C.; Cuevas, E.; Milán, J.; Cárdenas, O.; Barrón, J. Solid state fermentation process for producing chickpea (*Cicer arietinum* L.) tempeh flour. Physicochemical and nutritional characteristics of the product. *J. Sci. Food Agric.* **2014**, *84*, 271–278. [CrossRef]
54. Blanco, A. Importance of some factors on digestibility of black beans (*Phaseolus. vulgaris*) and of its amino acids in humans adults. *Guatemala USAC/INCAP* **1983**, *xi*, 134.

Sample Availability: Samples of the compounds are not available from the authors.

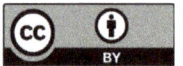

© 2017 by the authors. Licensee MDPI, Basel, Switzerland. This article is an open access article distributed under the terms and conditions of the Creative Commons Attribution (CC BY) license (http://creativecommons.org/licenses/by/4.0/).

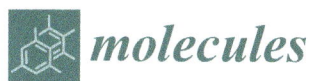

Article

Antioxidant Potential of Fruit Juice with Added Chokeberry Powder (*Aronia melanocarpa*)

Jana Šic Žlabur, Nadica Dobričević, Stjepan Pliestić, Ante Galić *, Daniela Patricia Bilić and Sandra Voća

Department of Agricultural Technology, Storage and Transport, Faculty of Agriculture, University of Zagreb, Svetošimunska Cesta 25, 10 000 Zagreb, Croatia; jszlabur@agr.hr (J.Š.Ž.); ndobricevic@agr.hr (N.D.); spliestic@agr.hr (S.P.); dpbilic@gmail.com (D.P.B.); svoca@agr.hr (S.V.)
* Correspondence: agalic@agr.hr; Tel.: +385-1239-3683

Received: 9 November 2017; Accepted: 1 December 2017; Published: 5 December 2017

Abstract: The purpose of this study was to determine the possibility of using chokeberry powder as a supplement in apple juice to increase the nutritional value of the final product with the aim of developing a new functional food product. Also, to determine the influence of ultrasound assisted extraction on the bioactive compounds content, nutritional composition and antioxidant potential of apple juice with added chokeberry powder. The juice samples with added chokeberry powder had higher antioxidant capacity, irrespective of the extraction technique used. Apple juice samples with added chokeberry powder treated with high intensity ultrasound had significantly higher content of all analyzed bioactive compounds. The application of high intensity ultrasound significantly reduced the extraction time of the plant material. A positive correlation between vitamin C content, total phenols, flavonoids and anthocyanins content and antioxidant capacity was determined in juice samples with added chokeberry powder treated with high intensity ultrasound.

Keywords: anthocyanins; polyphenolic compounds; classic extraction; ultrasound assisted extraction; antioxidant capacity

1. Introduction

Fresh berries, including various chokeberry products, have recently gained great popularity among consumers primarily because their high health value. According to the ORAC scale, chokeberry possesses the highest antioxidant activity value among other berry and fruit species [1–3]. By nutritional composition, fresh chokeberry is a rich source of bioactive compounds such as vitamin C, polyphenolic compounds, flavonoids and anthocyanins. The dark red coloration of chokeberry fruit is a result of the presence of anthocyanin, because of which chokeberry can be used as a natural dye. The most common chokeberry products are powder, syrup, juice, fruit jelly, fruit tea, liquor and wine. Consumption of juices and other chokeberry products is often limited due to its unique bitter, astringent taste so they are rarely used in their original form, but are more often added to other fruit products [4]. One of the possibility of chokeberry powder application is addition to various juices of other fruit species frequently to increase the organoleptic (specifically product color) and nutritional characteristics of the final product. In daily consumption one of the most popular fruit juices is apple juice while in food industry apple juice is often used as a base element in the preparation of other fruit products mainly because it's rich content of phytochemicals with strong antioxidant activity [5]. Based on the significant bioactive compounds content and high antioxidant activity, apple juice enriched with chokeberry powder potentially presents a new product type that may be categorized as a functional food.

Nowadays, in the field of food technology and biotechnology, new processes are evolving with the main aim of preserving organoleptic and nutritional qualities of the final product. Also, consumer demands are increasingly focused on high-quality, health and hygienically proper products, so the above-mentioned technology processes are focused to the principles of green chemistry, respectively environmentally and health-friendly chemical processes [6]. High intensity ultrasound recently found a great potential in processing technologies such as: drying, filtration, extraction, inactivation of microorganisms, homogenization, etc. [7]. High intensity ultrasound is characterized by the use of high intensity acoustic waves (typically in the range from 10 to 1000 W/cm^2) and the frequencies between 18 and 100 kHz [7,8] during which in the liquid medium occurs phenomenon of transient cavitation. Ultrasound assisted extraction (UAE) is one of the most applicable and numerous researches cites it's efficiency and other positive benefits such as reduced time of extraction, increased yield of different chemical compounds (polyphenols, vitamins) and significant energy savings [9–11].

The aim of this study was to determine the possibility of using the chokeberry powder as a supplement in apple juice to increase the nutritional value of the final product with a potential view to developing a new functional food product. Also, to determine the influence of ultrasound assisted extraction on the bioactive compounds content, nutritional composition and antioxidant potential of apple juice with added chokeberry powder.

2. Results

2.1. Basic Chemical Composition

The basic chemical composition results of raw apple juice (sample A), fruit juice samples with added chokeberry powder extracted classically (B1 to B7) and by those exposed to high intensity ultrasound (C1 to C6) are shown in Table 1.

Table 1. Basic chemical composition of juice samples with added chokeberry powder extracted classically and by ultrasound.

Treatment	Density (g cm^{-3}) $p \leq 0.0001$	TSS (%) $p \leq 0.0001$	TA (%) $p \leq 0.0001$	pH NS
		Control Sample		
A	1.0490 [g] ± 0.001	12.89 [f] ± 0.01	15.52 [f] ± 0.04	3.35 ± 0.01
		Classic Extraction		
B1	1.0530 [f] ± 0.001	13.80 [e] ± 0.01	17.31 [de] ± 0.05	2.89 ± 0.70
B2	1.0527 [f] ± 0.001	13.73 [e] ± 0.01	17.10 [e] ± 0.07	3.37 ± 0.01
B3	1.0539 [e] ± 0.001	13.99 [d] ± 0.01	17.29 [de] ± 0.19	3.38 ± 0.01
B4	1.0539 [e] ± 0.001	14.02 [cd] ± 0.01	17.52 [cd] ± 0.24	3.38 ± 0.01
B5	1.0547 [abc] ± 0.001	14.22 [a] ± 0.01	17.70 [abc] ± 0.01	3.37 ± 0.01
B6	1.0543 [cde] ± 0.001	14.12 [abcd] ± 0.01	17.54 [bcd] ± 0.22	3.38 ± 0.01
B7	1.0540 [de] ± 0.001	14.06 [bcd] ± 0.01	17.65 [abc] ± 0.06	3.38 ± 0.01
		Ultrasonic Extraction		
C1	1.0532 [f] ± 0.001	13.75 [e] ± 0.12	17.29 [de] ± 0.01	3.30 ± 0.03
C2	1.0541 [de] ± 0.001	14.01 [d] ± 0.08	17.66 [abc] ± 0.04	3.37 ± 0.01
C3	1.0545 [abcd] ± 0.001	14.09 [abcd] ± 0.08	17.71 [abc] ± 0.08	3.37 ± 0.01
C4	1.0543 [bcde] ± 0.001	14.06 [bcd] ± 0.02	17.59 [abcd] ± 0.14	3.37 ± 0.01
C5	1.0548 [ab] ± 0.001	14.16 [abc] ± 0.07	17.87 [ab] ± 0.04	3.35 ± 0.01
C6	1.0549 [a] ± 0.001	14.20 [ab] ± 0.04	17.93 [a] ± 0.05	3.37 ± 0.02

TSS—total soluble solids; TA—total acid content; NS—not significant. Different letters indicate significant differences between means.

ANOVA assay showed high significant statistical differences ($p \leq 0.0001$) between all analyzed samples (A, B, C) depending on the extraction method. The solution density of the analyzed juice samples with added classically extracted chokeberry powder amounted on average to 1.0538 g cm^{-3}, while for juice samples extracted by ultrasound the average density was 1.0543 g cm^{-3}. One of the major consequences of high intensity ultrasound is a transient cavitation phenomenon which increases the temperature in the system affecting a range of physical properties of the treated solutions, including density [8]. In juice samples with added chokeberry powder treated by ultrasound for longer time periods (15–30 min) the highest density values were determined, which was expected considering the recorded temperature increase of the system (Figure 1).

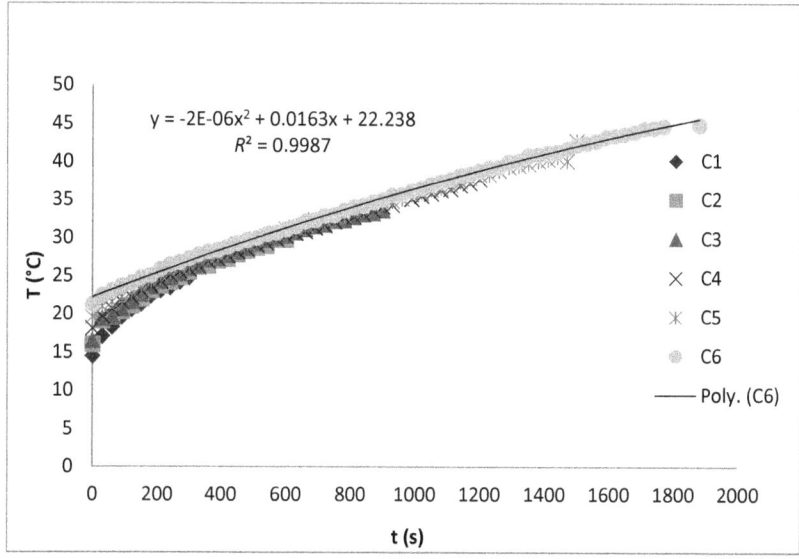

Figure 1. Temperature change in juice samples during ultrasonic treatment.

The average amount of total soluble solids (TSS) in juice samples with added chokeberry powder extracted classically was 13.99%, while in juice samples treated by ultrasound the average content was 14.05%. In general, the total soluble solids content in juice samples with added chokeberry powder shows an increasing trend in all the varied time periods, regardless of the extraction method. Extraction method, including high intensity ultrasound treatment, did not significantly affect the TSS in analyzed juice samples. In juice samples with added chokeberry powder extracted classically the average total acid (TA) content was 17.44%, while in samples treated by ultrasound the average TA was 17.68%, which for both extraction methods was approximately 2% higher than the control sample (A) value. TA content does not show significant differences depending on the extraction method (classic and ultrasound). It is important to emphasize that the addition of chokeberry powder in apple juice significantly increased the TA content regardless of the extraction method which was expected given the high vitamin C content determined in juice samples with added chokeberry powder. According to the Tolić et al. [4] TA content in chokeberry ranges from 0.29% to 1.32%, Kulling and Rawel [1] cite values in a range from 0.86% to 0.99%, while Jeppsson [12] and Šnebergová et al. [13] cite TA values in fresh berries in the range from 0.67% to 1.19%. pH-values of analyzed juice samples treated classically or by ultrasound of high intensity did not differ significantly, i.e., the pH-values of control sample as well as samples with added chokeberry powder extracted classically (B1–B7) and by ultrasound (C1–C6) are not significantly different ($p \leq 0.5321$). The average pH-value of all classically treated samples is 3.35 while for samples treated by ultrasound it is 3.36, which in comparison with the control sample (A) is a negligible difference.

2.2. Bioactive Compounds Content

The bioactive compounds content results of juice samples with added chokeberry powder are shown in Table 2. High significant statistical differences ($p \leq 0.0001$) were determined between all analyzed juice samples (A, B, C) depending on the method and time period of extraction. Fresh chokeberry fruit, as well as different chokeberry products such as juice and powder are rich sources of vitamin C [1,14,15], which has also been confirmed in this study. Namely, the determined vitamin C content in control sample (A) was 13.16 mg 100 g^{-1} while in juice samples with added chokeberry powder it was significantly higher, regardless of extraction method, with the exception of sample B1 which didn't significantly differ in vitamin C content from control sample (Table 2). The duration of the extraction period in both extraction methods (classic and ultrasound) significantly affected the vitamin C yield increase; thus classic extraction from 5 min to 24 h and ultrasound extraction from 5 to 30 min increased the vitamin C content about 3-fold. The highest vitamin C content was determined in the juice sample treated by ultrasound of high intensity for 30 min (C6) which is a 49% higher value compared with the same time period of classic extraction (sample B6), and a 16% higher value compared with sample B7 (24 h of classic extraction).

Table 2. The content of bioactive compounds in juice samples with added chokeberry powder extracted classically and by ultrasound.

Treatment	Vitamin C (mg 100 g^{-1}) $p \leq 0.0001$	TPC (mg L^{-1}) $p \leq 0.0001$	TFC (mg L^{-1}) $p \leq 0.0001$	TAC (mg L^{-1}) $p \leq 0.0001$	Antioxidant Capacity (µmol TE L^{-1}) $p \leq 0.0001$
			Control Sample		
A	13.16 ^{i} ± 0.88	512.64 ^{k} ± 0.09	205.89 ^{m} ± 0.40	ND	2164.54 ^{e} ± 0.01
			Classic Extraction		
B1	12.83 ^{i} ± 0.86	828.04 ^{i} ± 0.70	328.99 ^{l} ± 0.91	687.88 ^{h} ± 3.04	2208.62 ^{cd} ± 0.03
B2	15.5 ^{hi} ± 1.68	829.23 ^{i} ± 0.51	360.47 ^{i} ± 0.59	714.02 ^{gh} ± 0.87	2213.79 ^{bcd} ± 0.01
B3	17.46 ^{gh} ± 0.85	831.16 ^{hi} ± 0.29	390.18 ^{f} ± 1.16	846.25 ^{fg} ± 0.87	2215.59 ^{bcd} ± 0.01
B4	20.57 ^{fg} ± 5.54	838.54 ^{gh} ± 0.19	350.62 ^{k} ± 0.43	919.12 ^{ef} ± 3.04	2228.86 ^{abc} ± 0.01
B5	22.49 ^{ef} ± 4.29	840.81 ^{g} ± 0.21	353.67 ^{j} ± 0.95	927.42 ^{ef} ± 1.73	2233.81 ^{abc} ± 0.01
B6	28.76 ^{d} ± 3.39	851.30 ^{f} ± 0.70	381.25 ^{h} ± 0.80	991.08 ^{e} ± 9.13	2237.36 ^{abc} ± 0.04
B7	36.78 ^{bc} ± 0.88	761.11 ^{j} ± 0.80	421.22 ^{e} ± 4.59	1579.94 ^{bc} ± 18.26	2189.05 ^{de} ± 0.01
			Ultrasonic Extraction		
C1	15.57 ^{hi} ± 0.98	861.71 ^{e} ± 14.94	384.51 ^{g} ± 6.41	747.23 ^{gh} ± 15.65	2234.94 ^{abc} ± 0.01
C2	24.07 ^{ef} ± 3.92	894.04 ^{d} ± 14.64	443.01 ^{d} ± 1.15	997.54 ^{e} ± 56.53	2235.49 ^{abc} ± 0.01
C3	25.03 ^{de} ± 0.69	912.98 ^{c} ± 4.19	444.08 ^{d} ± 6.10	1393.90 ^{d} ± 0.44	2238.24 ^{ab} ± 0.01
C4	33.03 ^{c} ± 0.98	934.82 ^{b} ± 2.43	446.98 ^{c} ± 1.81	1452.02 ^{cd} ± 133.94	2239.55 ^{ab} ± 0.02
C5	40.87 ^{ab} ± 1.62	934.60 ^{b} ± 5.52	456.70 ^{b} ± 0.99	1707.86 ^{ab} ± 71.31	2241.84 ^{a} ± 0.01
C6	42.81 ^{a} ± 2.71	955.03 ^{a} ± 7.09	482.44 ^{a} ± 0.91	1823.79 ^{a} ± 77.85	2250.31 ^{a} ± 0.01

TPC—total phenol content; TFC—total flavonoid content; TAC—total anthocyanin content; ND—not determined. Different letters indicate significant differences between means.

Temperature increase during ultrasonic treatment enhances the diffusion process [16] while at the same time does not cause vitamin C degradation in the juice samples. Chokeberry is also characterized by high content of polyphenols, anthocyanins and flavonoids [4]. The total phenols content between all the studied juice samples (A, B, C) was significantly statistically different ($p \leq 0.0001$). Addition of chokeberry powder significantly increased the total phenol content regardless of the extraction method (classical and ultrasound, Table 2). Total phenol content in juice samples in which chokeberry powder after classical and ultrasound extraction shows an increasing trend for all the varied time periods. The most significant differences in the content of total phenols were determined in juice samples treated by ultrasound for 30 min: compared to the control sample (A) the total phenol increase was as high as 86%, in comparison with the juice sample B6 (classic extraction for 30 min) which increase was 12% and 25% in comparison with the juice sample B7 in which the powder was extracted classically for 24 h. The positive effect of high intensity ultrasound on the phenolic compounds extraction is in accordance with other literature data which emphasizes the significant efficacy of high intensity ultrasound on the extraction of different chemical compounds with various molecule structures [10,11,17,18]. In chokeberry fruits flavonoids (quercetin glycosides) are the most common from the group of polyphenols [2,14,15,19–23]. In all analyzed juice samples high statistical differences ($p \leq 0.0001$) of flavonoids content were determined (Table 2). Significant difference was determined between the juice sample with added chokeberry powder extracted by ultrasound for 30 min (C6) and the juice sample extracted classically for 24 h (B7). The determined difference between samples C6 and B7 amounted to 15%. Also, other scientific studies have proven the significant efficiency of high intensity ultrasound in the extraction of flavonoids [9–11]. Dark red chokeberry coloration is the result of the presence of anthocyanin which is primarily known for its strong antioxidant activity. According to the results from Table 2 juice samples with added chokeberry powder extracted with ultrasound for 30 min (C6) had 84% higher anthocyanin content compared to the juice sample extracted classically for the same time period (B6). Anthocyanin yield increased significantly depending on the extraction time, from 5 min to 24 h. Also, an increasing trend of anthocyanin content was recorded in the juice samples treated by high intensity ultrasound.

Other authors have presented results contrary to those shown in this study, emphasizing the degradation effect of high intensity ultrasound on the total anthocyanins content [24–27]. The main factors of high intensity ultrasound causing degradation of anthocyanins content are the amplitude and the extraction time. At higher levels of ultrasonic amplitude and prolonged time periods a higher degradation level of anthocyanins content was determined [28–30]. Also, another important factor of the ultrasound effect is the temperature increase; high temperatures have a significant impact on the anthocyanin reduction [27,28]. In this study, relatively low ultrasound power levels as well as a not-so-significant temperature increase in the system (max 44.8 °C, Figure 1) did not cause a significant reduction of the analyzed bioactive compounds content. Besides total bioactive compounds content, the content of the most common individual anthocyanins and other compounds from the group of polyphenols were analyzed (Table 3). High significant statistical differences ($p \leq 0.0001$) for all analyzed individual polyphenolic compounds depending on the method and extraction time were determined. The addition of chokeberry powder to apple juice, besides anthocyanins, significantly increased the content of other studied polyphenols, specifically the content of chlorogenic acid and quercetin. Extraction time from 5 min to 24 h positively influenced the yield increase of all analyzed compounds in both applied extraction methods, classic and ultrasound. High intensity ultrasound showed a positive effect on the yield of the analyzed individual anthocyanins: cy 3-galactoside, cy 3-glucoside, cy 3-arabinoside i cy 3-xyloside. Namely, comparing the juice sample with added chokeberry powder extracted classically for a time period of 30 min (B6) and the juice sample extracted for the same time period by high intensity ultrasound (C6) increases of cy 3-galactoside and cy 3-arabinoside by 2 times, cy 3-glucoside by 46%, and cy 3 xyloside by 86% were determined. Also, it is important to emphasize that a higher yield of all analyzed individual anthocyanins was identified in the sample C6 compared to the sample B7in which the extraction of mentioned anthocyanins lasted significantly longer (24 h) in the order of: cy 3-galactoside 19%, cy 3-glucoside 11%, cy 3-arabinoside 24% and cy 3-xyloside 18%. The positive impact of high intensity ultrasound and time period of extraction is also determined for other studied individual polyphenolic compounds. Chlorogenic acid content in sample C6 was 90% higher compared to sample B6 (classically extracted for 30 min), the epicatechin content increased by 98%, quercetin by 94% while the myricetin content did not change significantly.

Table 3. The anthocyanin profile and content of other polyphenols (mg L^{-1}) determined in juice samples with added chokeberry powder.

Treatment	Cyanidin 3-Galactoside $p \leq 0.0001$	Cyanidin 3-Glucoside $p \leq 0.0001$	Cyanidin 3-Arabinoside $p \leq 0.0001$	Cyanidin 3-Xyloside $p \leq 0.0001$	Chlorogenic Acid $p \leq 0.0001$	Epicatechin $p \leq 0.0001$	Quercetin $p \leq 0.0001$	Myricetin $p \leq 0.0001$
				Control Sample				
A	ND	ND	ND	ND	6.23 [k]	0.03 [h]	0.04 [l]	ND
				Classic Extraction				
B1	34.34 [m]	2.10 [i]	4.37 [l]	2.30 [h]	6.47 [j]	0.05 [h]	0.08 [k]	0.80 [d]
B2	36.32 [l]	2.10 [i]	4.37 [l]	2.30 [h]	6.47 [j]	1.22 [g]	0.28 [j]	0.80 [d]
B3	44.84 [j]	2.22 [h]	5.54 [j]	2.61 [g]	7.71 [i]	1.22 [g]	0.58 [h]	0.92 [c]
B4	47.67 [i]	2.34 [g]	6.12 [i]	2.61 [g]	7.71 [i]	1.22 [g]	1.18 [g]	0.92 [c]
B5	49.09 [h]	2.34 [g]	6.26 [h]	2.92 [f]	8.34 [h]	2.39 [f]	1.28 [f]	0.92 [c]
B6	55.62 [g]	2.58 [f]	7.28 [g]	3.22 [e]	8.96 [g]	2.99 [e]	1.38 [e]	1.04 [b]
B7	93.93 [c]	3.42 [b]	12.67 [c]	5.07 [b]	13.33 [d]	3.58 [d]	2.18 [c]	1.16 [a]
				Ultrasonic Extraction				
C1	42.56 [k]	2.22 [h]	5.09 [k]	2.30 [h]	6.47 [j]	0.05 [h]	0.08 [k]	0.80 [d]
C2	65.27 [f]	2.70 [e]	8.45 [f]	3.53 [d]	10.83 [f]	2.99 [e]	0.39 [i]	0.80 [d]
C3	85.98 [e]	3.18 [d]	11.51 [e]	4.45 [c]	12.08 [e]	2.99 [e]	1.78 [d]	0.92 [c]
C4	90.81 [d]	3.30 [c]	12.53 [d]	5.07 [b]	13.95 [c]	4.16 [c]	2.58 [b]	0.92 [c]
C5	110.39 [b]	3.78 [a]	15.44 [b]	5.99 [a]	15.82 [b]	5.34 [b]	2.58 [b]	1.04 [b]
C6	111.52 [a]	3.78 [a]	15.73 [a]	5.99 [a]	17.07 [a]	5.93 [a]	2.68 [a]	1.04 [b]

ND—not determined. Different letters indicate significant differences between means.

2.3. Antioxidant Capacity

Among all studied juice samples significant statistical differences ($p \leq 0.0001$) for antioxidant capacity were determined (Table 2). The lowest antioxidant capacity was determined in control sample (A) which is expected given that mentioned sample does not contain chokeberry powder. Time period as well as extraction technique showed a positive impact on the increase of antioxidant capacity in all juice samples, except for sample B7 in which a lower antioxidant capacity in comparison with samples B1 to B6 was determined. The mentioned results suggest that too long an extraction period can cause an opposite effect on bioactive compounds content, and particularly antioxidant capacity. The antioxidant activity of plant species is directly correlated with the content of vitamins, pigments and various plant phenolic phytochemicals, such as flavonoids, glycosides, alkaloids and others [10,31]. By statistical analysis of the correlations, a relationship between the two variables was observed: between the bioactive compounds content (vitamin C, total phenols, total flavonoids and total anthocyanins) and antioxidant capacity in the juice samples treated classically (B1 to B7) and juice samples treated by high intensity ultrasound (C1 to C6) (Table 4). In the classic treatments of the chokeberry powder the significance of the coefficient was determined between the content of total phenols and antioxidant capacity, while for the other observed parameters the significance was not determined. The significance of correlation coefficient was determined between all chemical parameters and antioxidant capacity in juice samples with added chokeberry powder treated with high intensity ultrasound for which correlation coefficient (r) were: $r = 0.79$ (total flavonoids), $r = 0.82$ (total phenols), $r = 0.83$ (vitamin C), $r = 0.86$ (total anthocyanins). Obtained results suggest that juice samples with higher determined vitamin C, total phenols, flavonoids and total anthocyanins content showed higher antioxidant capacity. Juice samples treated with high intensity ultrasound for 30 min had the highest content of all studied biologically active compounds and thus the highest antioxidant capacity. Based on the results of correlation coefficients it can be concluded that a stronger positive correlation exists between the analyzed bioactive compounds and antioxidant capacity in juices samples treated by ultrasound compared with the juice samples in which the chokeberry powder was extracted classically.

Table 4. Correlation coefficient (*r*) between the analyzed chemical compounds and antioxidant capacity (mmolTE L^{-1}) in the apple juice samples with added chokeberry powder treated classical and by ultrasound.

Chemical Parameter	Correlation Coefficient (*r*)
Classic Extraction	
Vitamin C	−0.22 NS
Total phenols	0.90 ***
Total flavonoids	−0.44 NS
Total anthocyanins	−0.48 NS
Ultrasonic Extraction	
Vitamin C	0.83 *
Total phenols	0.82 *
Total flavonoids	0.79 *
Total anthocyanins	0.86 *

NS—not significant; ***—$p \leq 0.0001$; *—$0.01 \leq p \leq 0.05$.

3. Materials and Methods

3.1. Plant Material

Chokeberry fruits (*Aronia melanocarpa*) were obtained from the Department of Pomology, Croatian Centre for Agriculture, Food and Rural Affairs (Zagreb, Croatia). Berry harvest was carried out at optimum fruit maturity, which occurs around the end of August. After the harvest the fruits were transported to the laboratory of the Department of Agricultural Technology, Storage and Transport, Faculty of Agriculture, University of Zagreb where they were washed and fruits with any mechanical damages and spoilage were discarded.

3.2. Chokeberry Powder Preparation

Fruit juice was isolated from the chokeberry fruits by a thermal heating process. The remaining fruit pulp was dried by a process of convective drying in a laboratory dryer (INKO ST 40, Zagreb, Croatia) at 60 °C until a water content of 10% was achieved. Dried chokeberry pulp was milled to a powder by a laboratory mill (IKA MF-10, Staufen, Germany) and stored in dark glass packaging in a dark, dry place. Total dry matter content of dried chokeberry powder was determined by a standard method of drying at 105 °C [30] and amounted to 9.65%. Apple juice was purchased in a local market for research purposes. The apple juice was RICO brand (Darda, Croatia) produced from 'Golden Delicious' cultivar apples by a pressing process.

3.3. Sample Preparation for the Classic Extraction

The experimental design of classical extraction is shown in Table 5. A previously weighed amount of chokeberry powder (2.5 g ± 0.0001 g) was placed in a 250 mL laboratory flask. On this chokeberry powder, room temperature (21.4 °C) apple juice (100 mL) was added. These samples were allowed to stand at room temperature for: 5 min (sample B1), 10 min (sample B2), 15 min (sample B3), 20 min (sample B4), 25 min (sample B5), 30 min (sample B6) and 24 h (sample B7). After each time period, the samples were filtered through Whatman filter paper (pore size 8–12 µm) to remove chokeberry powder and to stop further extraction.

3.4. Sample Preparation for Ultrasonic Extraction

The experimental design for ultrasonic assisted extraction is shown in Table 5. Prior to ultrasonic treatment, chokeberry powder (2.5 g ± 0.0001 g) was weighed into a glass beaker (250 mL) and room temperature (21.4 °C) apple juice (100 mL) was added. Immediately after the juice addition ultrasonic treatment was carried out, during which the time periods were varied as follows: 5 min (sample C1), 10 min (sample C2), 15 min (sample C3), 20 min (sample C4), 25 min (sample C5) and 30 min (sample C6). After each time period samples were filtered. Ultrasonic extraction was carried out in an ultrasonic bath (Bandelin RK 103H, Berlin, Germany) at a frequency of 35 kHz and a nominal maximum power of 140 W. Also, during each ultrasonic treatment the temperature of the samples was measured at 30 s time intervals with an infrared thermometer (Uni-Trend Technology UT 300C, Dongguan, China). This data is shown in Figure 1.

Table 5. Experimental design of classic and ultrasound extraction.

Extraction Method	Solvent	Solvent Volume (mL)	Time	Ultrasonic Bath	Sample
Classic	Apple juice	100	5 min	-	B1
Classic	Apple juice	100	10 min	-	B2
Classic	Apple juice	100	15 min	-	B3
Classic	Apple juice	100	20 min	-	B4
Classic	Apple juice	100	25 min	-	B5
Classic	Apple juice	100	30 min	-	B6
Classic	Apple juice	100	24 h	-	B7
UAE	Apple juice	100	5 min	35 kHz 140 W	C1
UAE	Apple juice	100	10 min	35 kHz 140 W	C2
UAE	Apple juice	100	15 min	35 kHz 140 W	C3
UAE	Apple juice	100	20 min	35 kHz 140 W	C4
UAE	Apple juice	100	25 min	35 kHz 140 W	C5
UAE	Apple juice	100	30 min	35 kHz 140 W	C6

3.5. The Determination of Basic Chemical Composition and Bioactive Compounds Content

The following chemical analysis for determination of basic chemical composition were carried out: solution density (g cm^{-3}) by a digital densitometer (Mettler–Toledo Densito 30PX, Schwerzenbach, Switzerland), total soluble solids content (%) by a digital refractometer (Mettler–Toledo Refracto 30PX) [30], total acid content (%) by potentiometric titration [30], pH–value by a digital pH–meter (Mettler–Toledo SevenMulti, Schwerzenbach, Switzerland) [30]. For determination of total content of specific bioactive compounds following analysis were carried out: total phenols and flavonoids content (mg L^{-1}) were obtained according to [31], total anthocyanins (mg L^{-1}) by bisulfite bleaching [32]. The antioxidant capacity was determined by ABTS method [33].

3.6. Vitamin C Determination (HPLC Method)

The analytical HPLC system employed consisted of a 920 LC system (Varian, Melbourne, Middelburg, Australia) equipped with Galaxie software (Varian, Melbourne, Australia), a multiple UV wavelength detector, auto-injector, autosampler and quaternary pump. Separation was done on Nucleosil C-18, 5 µm (250 × 4.6 mm I.D.) column with a Nucleosil C-18 guard column, 5 µm (10 × 4.6 mm I.D.). Juice samples were filtered through Nylon filter (0.45 µm) and directly injected into vials. The HPLC method for identification of vitamin C content was performed according to the Odriozola-Serrano et al. [34]. The employed mobile phase was sulfuric acid solution 0.01% (pH 2.6) at a flow rate of 1 mL min^{-1} with isocratic elution. Operating conditions were: column temperature 20 °C, injection volume 10 µL of the standards and extract samples. The detector was set at 245 nm. For identification a standard of vitamin C (Sigma Aldrich, St. Louis, MO, USA; Steinheim, Germany) was used.

3.7. HPLC Determination of Individual Anthocyanins and Polyphenols

For the HPLC determination of individual anthocyanins and polyphenols the same Varian 920 LC HPLC equipment as for vitamin C determination was used. Juice samples were filtered through a nylon filter (0.45 µm) and directly injected into vials. The HPLC methods for identification of individual anthocyanins and polyphenols were performed according to the Jakobek et al. [35]. For anthocyanin analysis, mobile phase A was 0.5% (v/v) water solution of phosphoric acid while mobile phase B was 100% HPLC grade methanol (Sigma Aldrich). Separation was optimized by gradient mobile condition as follows: linear from 3% to 65% B 0-38 min and 65% B 38–45 min with flow rate 1 mL min^{-1}. The UV-Vis detector was set to monitor spectra from 190 to 600 nm while detection wavelength was 520 nm. For polyphenol analysis, mobile phase A was 0.1% (v/v) water solution of phosphoric acid while mobile phase B was 100% HPLC grade methanol (Sigma Aldrich). Gradient elution was performed as follows: linear 5–80% B from 0 to 30 min; 80% B from 30 to 33 min; linear 80–5% B, 33–35 min with flow rate 0.8 mL min^{-1}. For both, anthocyanins and polyphenols determination operating conditions were: column temperature 20 °C, injection volume 10 µL of the standards and extract samples. The UV-Vis detector was set to monitor spectra from 190–600 nm while the detection wavelength was 360 nm. For identification the following standards were used: cyanidin 3-glucoside, cyanidin 3-arabinoside, cyanidin 3-galactoside, cyanidin 3-xyloside, myricetin, quercetin, chlorogenic acid and epicatechin (Sigma Aldrich). Individual anthocyanins and polyphenols were quantified using calibration curves and expressed as mg L^{-1}.

3.8. Statistical Analysis

The obtained data were statistically analyzed in the software package SAS, version 9.3 [36]. Duncan's test for significant difference (1%) was used. Results were subjected to one-way analysis of variance (ANOVA). The mean values were compared by *t*-test (LSD) and considered significantly different at $p \leq 0.0001$. Correlation analysis was performed to investigate the nature and intensity of relation between two variables: the vitamin C content, total phenol, total flavonoid, total anthocyanin and antioxidant capacity. The correlation value was numerically expressed by Pearson correlation coefficient (*r*), while the coefficient significance was expressed by *p* value: * $0.01 < p < 0.05$; ** $p < 0.01$; *** $p < 0.0001$, not significant at $p > 0.05$.

4. Conclusions

Based on the results, can be concluded that addition of chokeberry powder increases the basic chemical composition parameters (density, total soluble solids, total acidity and pH) and bioactive compound levels (vitamin C, total phenols, total flavonoids, total anthocyanins) in juice samples regardless of the extraction method (conventional or high intensity ultrasound). Juice samples with added chokeberry powder also had higher values of antioxidant capacity regardless of the extraction method. High intensity ultrasound effects a significant increase of all studied nutritional parameters: vitamin C, total phenols, total flavonoids and total anthocyanins. The application of high intensity ultrasound significantly reduces the time required for extraction of the plant material given that after 30 min a significantly higher content of all analyzed bioactive compounds was achieved. A positive correlation between the content of bioactive compounds (vitamin C, total phenols, total flavonoids, total anthocyanins) and antioxidant capacity in juice samples treated with high intensity ultrasound was determined. Based on the stated evidence, must be emphasized that apple juice with added chokeberry powder, represents a highly nutritional valuable product with numerous potential benefits for human health due to its determined rich content of bioactive compounds and significant antioxidant capacity. Also, further research on this potential new product, especially studies oriented to determining the organoleptic characteristics of such a product are desirable to address various consumer and market demands.

Acknowledgments: The authors thank the financial support from University of Zagreb within the project: "Antioxidant potential of fruit juice with added chokeberry powder".

Author Contributions: J.Š.Ž. and D.P.B. designed and wrote the manuscript. J.Š.Ž., D.P.B., A.G., S.V. performed data and statistical analysis. N.D. and S.P. contributed to writing of the manuscript. All authors read and approved the final manuscript.

Conflicts of Interest: The authors declare no conflict of interest.

References

1. Kulling, S.E.; Rawel, H.M. Chokeberry (*Aronia melanocarpa*)—A review on the characteristic components and potential health effects. *Planta Med.* **2008**, *74*, 1625–1634. [CrossRef] [PubMed]
2. Ciocoiu, M.; Badescu, L.; Miron, A.; Badescu, M. The Involvement of a Polyphenol-Rich Extract of Black Chokeberry in Oxidative Stress on Experimental Arterial Hypertension. *J. Evid. Based Complement. Altern. Med.* **2013**, *2013*, 1–9. [CrossRef] [PubMed]
3. Horszwald, A.; Julien, H.; Andlauer, W. Characterisation of Aronia powders obtained by different drying processes. *Food Chem.* **2013**, *141*, 2858–2863. [CrossRef] [PubMed]
4. Tolić, M.T.; Landeka Jurčević, I.; Panjkota Krbavčić, I.; Marković, K.; Vahčić, N. Phenolic Content, Antioxidant Capacity and Quality of Chokeberry (*Aronia melanocarpa*) Products. *Food Technol. Biotech.* **2015**, *53*, 171–179. [CrossRef] [PubMed]
5. Juarez-Enriquez, E.; Salmerón, I.; Gutierrez-Mendez, N.; Ortega-Rivas, E.; Lacroix, M. Ultraviolet Irradiation Effect on Apple Juice Bioactive Compounds during Shelf Storage. *Foods* **2016**, *5*, 10. [CrossRef] [PubMed]
6. Mustafa, A.; Turner, C. Pressurized liquid extraction as a green approach in food and herbal plants extraction: A review. *Anal. Chim. Acta* **2011**, *703*, 8–18. [CrossRef] [PubMed]
7. Knorr, D.; Zenker, M.; Heinz, V.; Lee, D.U. Applications and potential of ultrasonics in food processing. *Trends Food Sci. Tech.* **2004**, *15*, 261–266. [CrossRef]
8. Bosiljkov, T.; Tripalo, B.; Ježek, D.; Brnčić, M.; Karlović, S.; Dujmić, F. Influence of High Intensity Ultrasound Treatments on Physical Properties of Sheep Milk. *Croat. J. Food Technol. Biotechnol. Nutr.* **2012**, *7*, 44–48.
9. Koubaa, M.; Roselló-Soto, E.; Šic Žlabur, J.; Režek Jambrak, A.; Brnčić, M.; Grimi, N.; Boussetta, N.; Barba, F.J. Current and New Insights in the Sustainable and Green Recovery of Nutritionally Valuable Compounds from *Stevia rebaudiana* Bertoni. *J. Agric Food Chem.* **2015**, *12*, 6835–6846. [CrossRef] [PubMed]
10. Šic Žlabur, J.; Voća, S.; Dobričević, N.; Pliestić, S.; Galić, A.; Boričević, A.; Borić, N. Ultrasound-assisted extraction of bioactive compounds from lemon balm and peppermint leaves. *Int. Agrophys.* **2016**, *30*, 95–104. [CrossRef]
11. Šic Zlabur, J.; Voća, S.; Dobričević, N.; Rimac Brnčić, S.; Dujmić, F.; Brnčić, M. Optimization of ultrasound assisted extraction of functional ingredients from *Stevia rebaudiana* Bertoni leaves. *Int. Agrophys.* **2015**, *29*, 231–237. [CrossRef]
12. Jeppsson, N. The effects of fertilizer rate on vegetative growth, yield and fruit quality, with special respect to pigments, in black chokeberry (*Aronia melanocarpa*) cv. 'Viking'. *Sci. Hort.* **2000**, *83*, 127–137. [CrossRef]
13. Šnebergrová, J.; Čížková, H.; Neradová, E.; Kapci, B.; Rajchl, A.; Voldřich, M. Variability of Characteristic Components of Aronia. *Czech J. Food Sci.* **2014**, *32*, 25–30.
14. Benvenuti, S.; Pellati, F.; Melegari, M.; Bertelli, D. Polyphenols, anthocyanins, ascorbic acid, and radical scavenging activity of Robus, Ribes and Aronia. *J. Food Sci.* **2004**, *69*, 164–169.
15. Szajdek, A.; Borowska, E.J. Bioactive Compounds and Health-Promoting Properties of Berry Fruits: A Review. *Plant Foods Hum. Nutr.* **2008**, *63*, 147–156. [CrossRef] [PubMed]
16. Lovrić, T. *Procesi u Prehrambenoj Industriji s Osnovama Prehrambenog Inžinjerstva [Processes in the Food Industry with Fundamentals of Food Engineering]*; Hinus: Zagreb, Croatia, 2003.
17. Pingret, D.; Fabiano-Tixier, A.S.; Le Bourvellec, C.; Renard, M.G.C.C. Lab and pilot scale ultrasound-assisted water extraction of polyphenols from apple pomace. *J. Food Eng.* **2012**, *111*, 73–81. [CrossRef]
18. Puri, M.; Sharma, D.; Barrow, C.J.; Tiwari, A.K. Optimization of novel method for the extraction of steviosides from *Stevia rebaudiana* leaves. *Food Chem.* **2012**, *132*, 1113–1120. [CrossRef]
19. Slimestad, R.; Solheim, H. Anthocyanins from black currants (*Ribes nigrum* L.). *J. Agric. Food Chem.* **2002**, *50*, 3228–3231. [CrossRef] [PubMed]
20. Oszmiański, J.; Wojdyło, A. *Aronia melanocarpa* phenolics and their antioxidant activity. *Eur. Food Res. Technol.* **2005**, *22*, 809–813. [CrossRef]
21. Jakobek, L.; Šeruga, M.; Novak, I.; Medvidović-Kosanović, M. Flavonols, phenolic acids and antioxidant activity of some red fruits. *Dtsch. Lebensmitt. Rundsch.* **2007**, *103*, 369–378.
22. Olas, B.; Wachowicz, P.; Nowak, P.; Kedzierska, M.; Tomczak, A.; Stochmal, A.; Oleszek, W.; Jeziorski, A.; Piekarski, J. Studies on antioxidant properties of polyphenol-rich extract from berries of *Aronia melanocarpa* in blood platelets. *J. Physiol. Pharmacol.* **2008**, *59*, 823–835. [PubMed]

23. Taheri, R. Polyphenol Composition of Underutilized Aronia Berries and Changes in Aronia Berry Polyphenol Content through Ripening. Master's Thesis, University of Connecticut, Storrs, CT, USA, 2013. Available online: http://digitalcommons.uconn.edu/gs_theses/436 (accessed on 5 February 2016).
24. Tiwari, B.K.; O'Donnell, C.P.; Muthukumarappan, K.; Cullen, P.J. Effect of ultrasound processing on quality of fruit juices. *Stewart Postharvest Rev.* **2008**, *4*, 1–6.
25. Tiwari, B.K.; O'Donnell, C.P.; Patras, A.; Cullen, P.J. Anthocyanin and ascorbic acid degradation in sonicated strawberry juice. *J. Agric. Food Chem.* **2008**, *56*, 10071–10077. [CrossRef] [PubMed]
26. Ciccolini, L.; Taillandier, P.; Wilhem, A.M.; Delmas, H.; Strehaiano, P. Low frequency thermo-ultrasonication of Saccharomyces cerevisiae suspensions: Effect of temperature and of ultrasonic power. *Chem. Eng. J.* **1997**, *65*, 145–149. [CrossRef]
27. Sadilova, E.; Carle, R.; Stintzing, F.C. Thermal degradation of anthocyanins and its impact on color and in vitro antioxidant capacity. *Mol. Nutr. Food Res.* **2007**, *51*, 1461–1471. [CrossRef] [PubMed]
28. Patras, A.; Brunton, N.P.; O'Donnell, C.; Tiwari, B.K. Effect of thermal processing on anthocyanin stability in foods; mechanisms and kinetics of degradation. *Trends Food Sci. Technol.* **2010**, *21*, 3–11. [CrossRef]
29. Leja, M.; Mareczek, G.; Wyzgolik, G.; Klepacz-Baniak, J.; Czekońska, K. Antioxidative properties of bee pollen in selected plants pecies. *Food Chem.* **2007**, *100*, 237–240. [CrossRef]
30. AOAC. *Official Methods of Analysis*, 16th ed.; Method Number: 942.15; Association of Official Analytical Chemists: Washington, DC, USA, 1995.
31. Shukla, S.; Mehta, A.; Mehta, P.; Bajpai, V.K. Antioxidant ability and total phenolic content of aqueous leaf extract of *Stevia rebaudiana* Bert. *Exp. Toxicol. Pathol.* **2012**, *64*, 807–811. [CrossRef] [PubMed]
32. Ough, C.S.; Amerine, M.A. *Methods for Analysis of Musts and Wines*; John Wiley and Sons: New York, NY, USA, 1988.
33. Re, R.; Pellegrini, N.; Proteggente, A.; Pannala, A.; Yang, M.; Rice-Evans, C.A. Antioxidant activity applying an improved ABTS radical cation decolorization assay. *Free Radic. Biol. Med.* **1999**, *26*, 1231–1237. [CrossRef]
34. Odriozola-Serrano, I.; Hernández-Jover, T.; Martín-Belloso, O. Comparative evaluation of UV-HPLC methods and reducing agents to determine vitamin C in fruits. *Food Chem.* **2007**, *105*, 1151–1158. [CrossRef]
35. Jakobek, L.; Šeruga, M.; Medvidović-Kosanović, M.; Novak, I. Antioxidant Activity and Polyphenols of Aronia in Comparison to other Berry Species. *Agric. Conspec. Sci.* **2007**, *72*, 301–306.
36. SAS/STAT. *SAS Software*; Version 9.3; SAS Institute: Cary, NC, USA, 2010.

Sample Availability: Samples B1–B7 and C1–C6 are available from the authors.

© 2017 by the authors. Licensee MDPI, Basel, Switzerland. This article is an open access article distributed under the terms and conditions of the Creative Commons Attribution (CC BY) license (http://creativecommons.org/licenses/by/4.0/).

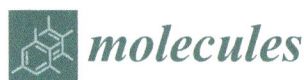

Communication

Antioxidant Properties of Four Commonly Consumed Popular Italian Dishes

Alessandra Durazzo [1,*], Massimo Lucarini [1,*], Antonello Santini [2], Emanuela Camilli [1], Paolo Gabrielli [1], Stefania Marconi [1], Silvia Lisciani [1], Altero Aguzzi [1], Loretta Gambelli [1], Ettore Novellino [2] and Luisa Marletta [1]

[1] CREA Research Centre for Food and Nutrition, Via Ardeatina 546, 00178 Rome, Italy; emanuela.camilli@crea.gov.it (E.C.); paolo.gabrielli@crea.gov.it (P.G.); stefania.marconi@crea.gov.it (S.M.); silvia.lisciani@crea.gov.it (S.L.); altero.aguzzi@crea.gov.it (A.A.); loretta.gambelli@crea.gov.it (L.G.); luisa.marletta@crea.gov.it (L.M.)
[2] Department of Pharmacy, University of Napoli Federico II, Via D. Montesano 49, 80131 Napoli, Italy; asantini@unina.it (A.S.); ettore.novellino@unina.it (E.N.)
* Correspondence: alessandra.durazzo@crea.gov.it (A.D.); massimo.lucarini@crea.gov.it (M.L.); Tel.: +30-065-149-4430 (A.D.); +30-065-149-4446 (M.L.)

Received: 11 March 2019; Accepted: 16 April 2019; Published: 19 April 2019

Abstract: Four popular dishes belonging to Italian cuisine and widely consumed in the country were experimentally prepared in a dedicated lab-kitchen following a validated and standardized protocol. This study provides their antioxidant properties evaluating the contribution of extractable and non-extractable bioactive compounds, and identifying the assessment of interactions between their natural active compounds and the food matrix. Ferric reducing antioxidant power (FRAP) values in aqueous-organic extract ranged from the highest antioxidant activity in *torta di mele* (10.72 µmol/g d.m.) to that in *besciamella* (2.47 µmol/g d.m.); in residue, *pasta alla carbonara* reached the highest value (73.83 µmol/g d.m.) following by that in *pasta alla amatriciana* (68.64 µmol/g d.m.). Total polyphenol content (TPC) ranged in aqueous-organic extracts between 36.50 and 64.28 mg/100 g d.m. and in residue from 425.84 to 1747.35 mg/100 g d.m. Our findings may contribute to the updating of the Italian Food Composition Database, by providing for the first time a value for the antioxidant properties. This could contribute to encourage the consumption of recipes rich in key nutrients and bioactive molecules. This information is useful and important for determining the association between diet and a healthy status.

Keywords: Italian popular recipes; food composition database; antioxidant properties; extractable compounds; non-extractable compounds; ferric reducing antioxidant power (FRAP); total polyphenol content (TPC)

1. Introduction

The study of food bioactivity and epidemiological investigations are increasing, emphasizing the perspective of considering the whole food matrix of interest for the risk of disease onset. Following the evolution of nutrition science, currently, researchers are trying to identify the concept of "optimal nutrition" also by studying not only the characteristics and functions of the individual foods or food components, but also their combination in composite foods, dishes, meals, and diets, in order to understand their overall impact on health.

There are only a few foods which are consumed raw, mainly vegetables and fruit, while most foods are heat-treated using different methods chosen according to the matrix, the type of food preparation, and the recipe to prepare them. This aspect is affected by various cultures and culinary traditions. Cooked foods and composed dishes are in fact the most consumed in our daily diet, but there is still little information concerning them, both in terms of their nutritional characteristics and their potential functions, whereas numerous data are available in the literature on the single ingredients, without taking into account either the formulation or the effects of technological process [1]. The interactions between single food components and/or between the different ingredients of a composite dish can play an important role, amplifying the importance of the concept of "food synergy" on health [2]; studies on technological and cooking treatments during the preparation of a recipe also highlight how they can influence their total characteristics, influencing and reflecting the state of health and well-being of consumers. It is well known that the physical, organoleptic, and chemical changes produced in food by heat treatments influence different parameters such as sensorial characteristics, nutrients content, quality and availability, bioactivity, and phytochemical composition [3–6].

To accurately estimate the dietary intake of the population and prevent cardiovascular disease, cancer, diabetes, etc., in recent years, the focus has increasingly been on studying the nutritional characteristics of foods and traditional recipes that are ready for consumption [7–13], also with the purpose of formulating dietary recommendations [14,15]. This seems to suggest that there is a need to have comprehensive datasets and databases that include composite and processed foods and food preparations as well as accurate dietary information to investigate the links between diet and health. Currently available data are still limited for two reasons: the scarcity of information on the nutritional composition of commonly consumed foods, in particular processed foods and composite dishes [16], and the deficit of up-to-date knowledge about population dietary habits in different contexts. Food composition databases (FCDBs) are used as the main tool to assess the dietary intake of individuals and groups of people at the regional, national, and international levels [17–20]. In addition to providing dietary information, consumed food characteristics and their overall nutritional role are also addressed to preserve important cultural elements, such as the great variety of traditional Italian cuisine that distinguishes the gastronomy of the country and reflects both the history and the local characteristics [21].

Specific research projects, such as the European Food Information Resource (EuroFIR) network [22] and the Italian national project Food Quality and Functional (QUALIFU) [23], were created and developed precisely to study, protect, and maintain the significant culture and culinary traditions of a country; Italy, particularly rich with various traditional foods and dishes, has taken part in these projects, and several national traditional recipes widely consumed have been studied, since they play an important role in preserving the local and regional food cultures.

In this framework, the aim of the present work is to provide new information on the antioxidant properties of some Italian recipes with respect to a previous work [12], in terms of extractable and non-extractable compounds, to examine any healthy aspects and identify their potential beneficial role.

The total antioxidant properties contribute to an assessment of interactions between natural active compounds and other food matrix components of foods, and this can be considered as a first step and as preliminary action towards the comprehension of potential beneficial properties of food matrices from the perspective of healthy food choices [24]. Each food matrix has its own antioxidant capacity that derives from the combined action of carotenoids, lignans, polyphenols, vitamins C and E, etc. Natural antioxidants can show different physiological properties, such as anti-inflammatory, antimicrobial, anti-allergic, anti-atherogenic, anti-thrombotic, cardio-protective, and vasodilatory effects [24–33]. With respect to antioxidant chemicals, it is worth mentioning that the current review of Yeung et al. [34], based on a scientific literature landscape analysis of works since 1991, concluded that a transition of the scientific interest, shifting from research focused on antioxidant vitamins and minerals to research on antioxidant phytochemicals (plant secondary metabolites), has been observed. In particular, the scientific community recently reached consensus on the distinction between extractable and non-extractable antioxidants: a development and assessment of methodologies was achieved [35]. Antioxidants occur in two forms [35,36]: as easily extractable compounds -free forms that are soluble in aqueous-organic solvents- and as less extractable compounds -bound forms that remain in the residue of aqueous-organic extract-. Their incidence in foodstuffs as raw, cooked, and processed food products was studied [37–48]. As remarked previously by Durazzo [35], due to the presence of multiple aspects and factors, it has become difficult to carry out a categorization of the main trends of the contribution of extractable and non-extractable compounds to the total antioxidant properties of major food groups. Generally, it is thought that the analysis of antioxidants in plant foods that remain in residues is necessary. Particular attention in fact should be paid to high fat food matrices [49] and to complex food matrices [12].

The assessment of bioactive compounds to dietary intake is a key issue. Additionally, a proper assessment of the contribution of extractable and non-extractable compounds to the dietary intake is required. Most of the studies available in the literature present daily intakes of extractable polyphenols, whereas little research has been done on the intake of non-extractable polyphenols [50–54], an important fraction contributing to total polyphenol intake [55]. Saura-Calixto et al. [50] estimated the amount of total polyphenols (as extractable and non-extractable polyphenols) consumed in a whole diet (Spanish Mediterranean diet) and their intestinal bioaccessibility: the amount of non-extractable polyphenols was almost double compared to extractable polyphenols. Pérez-Jiménez and Saura-Calixto [51] evaluated non-extractable polyphenols for the 24 most consumed fruit and vegetables in four European countries (France, Germany, The Netherlands, and Spain): macromolecular antioxidants, made up of hydrolysable polyphenols and polymeric proanthocyanidins, are the major contributors (mean value 57%) to the total polyphenol content of fruit and vegetables, and the intake of non-extractable polyphenols was estimated at about 200 mg. In particular, the authors reported that Spain had the highest daily per capita non-extractable polyphenols intake from fruit, whereas the Netherlands had the highest intake derived from vegetable consumption [51]. It is worth mentioning the work of Koehnlein et al. [52] on estimation of the total dietary antioxidant capacity (TDAC) in the Brazilian population: TDAC, evaluated as the ferric-reducing antioxidant power and as the Trolox equivalent antioxidant capacity, was 10.3 and 9.4 mmol/d, respectively. In a further work [53], the same authors compared the phenolic content and the total antioxidant capacity of the 36 most popular Brazilian foods submitted to aqueous extraction or in vitro digestion: after in vitro digestion, cereals, legumes, vegetables, tuberous vegetables, chocolate, and fruits showed higher phenolic contents and higher antioxidant activities than those obtained by aqueous extraction. The digestion caused a reduction in phenolic contents and the antioxidant activities of beverages (red wine, coffee, and yerba mate) [53]. Another work to mention is the research of Faller et al. [54] on the chemical and cellular antioxidant activity of feijoada, a typical Brazilian dish, coupled with an in vitro digestion: bound and residue contributions to total phenolics were 20.9% and 32.2%, respectively, suggesting that phenolics are capable of reaching the colon after the intake.

The overall goal is the development of specified and dedicated databases as well as the inclusion of extractable and non-extractable compounds in current comprehensive and harmonized FCDBs for a better and correct dietary intake assessment. Studies direction [56,57] on this are carried out in eBASIS BioActive Substances in Food Information System [58–60]: search protocols and data collection systems are developed to enable the expansion of eBASIS with new quality evaluated data on extractable and non-extractable antioxidants, producing a valuable unique resource [56,57].

The present study evaluates the contribution of extractable and non-extractable bioactive compounds on the antioxidant properties of four popular Italian dishes commonly consumed, previously characterized by their nutrient content [13], to better understand their nutritional role and provide additional dietary information to be included in the next update of the Italian National Food Composition Database (FCDB) of the CREA Research Centre for Food and Nutrition.

2. Results and Discussion

In our study, the antioxidant properties of the whole matrix as consumed were studied due to the complexity of the examined matrices. The changes in antioxidants and the interactions between components are correlated to the phytochemical structure and concentration, to the typology of food matrixes, to the preparation procedure, and to the typology and time of cooking [61–64].

In Table 1, Ferric Reducing Antioxidant Power (FRAP) values (μmol/g d.m.) and Total Polyphenol Content (TPC) (mg/100 g d.m.) were reported for selected popular Italian dishes.

Table 1. Ferric Reducing Antioxidant Power (FRAP) and Total Polyphenol Content (TPC) of popular Italian dishes *.

	FRAP (μmol/g d.m.)		TPC (mg/100 g d.m.)	
	Aqueous-Organic Extract	Residue	Aqueous-Organic Extract	Residue
Pasta alla amatriciana	4.01 ± 0.67 [b]	68.64 ± 4.43 [c]	60.87 ± 5.48 [c]	1447.59 ± 70.33 [c]
Pasta alla carbonara	2.62 ± 0.53 [a]	73.83 ± 3.52 [d]	36.50 ± 6.31 [a]	1747.35 ± 72.91 [d]
Besciamella	2.47 ± 0.17 [a]	52.98 ± 1.22 [b]	51.90 ± 3.38 [b]	1173.44 ± 73.07 [b]
Torta di mele	10.72 ± 0.80 [c]	18.24 ± 5.09 [a]	64.28 ± 2.39 [c]	425.84 ± 63.86 [a]

* Mean ± S.D.; ANOVA and Tukey's HSD test: by column, means followed by different letters are significantly different ($p < 0.05$).

FRAP values in aqueous-organic extract decreased in the following order: *torta di mele* > *pasta alla amatriciana* > *pasta alla carbonara* = *besciamella*; in residue, *pasta alla carbonara* reached the highest value followed by *pasta alla amatriciana*. The FRAP values of pasta-based dishes confirmed the value reported in our previous work [12] for another dish, the *spaghetti alle vongole*, namely 4.20 μmol/g d.m. and 64.22 μmol/g d.m. in aqueous-organic extract and residue, respectively. In general, the antioxidant properties of cereals and derivatives thereof have been well documented over the years [42,65,66]; with reference to antioxidants in pasta, one of most popular staple foods, the effect of cooking [67,68] as well as new formulations and functional products have been studied [69–72]. In this regard, it is worth mentioning the work of Ioannou et al. [63], since they remarked how the addition of ingredients with high antioxidant activity to a complex preparation can contribute to increases in total antioxidant capacity, but not in a proportional way.

Besciamella belongs to the category of the white sauces, and it is an example of milk-based dishes. In recent years, emerging studies on the antioxidant properties of milk [73,74] as well as dairy products [75,76] have been carried out. For instance, Manzi and Durazzo [74], by evaluating the antioxidant properties of industrial heat-treated milk, namely UHT, microfiltered, and high quality pasteurized milk, showed that UHT milk has the highest total polyphenol content, DPPH, and FRAP values. The authors [74] explained that the behavior of UHT milk is probably related to the development of antioxidant compounds, formed during the Maillard reaction occurring when milk treatment is performed at high temperatures (≥135 °C for at least 1 s) according to previous authors [77–79].

Torta di mele belongs to the subcategory of fruit cake comprised among the desserts, and evidenced the highest FRAP value in aqueous-organic extract and the lowest value in the residue with respect to other items. This seems to reflect the high content of organic acids in the apples used in the preparation of this dessert [80,81]. For instance, for apple, in Phenol Explorer Databases the total polyphenol content was 131.80 mg/100 g FW, as mean of 53 original content values extracted from eight published papers [82].

Table 2 shows and summarizes the contribution of extractable and non-extractable compounds to the antioxidant properties of all Italian dishes we investigated grouped by category, in this work and in a previous one [12].

For the four new dishes studied, the extractable antioxidants (aqueous-organic extracts) were minor contributors to the total antioxidant activity; consequently, the hydrolysable polyphenols (residues) contributed significantly more: for *pasta alla amatriciana*, *pasta alla carbonara*, and *besciamella* the extractable antioxidants contribute less than 6% and non-extractable compounds contribute in a range from 94 to 97%, whereas for *torta di mele* the percentages of contributions were 37% and 63%, respectively, for extractable polyphenols and hydrolysable polyphenols.

Table 2. Contribution % of extractable and non-extractable compounds to antioxidant properties of popular Italian dishes *.

Italian Dishes	Aqueous-Organic Extract	Residue
Sauces		
Besciamella	4	96
First Courses		
Spaghetti alle vongole *	6	94
Pasta alla amatriciana	6	94
Pasta alla carbonara	3	97
One Dish Meals		
Pomodori al riso *	15	85
Gâteau di patate *	11	89
Side Courses		
Carciofi alla romana *	58	42
Desserts		
Pan di Spagna *	5	95
Torta di mele	37	63

* Data derived from Durazzo et al. [12].

Regarding total polyphenol content evaluation, as reported in Table 1, TPC values ranged in aqueous-organic extracts between 36.50 and 64.28 mg/100 g d.m. and in residue from 425.84 to 1747.35 mg/100 g d.m. Hydrolysable polyphenols represent consequently a significant fraction, by accounting in the range between 87% (*torta di mele*) and 98% (*pasta alla carbonara*) of total polyphenols. A good Pearson correlation between TPC values with FRAP ones was found in aqueous-organic extract (r = 0.6798) and in residues (r = 0.9909). For instance, *pasta alla carbonara* showed the lowest values in aqueous-organic extract and the highest value in residue both in FRAP and TPC, whereas *torta di mele* showed the opposite behavior.

3. Materials and Methods

3.1. Recipes: Identification of Standard Recipe, Sampling and Dish Preparation

Four recipes (Table 3), all identified from survey Italian National Food Consumption Survey INRAN-SCAI 2005-2006 [83], and selected in the QUALIFU project [23], were experimentally prepared [13] in a dedicated lab-kitchen following a validated and standardized protocol developed within the EuroFIR Network [84]; three preparations represented some popular, most commonly consumed Italian dishes: *pasta alla amatriciana*; *pasta alla carbonara*, and *torta di mele*; one sauce, the *besciamelle*, was selected and studied for its great use in other traditional food preparations (lasagna, vegetables au gratin, baked pasta, salted cakes, etc.). The different ingredients included were pasta, cured meat, milk, cheeses, eggs, vegetables, fruits, extra virgin olive oil, and butter, thus covering a wide range of antioxidant properties. Our previous studies on traditional Italian dishes were focused on determining proximate composition and a dietary intake evaluation [12,13] and aimed at applying an integrated and emerging (analytical) approach to classifying dishes [85,86]. The present study focuses on the health-beneficial properties of selected traditional Italian dishes with the aim of extending and triggering interest to this type of research, which connects the nutritional aspects to health-beneficial properties and traditionally consumed foods.

Table 3. Italian popular dishes: ingredients, method and time cooking.

Original Name	Food Name	Ingredients (g/100 g)	Cooking	Timing (min.)
Pasta alla amatriciana	Amatriciana pasta	Short pasta (37.5), tomato pulp (37.5), Amatrice cheek lard diced (16), Amatrice Pecorino cheese PAT (hard cheese from sheep) (7.5), extra virgin olive oil (1.1), salt (0.3), chili pepper (0.1).	Boiling, pan-frying, and simmering	25
Pasta alla carbonara	Carbonara pasta	Short pasta (47.3), bacon cubes (20.3), Roman Pecorino cheese PDO (hard cheese from sheep) (13.6), eggs (16.6), extra virgin olive oil (1.4), salt (0.4), black pepper (0.4).	Boiling and pan-frying	13
Besciamella	Béchamel sauce	Milk (83), butter (8), flour (8), salt (0.5).	Simmering gently	33
Torta di mele	Apple Pie	Apples (37.7), sugar (15), wheat flour (18), butter (9.3), eggs (9.2), whole milk (7.5), baking powder (1), vanilla (0.03), grated lemon peel (0.2), lemon juice (2.4).	Baking	30

In detail, at first a document collection was carried out from the most popular and traditional cookbooks in Italy (Il cucchiaio d'argento; La cucina italiana, etc.) for every recipe selected; therefore, for every dish one "standard recipe" was identified and one "preparation protocol" was drafted in detail identifying ingredients, quantities, preparation techniques, type, temperature, and time cooking; dishes production had been carried out according to the standard procedures developed within the EuroFIR network.

The sampling plan had taken into account the collection of simple ingredients at various retail stores and supermarkets in Rome; to represent the variability of the ingredients, the main brands and cultivars of the same product were considered and purchased: 8 brands of pasta and tomato pulp, 7 brands of eggs, 6 brands of bacon, 4 samples of Amatrice cheek lard and Pecorino cheese, 4 brands of extra virgin olive oil, and 2 brands of wheat flour, butter, and milk. Each brand (primary sample) for every ingredient (secondary sample) was properly prepared, weighed, and then combined to make a composite sample (pool) before use for the preparation of the final dish (laboratory sample). This was weighed, assembled, and cooked in a laboratory and dedicated kitchen at the CREA Research Centre for Food and Nutrition by trained persons according to the preparation protocol of the standard recipe, applying methods and utensils commonly used in households. The recipes, once completed and cooked, were homogenized, frozen at −30 °C, and lyophilized. For each type of dish, two independent batches (laboratory sample) were prepared and on each one the analysis were performed in triplicate.

3.2. Evaluation of Antioxidant Properties by Ferric Reducing Antioxidant Power (FRAP) and Total Polyphenol Content (TPC)

3.2.1. Extraction Procedure

Extractable and non-extractable polyphenols were extracted as described by Durazzo et al. [12]. Aqueous-organic extracts (extractable antioxidants) and their residues (non-extractable antioxidants) were isolated and studied.

In particular, among non-extractable antioxidants, attention was paid to hydrolysable polyphenols, which were isolated and determined following a specific and suitable acid hydrolysis procedure as reported below.

Aqueous-Organic Extract

On the basis of dish ingredients and available literature data, a quantity of 3–5.5 g of each sample was placed in a test tube, and 20 mL of acid methanol/water (50:50 *v/v*, pH 2) were added. The tubes were vortexed at room temperature for 3 min and then mildly shaken for 1 h in a water bath at room temperature. The tubes were then centrifuged at 2500 rpm for 10 min and the supernatants were recovered. Twenty milliliters of acetone/water (70:30 *v/v*) mixture were added to the residues. All operations (vortexing, shaking, centrifugation) were then repeated. Methanolic and acetonic extracts were combined and centrifuged at 2800 rpm for 15 min. The resulting supernatant was transferred into tubes and directly used for the determination of FRAP and TPC.

Residue

The residues remaining after the previously described extraction were left in a ventilated and heated apparatus (max temperature 25 °C) until dry. Briefly, about 200–450 mg of the residue, respectively, were mixed with 20 mL of methanol and 2 mL of concentrated sulfuric acid (18 M). The samples were gently stirred for 1 min and were shaken in a water bath at 85 °C for 20 h; samples were then centrifuged (2500 g for 10 min), and the supernatant was recovered. After two washings, with minimum volumes of distilled water and recentrifuging where necessary, the final volume was 50 mL. The tube was centrifuged at 2800 rpm for 20 min, and the resultant supernatant was directly used for the determination of FRAP and TPC.

3.2.2. Antioxidant Assays

Several methods have been proposed for evaluating the antioxidant properties of single compounds and foods [87]. The most common are (i) the Folin–Ciocalteu assay used widely to determine the total phenolics; (ii) the Trolox equivalent antioxidant capacity (TEAC); (iii) the oxygen radical absorbance capacity (ORAC); (iv) the total radical-trapping antioxidant parameter (TRAP); (v) the ferric-reducing antioxidant power (FRAP); and (vi) the 2,2-diphenyl-1-picrylhydrazyl (DPPH) radical scavenging activity assay [88–90]. All these methods are based on the measurement of the capacity of a food component or a food to scavenge specific free radicals or to reduce a target molecule.

These assays differ in their principles, mechanisms, and experimental conditions as well as in how their end points are measured, so different methods to estimate and/or determine the antioxidant activity of the compounds should be carried out. Three are the main mechanisms by which the antioxidants act, encompassing the direct reaction with radicals and the chelation of free metals (involved in reaction finally generating free radicals): the H atom transfer, the single electron transfer, and the metal chelation [91]. Literature data report that the use of at least two or three assays is strongly recommended for assessing antioxidant properties [92]. Prior et al. [93] proposed that procedures and applications for three assays should be considered for standardization: the oxygen radical absorbance capacity (ORAC) assay, the Folin–Ciocalteu method, and possibly the Trolox equivalent antioxidant capacity (TEAC) assay [93].

FRAP

The determination of the FRAP assay was carried out according to the methods of Benzie & Strain [94] and Pulido et al. [95], through the use of a Tecan Sunrise® plate reader spectrophotometer. The method is based on the reduction of the Fe^{3+}-TPTZ (2,4,6-tripyridyl-s-triazine) complex to a ferrous one at acidic pH value.

Total Polyphenol Content (TPC)

The TPC was determined using the Folin–Ciocalteu method [96]. Briefly, appropriate dilutions of extracts were oxidized with Folin–Ciocalteu reagent, and the reaction was neutralized with sodium carbonate. The absorbance of the resulting blue color was measured at a wavelength of 760 nm against an appropriate blank after 2 h of reaction at room temperature. Gallic acid was used as reference standard.

3.3. Statistical Analysis

All analyses were performed in triplicate. Data are presented as mean ± standard deviation (s.d.) of the analysis carried out on two preparations of every dish. Statistica for Windows (Statistical package; release 4.5; StatSoft Inc., Vigonza, PD, Italy) was used to perform one-way analysis of variance (ANOVA) and a post-hoc test: Tukey's honest significant difference (HSD) test.

4. Conclusions

In this study, antioxidant properties of four commonly consumed popular Italian dishes are provided for the first time. Our findings can contribute to the updating of the Italian FCDB by providing a value of antioxidant properties that are useful and important for study on the association between diet and a healthy status [97,98].

The innovative character of this research lays in the fact that the four dishes were experimentally prepared in a dedicated lab-kitchen following a validated and standardized protocol based on harmonized guidelines. The other key aspect is the study of antioxidant properties, in term of extractable and non-extractable antioxidants, applied to complex matrixes, i.e., food preparations and food composite dishes.

Our study highlighted the importance of evaluating the real nutritional information about foods as taken, since ingredients are often mixed and heat-treated to formulate/prepare dishes. The availability of these new and appropriate food composition data is needed in order to correctly evaluate the dietary intake of recipes rich in key nutrients and bioactive molecules, facilitating further nutrition-related studies, and can be used to encourage the consumption of certain recipes. Further studies in this direction are needed to provide a detailed nutritional overview of popular and traditional Italian dishes and are currently being carried out in our laboratories.

Author Contributions: A.D., M.L., A.S., E.N. and L.M. have conceived the work and wrote the manuscript. P.G., S.M., S.L., A.A., and L.G. have carried out the experimental study and A.D., M.L., A.S., E.C., E.N. and L.M. analyzed the data. All authors have made a substantial contribution to revise the work and approved it for publication.

Funding: This work was supported by the project QUALIFU-SIAGRO (MiPAAF D.M. 2087/7303/09, 28/01/2009).

Conflicts of Interest: The authors declare no conflict of interest.

References

1. Pennington, L. Food composition database for bioactive food components. *J. Food Compos. Anal.* **2002**, *15*, 419–434. [CrossRef]
2. Jacobs, D.R.; Tapsell, L.C. Food, not nutrients, is the fundamental unit in nutrition. *Nutr. Rev.* **2007**, *65*, 439–450. [CrossRef] [PubMed]
3. Naviglio, D.; Romano, R.; Pizzolongo, F.; Santini, A.; De Vivo, A.; Schiavo, L.; Nota, G.; Spagna Musso, S. Rapid determination of esterified glycerol and glycerides in triglycerides fats and oils by means of periodate method after transesterification. *Food Chem.* **2007**, *102*, 399–405. [CrossRef]
4. Pannico, A.; Schouten, R.E.; Basile, B.; Romano, R.; Woltering, E.J.; Cirillo, C. Non-destructive detection of flawed hazelnut kernels and lipid oxidation assessment using NIR spectroscopy. *J. Food Eng.* **2015**, *160*, 42–48. [CrossRef]
5. Cilla, A.; Bosch, L.; Barberá, R.; Alegría, A. Effect of processing on the bioaccessibility of bioactive compounds—A review focusing on carotenoids, minerals, ascorbic acid, tocopherols and polyphenols. *J. Food Compos. Anal.* **2018**, *68*, 3–15. [CrossRef]
6. Romano, R.; Giordano, A.; Le Grottaglie, L.; Manzo, N.; Paduano, A.; Sacchi, R.; Santini, A. Volatile compounds in intermittent frying by gas chromatography and nuclear magnetic resonance. *Eur. J. Lipid Sci. Technol.* **2013**, *115*, 764–773. [CrossRef]

7. D'Evoli, L.; Salvatore, P.; Lucarini, M.; Nicoli, S.; Aguzzi, A.; Gabrielli, P.; Lombardi-Boccia, G. Nutritional value of traditional Italian meat-based dishes: Influence of cooking methods and recipe formulation. *Int. J. Food Sci. Nutr.* **2009**, *60*, 38–49. [CrossRef]
8. Marletta, L.; Camilli, E.; Turrini, A.; Scardella, P.; Spada, R.; Piombo, L.; Khokhar, S.; Finglas, P.; Carnovale, E. The nutritional composition of selected ethnic foods consumed in Italy. *Nutr. Bull.* **2010**, *35*, 350–356. [CrossRef]
9. Lucarini, M.; D'Evoli, L.; Nicoli, S.; Aguzzi, A.; Gabrielli, P.; Lombardi-Boccia, G. Effect of cooking treatments on nutrient profile of dishes based on veal meat. *Italian J. Food Sci.* **2011**, *23*, 395–403.
10. Ramdath, D.D.; Hilaire, D.G.; Brambilla, A.; Sharma, S. Nutritional composition of commonly consumed composite dishes in Trinidad. *Int. J. Food Sci. Nutr.* **2011**, *62*, 34–46. [CrossRef]
11. Costa, H.S.; Albuquerque, T.G.; Sanches-Silva, A.; Vasilopoulou, E.; Trichopoulou, A.; D'Antuono, L.F.; Alexieva, I.; Boyko, N.; Costea, C.; Fedosova, K.; et al. New nutritional composition data on selected traditional foods consumed in Black Sea Area countries. *J. Sci. Food Agric.* **2013**, *93*, 3524–3534. [CrossRef]
12. Durazzo, A.; Lisciani, S.; Camilli, E.; Gabrielli, P.; Marconi, S.; Gambelli, L.; Aguzzi, A.; Lucarini, M.; Maiani, G.; Casale, G.; et al. Nutritional composition and antioxidant properties of traditional Italian dishes. *Food Chem.* **2017**, *218*, 70–77. [CrossRef] [PubMed]
13. Durazzo, A.; Camilli, E.; Marconi, S.; Lisciani, S.; Gabrielli, P.; Gambelli, L.; Aguzzi, A.; Lucarini, M.; Kiefer, J.; Marletta, L. Nutritional composition and dietary intake of composite dishes traditionally consumed in Italy. *J. Food Compos. Anal.* **2019**, *77*, 115–124. [CrossRef]
14. SINU, Società Italiana di Nutrizione Umana. *Livelli di Assunzione di Riferimento di Nutrienti ed Energia per la Popolazione Italiana*; (IV Revisione); SICS (Società Italiana di Comunicazione Scientifica e Sanitaria): Milano, Italy, 2014.
15. Finglas, P.; Roe, M.; Pinchen, H.; Astley, S. The contribution of food composition resources to nutrition science methodology. *Br. Nutr. Found. Nutr. Bull.* **2017**, *42*, 198–206. [CrossRef]
16. Ribeiro, P.; de Moris, T.B.; Colugnati, F.A.; Sigulem, D.M. Food composition tables: Laboratory comparative analysis. *Revista de Saude Publica* **2003**, *37*, 216–225. [CrossRef]
17. Gibson, R.S. *Principles of Nutritional Assessment*, 2nd ed.; Oxford University Press: New York, NY, USA, 2005.
18. Elmadfa, I.; Meyer, A.L. Importance of food composition data to nutrition and public health. *Eur. J. Clin. Nutr.* **2010**, *3*, 4–7. [CrossRef]
19. Church, S.M. The importance of food composition data in recipe analysis. *Nutr. Bull.* **2015**, *40*, 40–44. [CrossRef]
20. Howie, M. The nutritional value of food: A retailer's view on McCance and Widdowson's The Composition of Foods Data. *Br. Nutr. Found. Nutr. Bull.* **2015**, *40*, 104–106. [CrossRef]
21. Capatti, A.; Montanari, M. La cucina italiana. In *Storia di una Cultura*, 7th ed.; Laterza: Bari, Italy, 2006.
22. EuroFIR AISBL. EuroFIR—European Food Information Resource. Available online: http://www.eurofir.org (accessed on 10 January 2019).
23. Project Food Quality and Functional (QUALIFU). Available online: http://nut.entecra.it/441/qualita_alimentare_e_funzionale_qualifu.html (accessed on 10 January 2019).
24. Durazzo, A.; Lucarini, M. A Current shot and re-thinking of antioxidant research strategy. *Braz. J. Anal. Chem.* **2018**, *5*, 9–11. [CrossRef]
25. Andrew, R.; Izzo, A.A. Principles of pharmacological research of nutraceuticals. *Br. J. Pharmacol.* **2017**, *174*, 1177–1194. [CrossRef]
26. Santini, A.; Novellino, E.; Armini, V.; Ritieni, A. State of the art of Ready-to-Use Therapeutic Food: A tool for nutraceuticals addition to foodstuff. *Food Chem.* **2013**, *140*, 843–849. [CrossRef] [PubMed]
27. Santini, A.; Novellino, E. To Nutraceuticals and Back: Rethinking a Concept. *Foods* **2017**, *6*, 74. [CrossRef]
28. Santini, A.; Tenore, G.C.; Novellino, E. Nutraceuticals: A paradigm of proactive medicine. *Eur. J. Pharm. Sci.* **2017**, *96*, 53–61. [CrossRef] [PubMed]
29. Santini, A.; Novellino, E. Nutraceuticals: Shedding light on the grey area between pharmaceuticals and food. *Expert Rev. Clin. Pharmacol.* **2018**, *11*, 545–547. [CrossRef]
30. Santini, A.; Cammarata, S.M.; Capone, G.; Ianaro, A.; Tenore, G.C.; Pani, L.; Novellino, E. Nutraceuticals: Opening the debate for a regulatory framework. *Br. J. Clin. Pharmacol.* **2018**, *84*, 659–672. [CrossRef]
31. Daliu, P.; Santini, A.; Novellino, E. From pharmaceuticals to nutraceuticals: Bridging disease prevention and management. *Expert Rev. Clin. Pharmacol.* **2018**, *28*, 1–7. [CrossRef] [PubMed]

32. Daliu, P.; Santini, A.; Novellino, E. A decade of nutraceutical patents: Where are we now in 2018? *Expert Opin. Ther. Patents* **2018**, *28*, 875–882. [CrossRef] [PubMed]
33. Durazzo, A.; D'Addezio, L.; Camilli, E.; Piccinelli, R.; Turrini, A.; Marletta, L.; Marconi, S.; Lucarini, M.; Lisciani, S.; Gabrielli, P.; et al. From Plant Compounds to Botanicals and Back: A Current Snapshot. *Molecules* **2018**, *23*, 1844. [CrossRef]
34. Yeung, A.W.K.; Tzvetkov, N.T.; El-Tawil, O.S.; Bungǎu, S.G.; Abdel-Daim, M.M.; Atanasov, A.G. Antioxidants: Scientific Literature Landscape Analysis. *Oxid. Med. Cell. Longev.* **2019**, *2019*, 8278454. [CrossRef]
35. Durazzo, A. Study Approach of Antioxidant Properties in Foods: Update and Considerations. *Foods* **2017**, *6*, 17. [CrossRef]
36. Durazzo, A. Extractable and Non-extractable polyphenols: An overview. In *Non-Extractable Polyphenols and Carotenoids: Importance in Human Nutrition and Health*; Saura-Calixto, F., Pérez-Jiménez, J., Eds.; Royal Society of Chemistry: London, UK, 2018; pp. 1–37.
37. Ebun, O.; Santosh, K. Effect of domestic cooking on the polyphenolic content and antioxidant capacity of plantain (*Musa paradisiaca*). *World J. Dairy Food Sci.* **2011**, *6*, 189–194.
38. Pérez-Jiménez, J.; Torres, J.L. Analysis of non-extractable phenolic compounds in foods: The current state of the art. *J. Agric. Food Chem.* **2011**, *59*, 12713–12724. [CrossRef] [PubMed]
39. Durazzo, A.; Turfani, V.; Azzini, E.; Maiani, G.; Carcea, M. Phenols, lignans and antioxidant properties of legume and sweet chestnut flours. *Food Chem.* **2013**, *140*, 666–671. [CrossRef] [PubMed]
40. Durazzo, A.; Turfani, V.; Narducci, V.; Azzini, E.; Maiani, G.; Carcea, M. Nutritional characterisation and bioactive components of commercial carobs flours. *Food Chem.* **2014**, *153*, 109–113. [CrossRef]
41. Pérez-Jiménez, J.; Díaz-Rubio, M.E.; Saura-Calixto, F. Non-extractable polyphenols, a major dietary antioxidant: Occurrence, metabolic fate and health effects. *Nutr. Res. Rev.* **2013**, *26*, 118–129. [CrossRef] [PubMed]
42. Camelo-Méndez, G.A.; Bello-Pérez, L.A. Antioxidant Capacity of Extractable and Non-extractable Polyphenols of Pigmented Maize. *Food Biotechnol.* **2014**, *4*, 6–13.
43. Durazzo, A.; Gabrielli, P.; Manzi, P. Qualitative Study of Functional Groups and Antioxidant Properties of Soy-Based Beverages Compared to Cow Milk. *Antioxidants* **2015**, *4*, 523–532. [CrossRef]
44. Zambrano-Moreno, E.L.; Chávez-Jáuregui, R.N.; de Lurdes, P.M.; Wessel-Beaver, L. Phenolic content and antioxidant capacity in organically and conventionally grown eggplant (*Solanum melongena*) fruits following thermal processing. *Food Sci. Technol.* **2015**, *35*, 414–420. [CrossRef]
45. Olivas-Aguirre, F.J.; González-Aguilar, G.A.; Velderrain-Rodríguez, G.R.; Torres-Moreno, H.; Robles-Zepeda, R.E.; Vázquez-Flores, A.A.; de la Rosa, L.A.; Wall-Medrano, A. Radical scavenging and anti-proliferative capacity of three freeze-dried tropical fruits. *Int. J. Food Sci. Technol.* **2017**, *52*, 1699–1709. [CrossRef]
46. Peng, H.; Li, W.; Li, H.; Deng, Z.; Zhang, B. Extractable and nonextractable bound phenolic compositions and their antioxidant properties in seed coat and cotyledon of black soybean (*Glycinemax* (L.) Merr). *J. Funct. Foods* **2017**, *32*, 296–312. [CrossRef]
47. Sanz-Pintos, N.; Pérez-Jiménez, J.; Buschmann, A.H.; Vergara-Salinas, J.R.; Pérez-Correa, J.R.; Saura-Calixto, F. Macromolecular Antioxidants and Dietary Fiber in Edible Seaweeds. *J. Food Sci.* **2017**, *82*, 289–295. [CrossRef]
48. Song, Y.; Wei, X.Q.; Li, M.Y.; Duan, X.W.; Sun, Y.M.; Yang, R.L.; Su, X.D.; Huang, R.M.; Wang, H. Nutritional Composition and Antioxidant Properties of the Fruits of a Chinese Wild *Passiflora foetida*. *Molecules* **2018**, *23*, 459. [CrossRef] [PubMed]
49. Arranz, S.; Perez-Jimenez, J.; Saura-Calixto, F. Antioxidant capacity of walnut (*Juglans regia* L.): Contribution of oil and defatted matter. *Eur. Food Res. Technol.* **2008**, *227*, 425–431. [CrossRef]
50. Saura-Calixto, F.; Serrano, J.; Goni, I. Intake and Bioaccessibility of Total Polyphenols in a Whole Diet. *Food Chem.* **2007**, *101*, 492–501. [CrossRef]
51. Pérez-Jiménez, J.; Saura-Calixto, F. Macromolecular antioxidants or non-extractable polyphenols in fruit and vegetables: Intake in four European countries. *Food Res. Int.* **2015**, *74*, 315–323. [CrossRef]
52. Koehnlein, E.A.; Bracht, A.; Nishida, V.S.; Peralta, R.M. Total antioxidant capacity and phenolic content of the Brazilian diet: A real scenario. *Int. J. Food Sci. Nutr.* **2014**, *65*, 293–298. [CrossRef] [PubMed]
53. Koehnlein, E.A.; Koehnlein, É.M.; Corrêa, R.C.; Nishida, V.S.; Correa, V.G.; Bracht, A.; Peralta, R.M. Analysis of a whole diet in terms of phenolic content and antioxidant capacity: Effects of a simulated gastrointestinal digestion. *Int. J. Food Sci. Nutr.* **2016**, *67*, 614–623. [CrossRef] [PubMed]

54. Faller, A.L.K.; Fialho, E.; Liu, R.H. Cellular Antioxidant Activity of Feijoada Whole Meal Coupled with an in Vitro Digestion. *J. Agric. Food. Chem.* **2012**, *60*, 4826–4832. [CrossRef] [PubMed]
55. Pinto, P.; Santo, C.N. Worldwide (poly)phenol intake: Assessment methods and identified gaps. *Eur. J. Nutr.* **2017**, *56*, 1393–1408. [CrossRef] [PubMed]
56. Durazzo, A.; Plumb, J.; Lucarini, M.; Fernandez-Lopez, G.; Camilli, E.; Turrini, A.; Finglas, P.; Marletta, L. *Extractable and Non-Extractable Antioxidants at the Interface of eBASIS Structure: Database Development and Expansion*; EuroFIR Food Forum: Brussels, Belgium, 2018.
57. Plumb, J.; Fernandez-Lopez, G.; Durazzo, A.; Lucarini, M.; Mantur-Vierendeel, A.; Camilli, E.; Turrini, A.; Marletta, L.; Finglas, P. Compiling quality evaluated data on extractable and non-extractable antioxidants within the eBASIS database Bioavailability 2018 Conference, 10-13 September, Nowich. In Proceedings of the Bioavailability 2018, Norwich, UK, 10–13 September 2018.
58. eBASIS—Bioactive Substances in Food Information System. Available online: http://ebasis.eurofir.org/Default.asp (accessed on 8 January 2019).
59. Kiely, M.; Black, L.J.; Plumb, J.; Kroon, P.A.; Hollman, P.C.; Larsen, J.C.; Speijers, G.J.; Kapsokefalou, M.; Sheehan, D.; Gry, J.; et al. EuroFIR eBASIS: Application for health claims submissions and evaluations. *Eur. J. Clin. Nutr.* **2010**, *64*, S101–S107. [CrossRef] [PubMed]
60. Plumb, J.; Pigat, S.; Bompola, F.; Cushen, M.; Pinchen, H.; Nørby, E.; Astley, S.; Lyons, J.; Kiely, M.; Finglas, P. eBASIS (Bioactive Substances in Food Information Systems) and bioactive intakes: Major updates of the bioactive compound composition and beneficial bio effects database and the development of a probabilistic model to assess intakes in Europe. *Nutrients* **2017**, *9*, 320. [CrossRef]
61. Manzocco, L.; Calligaris, S.; Mastrocola, D.; Nicoli, M.C.; Lerici, C.R. Review of non-enzymatic browning and antioxidant capacity in processed foods. *Trends Food Sci. Technol.* **2001**, *11*, 340–346. [CrossRef]
62. Pinelo, M.; Manzocco, L.; Nunez, M.J.; Nicoli, M.C. Interaction among phenols in food fortification: Negative synergism on antioxidant capacity. *J. Agric. Food Chem.* **2004**, *52*, 1177–1180. [CrossRef]
63. Ioannou, I. Comparative study of antioxidant activity between basic and convenience foods. *J. Food Res.* **2012**, *1*, 143–156. [CrossRef]
64. Amarowicz, R.; Carle, R.; Dongowski, G.; Durazzo, A.; Galensa, R.; Kammerer, D.; Maiani, G.; Piskula, M.K. Influence of postharvest processing and storage on the content of phenolic acids and flavonoids in foods. *Mol. Nutr. Food Res.* **2009**, *53*, S151–S183. [CrossRef]
65. Durazzo, A.; Casale, G.; Melini, V.; Maiani, G.; Acquistucci, R. Total polyphenol content and antioxidant properties of Solina (*Triticum aestivum* L.) and derivatives thereof. *J. Food Sci.* **2016**, *28*, 221.
66. Turfani, V.; Narducci, V.; Durazzo, A.; Galli, V.; Carcea, M. Technological, nutritional and functional properties of wheat bread enriched with lentil or carob flours. *LWT–Food Sci. Technol.* **2017**, *78*, 361. [CrossRef]
67. Hirawan, R.; Ser, W.Y.; Arntfield, S.D.; Beta, T. Antioxidant properties of commercial, regular- and whole-wheat spaghetti. *Food Chem.* **2009**, *119*, 258–264. [CrossRef]
68. Durazzo, A.; Turfani, V.; Azzini, E.; Maiani, G.; Carcea, M. Antioxidant properties of experimental pastas made with different wholegrain cereals. *J. Food Res.* **2014**, *3*. [CrossRef]
69. Sant'Anna, V.; Christiano, F.D.P.; Marczak, L.D.F.; Tessaro, I.C.; Thys, R.C.S. The effect of the incorporation of grape marc powder in fettuccini pasta properties. *LWT-Food Sci. Technol.* **2014**, *58*, 497–501. [CrossRef]
70. Gull, A.; Prasad, K.; Kumar, P. Nutritional, antioxidant, microstructural and pasting properties of functional pasta. *J. Saudi Soc. Agric. Sci.* **2018**, *17*, 147–153. [CrossRef]
71. Ivanišováeva, I.; Košec, M.; Brindza, J.; Grygorieva, O.; Tokár, M. Green Barley as an Ingredient in Pasta: Antioxidant Activity and Sensory Characteristics Evaluation. *Contemp. Agric.* **2018**, *67*, 81–86. [CrossRef]
72. Palavecino, P.M.; Ribotta, P.D.; Leóna, A.E.; Bustosa, M.C. Gluten-free sorghum pasta: Starch digestibility and antioxidant capacity compared with commercial products. *J. Sci. Food Agric.* **2019**, *99*, 1351–1357. [CrossRef] [PubMed]
73. Kuhnen, S.; Moacyr, J.R.; Mayer, J.K.; Navarro, B.B.; Trevisan, R.; Honorato, L.A.; Maraschin, M.; Pinheiro Machado Filho, L.C. Phenolic content and ferric reducing—Antioxidant power of cow's milk produced in different pasture-based production systems in southern Brazil. *J. Food Sci. Agric.* **2014**, *94*, 3110–3117. [CrossRef]
74. Manzi, P.; Durazzo, A. Antioxidant properties of industrial heat-treated milk. *J. Food Measur. Charact.* **2017**, *11*, 1690–1698. [CrossRef]

75. Mattera, M.; Durazzo, A.; Nicoli, S.; Di Costanzo, M.G.; Manzi, P. Chemical, nutritional, physical and antioxidant properties of Pecorino d'abruzzo cheese. *Ital. J. Food Sci.* **2016**, *28*, 579–597.
76. Yilmaz-Ersan, L.; Ozcan, T.; Akpinar-Bayizit, A.; Sahin, S. Comparison of antioxidant capacity of cow and ewe milk kefirs. *J. Dairy Sci.* **2018**, *101*, 3788–3798. [CrossRef]
77. Calligaris, S.; Manzocco, L.; Anese, M.; Nicoli, M.C. Effect of heat-treatment on the antioxidant and and pro-oxidant activity of milk. *Int. Dairy J.* **2004**, *14*, 421–427. [CrossRef]
78. Zulueta, A.; Maurizi, A.; Frigola, A.; Esteve, M.J.; Coli, R.; Burini, G. Antioxidant capacity of cow milk, whey and deproteinized milk. *Int. Dairy J.* **2009**, *19*, 380–385. [CrossRef]
79. Cortés Yáñez, D.A.; Gagneten, M.; Leiva, G.E.; Male, L.S. Antioxidant activity developed at the different stages of Maillard reaction with milk proteins. *LWT* **2018**, *89*, 344–349. [CrossRef]
80. Bars-Cortina, D.; Macià, A.; Iglesias, I.; Romero, M.P.; Motilva, M.J. Phytochemical profiles of new red-fleshed apple varieties compared with traditional and new white-fleshed varieties. *J. Agric. Food Chem.* **2017**, *65*, 1684–1696. [CrossRef] [PubMed]
81. Kumar, P.; Sethi, S.; Sharma, R.R.; Singh, S.; Saha, S.; Sharma, V.K.; Verma, M.K.; Sharma, S.K. Nutritional characterization of apple as a function of genotype. *J. Food Sci. Technol.* **2018**, *55*, 2729–2738. [CrossRef] [PubMed]
82. Phenol-Explorer—Database on Polyphenol Content in Foods. Available online: http://phenol-explorer.eu/ (accessed on 15 January 2019).
83. Leclercq, C.; Arcella, D.; Piccinelli, R.; Sette, S.; Le Donne, C.; Turrini, A.; INRAN-SCAI 2005-06 Study Group. The Italian National Food Consumption Survey INRAN-SCAI 2005-06: Main results in terms of food consumption. *Public Health Nutr.* **2009**, *12*, 2504–2532. [CrossRef] [PubMed]
84. Finglas, P.M.; Berry, R.; Astley, S. Assessing and improving the quality of food composition databases for nutrition and health applications in Europe: The contribution of EuroFIR. *Adv. Nutr.* **2014**, *5*, 608–614. [CrossRef]
85. Durazzo, A.; Kiefer, J.; Lucarini, M.; Marconi, S.; Lisciani, S.; Camilli, E.; Gambelli, L.; Gabrielli, P.; Aguzzi, A.; Finotti, E.; et al. An innovative and integrated food research approach: Spectroscopy applications to milk and a case study of a milk-based dishes. *Braz. J. Anal. Chem.* **2018**, *5*, 12–27. [CrossRef]
86. Durazzo, A.; Kiefer, J.; Lucarini, M.; Camilli, C.; Marconi, S.; Gabrielli, P.; Aguzzi, A.; Gambelli, L.; Lisciani, S.; Marletta, L. Qualitative Analysis of Traditional Italian Dishes: FTIR Approach. *Sustainability* **2018**, *10*, 4112. [CrossRef]
87. Tabart, J.; Kevers, C.; Pincemail, J.; Defraigne, J.O.; Dommes, J. Comparative antioxidant capacities of phenolic compounds measured by various tests. *Food Chem.* **2009**, *113*, 1226–1233. [CrossRef]
88. Apak, R.; Özyürek, M.; Güçlü, K.; Çapanoglu, E. Antioxidant activity/capacity measurement. 1. Classification, physicochemical principles, mechanisms, and electron transfer (ET)-based assays. *J. Agric. Food Chem.* **2016**, *64*, 997–1027. [CrossRef] [PubMed]
89. Apak, R.; Özyürek, M.; Güçlü, K.; Çapanoglu, E. Antioxidant Activity/Capacity Measurement. 2. Hydrogen Atom Transfer (HAT)-Based, Mixed-Mode (Electron Transfer (ET)/HAT), and Lipid Peroxidation Assays. *J. Agric. Food Chem.* **2016**, *64*, 1028–1045. [CrossRef]
90. Apak, A.; Capanoglu, E.; Shahidi, F. *Measurement of Antioxidant Activity and Capacity: Recent Trends and Applications*; Wiley: New York, NY, USA, 2018; ISBN 978-1-119-13535-7.
91. Leopoldini, M.; Russo, N.; Toscano, M. The molecular basis of working mechanism of natural polyphenolic antioxidants. *Food Chem.* **2011**, *125*, 288–306. [CrossRef]
92. Schlesier, K.; Harwat, M.; Bohm, V.; Bitsch, R. Assessment of antioxidant activity by using different in vitro methods. *Free Radic. Res.* **2002**, *36*, 177–187. [CrossRef] [PubMed]
93. Prior, R.L.; Wu, X.; Schaich, K. Standardized methods for the determination of antioxidant capacity and phenolics in foods and dietary supplements. *J. Agric. Food Chem.* **2005**, *53*, 4290–4302. [CrossRef]
94. Benzie, I.F.F.; Strain, J.J. The ferric reducing ability of plasma (FRAP) as a measure of "antioxidant power": The assay. *Anal. Biochem.* **1996**, *239*, 70–76. [CrossRef]
95. Pulido, R.; Bravo, L.; Saura-Calixto, F. Antioxidant activity of dietary polyphenols as determined by a modified ferric reducing/antioxidant power assay. *J. Agric. Food Chem.* **2000**, *48*, 3396–3402. [CrossRef] [PubMed]
96. Singleton, V.L.; Orthofer, R.; Lamuela-Raventos, R.M. Analysis of total phenols and other oxidation substrates and antioxidants by means of Folin–Ciocalteu reagent. *Methods Enzymol.* **1999**, *299*, 152–178.

97. Nascimento-Souza, M.A.; Paiva, P.G.; Martino, H.S.D.; Ribeiro, A.Q. Dietary total antioxidant capacity as a tool in health outcomes in middle-aged and older adults: A systematic review. *Crit. Rev. Food Sci. Nutr.* **2018**, *58*, 905–912. [CrossRef] [PubMed]
98. Parohan, M.; Anjom-Shoae, J.; Nasiri, M.; Khodadost, M.; Khatibi, S.R.; Sadeghi, O. Dietary total antioxidant capacity and mortality from all causes, cardiovascular disease and cancer: A systematic review and dose-response meta-analysis of prospective cohort studies. *Eur. J. Nutr.* **2019**. [CrossRef]

Sample Availability: Samples of the compounds are available from the authors.

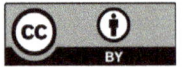

© 2019 by the authors. Licensee MDPI, Basel, Switzerland. This article is an open access article distributed under the terms and conditions of the Creative Commons Attribution (CC BY) license (http://creativecommons.org/licenses/by/4.0/).

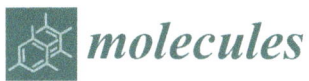

Perspective

Bio-Based Compounds from Grape Seeds: A Biorefinery Approach

Massimo Lucarini [1,*], Alessandra Durazzo [1], Annalisa Romani [2], Margherita Campo [2], Ginevra Lombardi-Boccia [1] and Francesca Cecchini [3]

1. CREA—Research Centre for Food and Nutrition, 00178 Roma, Italy; alessandra.durazzo@crea.gov.it (A.D.); g.lombardiboccia@crea.gov.it (G.L.-B.)
2. PHYTOLAB, University of Florence, 50019 Sesto Fiorentino, (Firenze), Italy; annalisa.romani@unifi.it (A.R.); margherita.campo@unifi.it (M.C.)
3. CREA—Research Centre for Viticulture and Enology, 00049 Velletri, Roma, Italy; francesca.cecchini@crea.gov.it
* Correspondence: massimo.lucarini@crea.gov.it; Tel.: +39-065-149-4446

Academic Editor: Derek J. McPhee
Received: 26 June 2018; Accepted: 26 July 2018; Published: 28 July 2018

Abstract: Food and agricultural waste represents a growing problem with negative effects on the economy, environment, and human health. Winemaking produces byproducts with high added value, which can be used for new productions in several application fields. From the perspective of biorefinery and circular economy, grape seeds could be exploited by extracting bioactive compounds with high added value before using biomass for energy purposes. The markets concerned are, in addition to the food, cosmetics, and pharmaceuticals sectors, which use bioactive compounds, the sector of biopolymeric materials and of energy for the production of biohydrogen and biomethane. Generally, bioactive components should be investigated through an integrated and multidisciplinary study approach based on emerging analytical techniques; in this context, attention is addressed towards green and sustainable procedures; an update of extraction techniques, innovative technologies, and chemometrics are described. Nowadays, processes so far tested on a pilot scale for grape waste are developed to enhance the extraction yields. Here, a picture of the Italian experience applied to the byproducts of the wine industry is given.

Keywords: biorefinery; circular economy; grape seed; bio-based; chemometrics

---

1. Introduction

Food and agricultural waste is a growing problem that, if not properly addressed, has negative effects on the economy, environment, and human health. Food and agricultural waste can not only be avoided but it is possible to intercept the opportunity to exploit the waste to define, for example, new bioproducts in a more complete view of biorefinery. It has been estimated that a third of all the food produced in the world is not consumed, making for a total of about 1.3 billion tons of waste a year [1,2].

In Italy, the economic value of food waste is around 8.5 billion euro per year [3], of which about 11% (equivalent to €180 million) takes place during industrial processing in the fruit and vegetables sector [4].

In Europe, viticulture plays a fundamental role, with a market dominated by Italy, France, and Spain. Vinification is wrongly considered a production with low environmental impact; instead, it requires considerable quantities of resources such as water, soil fertilizers, amendments, producing a huge amount of waste [5,6]. From an agronomic point of view, the vineyard area in Italy is about 5.2% of the Used Agricultural Surface (SAU), equivalent to 664,296 hectares at national level [7], with a wine production of 47 million hectoliters in the 2017 harvest (biggest wine producer by volume) [8,9].

Winemaking produces a series of byproducts, easily exploitable for new productions and in various supply chains.

During the winemaking process, the quality and quantity of these byproducts depend on a set of cofactors, but basically on the type of vinification [5,10–13]. Grape seeds represent the portion of fruit with the highest concentration of bioactive molecules; several studies reported that, among the different parts of grape fruit, seeds show the highest antioxidant activity, followed by the skin and pulp [14,15].

Grape seeds still have great biological potential that could be exploited by extracting bioactive compounds with high added value before using biomass for energy purposes to obtain extracts and semifinished products useful for agronomic, cosmetics, feed, food, nutraceutical, and pharmaceutical purposes.

Therefore, considering grape seeds as waste represents a double loss for the food industry, both for the disposal costs and for the loss of profits deriving from their recycling and exploitation.

From the processing of one ton of grapes, approximately 0.13 tons of pomace are produced, 0.06 tons of lees, 0.03 tons of pomace, and 1.65 m^3 of waste water [5,6]. Seeds can be easily recovered from pomace by separation and sifting technologies. Accounting for 8–20% of the weight of grapes processed by the wine industry [11,16], it can be estimated that in Italy there is an amount of seeds coming from the winemaking process that varies between 0.1 and 0.3 million tons [17,18].

The disposal of waste and byproducts led to strong environmental impact that can be estimated by assessing the carbon footprint that is slowly also spreading in the wine sector: the most widely used methodology is the Life Cycle Assessment (LCA) [12,19–25]; on the Italian level, the calculation of the emission of CO_2 equivalents due to the 2016 vinification waste was calculated on the basis of the "International Wine Carbon Calculator" [26] and was equal to 278,100 tons from lees, 834,300 tons from pomace, and 185,400 tons from stems [27]; in Italy in the 2016 harvest, 1300 tons of CO_2 equivalents were produced, which could be reduced by using these byproducts as raw material for other production chains, as underlined by Bevilacqua et al. [27].

The creation of an integrated model with a biorefinery approach applied to the oenological sector would therefore allow considering winemaking waste as co-products in a virtuous circular economy process aligned with European waste legislation and meeting or exceeding the Kyoto protocol goals [28].

2. The Biorefinery Concept

A biorefinery is a facility that provides for an integrated, efficient, and flexible conversion of biomass feedstocks through a combination of physical, chemical, biochemical, and thermochemical processes into multiple products. As a broad technological definition, biorefinery is intended as the conversion of all kinds of biomass (e.g., organic residues, energy crops, aquatic biomass) into a wide range of bio-based products, such as food and feed, chemicals, materials, fuels, power, and heat [29,30].

Biorefineries are considered the most complete way for the creation of an industry based on products derived from biological materials or able to enhance the different chemical components of biomass.

The concept of biorefinery is analogous to oil refineries but tends to exceed the limit of a purely energetic crop destination, proposing the use of plant biomass to extract chemicals to be used in several sectors. The biorefinery deals with separating the components of the biomass in its constituents to assign each of them to the use that allows obtaining the greatest yield in terms of biovalue. The biorefinery approach, applied to winemaking, provides for the optimal exploitation of byproducts in industrial sectors not in competition with that of wine.

Biorefinery outputs are classified into a biovalor hierarchy that indicates the value of biomass transformations (Figure 1) based on new circular agricultural or economic models. At the top of the pyramid there are substances for fine and pharmaceutical chemistry, useful for the synthesis of vaccines, antibiotics, and immunotherapy proteins. Further down the hierarchy of biorefinery products, there are food and feed products, followed by substances for the chemical industries, such as bioplastics, lubricants, solvents, adhesives, fibers, and dyes. At the bottom of the pyramid there are all the substances for the production of biogas by fermentation and biofuels in the field of energy sector.

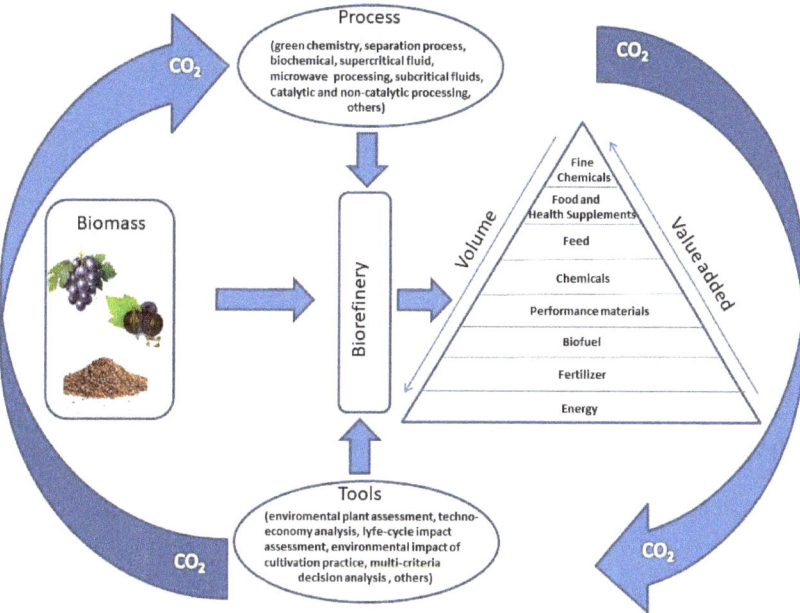

Figure 1. The biorefinery concept: a puzzle piece of circular bioeconomy.

The more suitable technologies for separation, fermentation, gasification, and chemical conversion must be identified, as well as for biomasses' pretreatment and storage.

In addition to territorial integration, favored by the reduced size of the plants compared to those of traditional petrochemicals, the availability of biomass requires the development of integration processes within the relationship with suppliers; this allows access to a limited supply range to qualified materials to be included in the production processes.

In terms of efficiency and sustainability, chemical products from biomass should be considered and certified on the basis of criteria referring to the entire life cycle of products [31]. According to estimates by international organizations, the transition to a green economy could generate from 15 to 60 million jobs (green jobs) globally in the next twenty years [32]. Communication also plays a role of primary importance: informing consumers about the safety aspects, as well as about the benefits that can arise from good planning of the valorization of biomass, will be even more than any other incentive paths [18].

3. High Value-Added Compounds in Grape Seed

The waste generated by the agroindustry should be considered for a biorefinery approach, as they meet different criteria, such as the quantity of raw material and the content in molecules with high added value [33–36]. The interest in grape seeds has increased, especially for their content in nutraceuticals, such as phenolic compounds (gallic acid, hydroxybenzoic and cinnamic acid derivatives, quercetin, kaempferol, monomeric flavan-3-ols, i.e., (+)-catechin, (−)-epicatechin, gallocatechin and epicathechin 3-O-gallate, procyanidin dimers, trimers, and more highly polymerized procyanidins) [37], unsaturated fatty acids [38–40], vitamin E, carotenoids, and phytosterols [41].

Several studies reported potential protective properties of grape seeds [42–48], i.e., the anticancer and chemopreventive efficacy of grape seed extract against various types of cancers [49–52]. The beneficial effects of grape seed on human health are due to the concerted and combined action of bioactive compounds; it is clear that the first step of bioactivity is linked to antioxidant properties [53,54].

Other than genetic traits of the grape cultivar, extrinsic factors as the year of production (i.e., the climatic condition from year to year), the site of production (such as the effect of geographic origin of grapes, soil composition, and fertilization), the degree of maturation, and postharvest practices strongly influence the levels of nutraceutical compounds [55–58]. Furthermore, processing technologies, as type of vinification and some related steps, e.g., fermentation, represent additional factors in determining the bioactive profile of grape seeds [59,60].

The identification, isolation, and quantification of functional grape seed components, as well as the assessment of their interactions, are necessary prerequisites for selecting adequate procedures in biorefinery. For this reason, particular attention should be paid towards fast and green procedures and alternative analytical techniques.

4. Green and Sustainable Procedures: Extraction Techniques, Innovative Technologies, and Chemometrics

Generally, studies on the evaluation of bioactive components should be integrated in a multidisciplinary and innovative study approach for food research: the combination of emerging analytical techniques and the application of statistical methods in food science led to the innovative challenge for modelling agrofood systems.

Sampling and extraction procedures are crucial processes for the recovery, isolation, and identification of bioactive compounds from grape seeds. The optimal extraction procedure should provide the maximum yield in terms of concentration of target compounds. Different variables should be considered—pretreatment of the sample, solvent/sample ratio, type of solvent, particle sizes, time and temperature of extraction, and so on [61,62].

Conventionally, several types of pressing machines and different conventional solvent extraction techniques have been applied in the analysis of bioactive compounds from food wastes. These techniques are generally based on the use of toxic compounds, restricting the application of grape seed extracts in biorefinery perspectives.

Nowadays, several extraction, processing, and preservation methodologies have been introduced, with particular regards to green and sustainable techniques for the separation of natural products from waste [36,63].

Examples of non-conventional techniques applied to *Vitis vinifera* waste [64] were given, like enzymatic treatment [65], microwave-assisted extraction [66], ultrasound-assisted extraction [67], and supercritical and subcritical fluid extraction [68–72].

The earliest works about laboratory extraction with supercritical CO_2, applied to grape byproducts such as skin, seeds, and stems [69], were followed by industrial-scale studies, with multipurpose biorefineries in which polyphenols and sugars extraction in supercritical CO_2 is accompanied by further processes for the recovery of fatty acids and the production of biogas [70]. Prado et al. [71] reviewed the supercritical fluid extraction of grape seed by describing process scale-up, chemical composition of extracts, and economic evaluation.

The food industry has recently utilized the ultrasound assisted extraction (UAE) process to extract bioactive compounds from plant and animal materials (e.g., polyphenolics, anthocyanins, aromatic compounds, polysaccharides, and functional compounds). This procedure increased the yields of extracted components, rates of extraction, and processing throughput. The optimization of this technology, which complements current methods, could allow for: modification of plant cell material to improve the bioavailability of micronutrients while retaining the natural-like quality; simultaneous extraction and encapsulation; quenching of radical sonochemistry, especially in aqueous systems;

avoiding degradation of labile compounds; potential use of radical sonochemistry to achieve targeted hydroxylation of polyphenolics and carotenoids and increase bioactivity [67].

Boussetta and colleagues [73] tested the effects of high-voltage electrical discharges (HVED) on the aqueous extraction of polyphenols from grape pomace at constant temperature in the range of 20–60 °C; HVED increased the extraction kinetics of total solutes and total polyphenols from grape pomace—whatever the method of conservation (fresh, sulphured and frozen)—by damaging both cell membranes and cell walls. The final yields of solutes, reached after HVED application followed by diffusion for 40 min, were more than two-fold higher than the values obtained after 240 min of conventional extraction under similar conditions. Thus, the main advantages of HVED application were the reduced extraction times and temperatures.

Pilot plant scale enzyme-assisted extraction of polyphenols from winery byproducts was optimized after preliminary laboratory tests [74]. Pectinolytic and cellulolytic enzymatic treatment of grape pomace causes the liquefaction of grape skins; this procedure enhances both the extraction yield of polyphenolic compounds and the extraction rates of flavonoids and stilbenes, in respect of those of sulfite extraction. Pre-extraction of pomace with hot water further increased yields of phenolic compounds [74]. A recent extraction method for recovery of phenols from grape seed was developed by Stambuk et al. [75] by application of pectinase, an example of enzyme-assisted extraction.

Spectroscopic techniques coupled to chemometrics could represent a valid green alternative to conventional methods for determination of bioactive compounds in foods and food waste; numerous advantages are given by the use of spectroscopic techniques, with respect to the conventional ones, e.g., simple sample preparation procedure, and short time for data collection and analysis.

Canbay and Bardakçı [76] have carried out structural analysis of grape seed oil and pulp by FT/IR spectrometry by highlighting peculiar functional groups and modes of vibration of main components. Hanganu et al. [77], using the Principal Component Analysis method to the spectral information, studied the application in authenticity control of grape seed oils from common genuine oils (sunflower, soybean, linseed, and rapeseed).

Recently, the spectroscopic technique has been applied to the study and quantification of bioactive compounds in grape seed. Nogales–Bueno et al. [78] have used near-infrared hyperspectral tools for the screening of extractable polyphenols in red grape skins. Further studies [79,80], by jointly applying ATR-FTIR and Raman spectroscopy to grape seed samples, studied and linked the more important spectral features to phenolic extractability and other attributes in grape skin and grape seed. Therefore, FTIR spectroscopy coupled with chemometrics can represent a valuable tool for monitoring the composition of byproducts, allocating them to the most suitable extraction process.

5. A Grape Seed Biorefinery: A Picture of Italian Experience

The conversion of winery waste into energy is a source of benefits for wine producers, able to reduce their energy costs by generating renewable energy. Power can be obtained: via biomass gasifiers that convert grape marc to syngas, which is then fed to an internal combustion engine to drive a generator; via biomass boilers used to supply heat to an absorption chiller for fermenter cooling; and via anaerobic digesters used to produce biogas that is directed to an internal combustion engine to drive a generator. Removing polyphenols from the vegetal material before the conversion into energy could be a further important method to increase yields of power due to the antimicrobial potential of these compounds that could inhibit the fermentation processes, and for obtaining new products environmentally and economically sustainable to place on the market. Methods for the recovery of anthocyanins from winery byproducts using sulfite-containing water are not completely suitable because sulfite cannot be removed quantitatively from the extracts, and pseudoallergic reactions caused by foods with added sulfites have been described [81,82]. Extraction with ecocompatible solvents, mainly water, eventually with low percentages of ethilic alcohol, is a suitable method to recover interesting and important bioactive compounds from vegetal matrices [83,84]. This technique, suitable for integration with other processes within biorefinery plants, is ecologically and economically sustainable, as water does not involve high costs, it can be more easily disposed of, and, above all, it can be recovered almost pure while concentrating the extracts to be reintroduced into the production process [85–87].

Experimental processes so far tested on a pilot scale in Italy for grape waste (leaves and skin) are based on aqueous extraction accompanied by additional biochemical or physical processes to enhance the extraction yields [85,86].

An example of an operating diagram for the extraction and purification/concentration of hydrolysable and condensed tannins from vegetal matrices is shown in Figure 2 [87]. The described plant, operating in Tuscany, is suitable for extraction with aqueous or hydroalcoholic solvents, and it can be used to obtain concentrated extracts and fractions of condensed tannins from grape seeds. All the purification and concentration steps are performed by physical processes using semipermeable membranes for micro- and nanofiltration; thus, the whole process can be green and environmentally friendly [85].

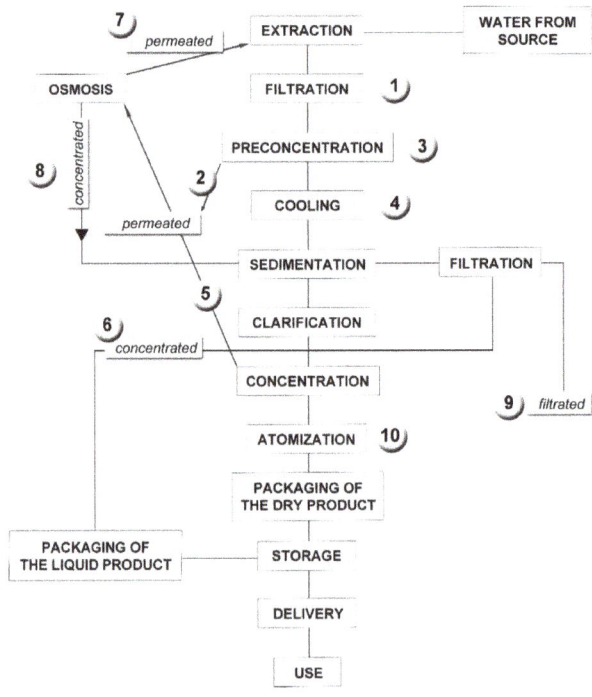

Figure 2. Operating diagram of extraction and fractionation plant from Reference [87], consisting of (**1**) filtered tannin broths; (**2**) permeate from nanofiltration Step 1; (**3**) concentrate from nanofiltration Step 1; (**4**) concentrate from nanofiltration Step 2; (**5**) permeate from nanofiltration Step 2; (**6**) concentrate from nanofiltration Step 3; (**7**) osmosis permeate; (**8**) osmosis concentrate; (**9**) settled fraction from clarification step; (**10**) spray-dried obtained from fraction 6.

The extraction plant works by extracting the vegetal matrices in 100% water or by using low percentages of alcohol. For wood or hard matrices such as grape seeds, yields of aqueous extraction can also be raised by working at high temperatures, compatibly with the stability of the active principles that have to be preserved: in subcritical water extraction processes at high temperatures (150 °C) of grape seeds, there have been observed high yields on procyanidins extraction, but also hydrolysis processes of galloylated compounds, and consequently increased concentrations of free gallic acid [83]. The extraction chamber is fed with 20 m³ of biomass and the extraction solvent can reach a temperature of 80 °C. The boiler is fed with the exhausted biomass that has already undergone the polyphenol extraction process, so that the plant can be entirely powered by cogeneration according to the specific process parameters and calorific values of the different matrices (wood matrices have an average calorific value of 2000–5000 Kcal/Kg; the boiler can exploit 10 tons of biomass each batch). The purification and concentration steps are performed by membrane technology, avoiding the use of the organic solvents usually employed in industrial purification processes. This methodology also allows, when necessary, for a selective concentration of specific subclasses of compounds with different chemical and biological properties. The final product is a concentrated extract or spray-dried powder obtained with an average yield of 5% with respect to the vegetal material.

Within the activities of the European project EVERGREEN (Environmentally friendly biomolecules from agricultural wastes as substitutes of pesticides for plant diseases control—LIFE13 ENV/IT/000461) grape seed waste, obtained after wine production and mechanical extraction of oil, was extracted and analyzed for the polyphenol compounds by HPLC/DAD/MS methods [42].

The grape seeds were isolated from marcs obtained after the winemaking process, and pretreated by drying at controlled temperature; the drying parameters were set according to the type of vegetable matrix, with particular attention to avoiding the degradation of the active ingredients. The vegetal material was put in perforated stainless steel baskets inside a drying chamber and maintained at a maximum temperature of 38 °C until its weight was stable. Two batches of seeds pretreatment were monitored in depth: the initial weights were 1260 Kg and 1560 Kg, respectively, and the respective dried weight was 554 Kg and 708 Kg (44% and 45% yields). The dried product was packed in polypropylene bags for food use and stored at room temperature, protected from light.

The dried grape seeds were used for oil mechanical extraction with a 15% yield. The cold-pressing process allows for obtaining totally solvent-free oil, together with an exhausted matrix that consists of the extruded solid after mechanical pressing. The grape seed residue post-oil extraction was considered for agronomical formulations according to the objectives of the Project, since it showed to contain still high levels of polyphenols—in particular condensed tannins.

For this purpose, both seeds and byproducts were characterized by laboratory extraction: for the grape seeds as such, exhaustive extraction in hydroalcoholic solvent (EtOH:H_2O 70:30, pH 2.5 by HCOOH addition) was performed; for the minced residue after oil extraction, both hydroalcoholic exhaustive extraction and aqueous extraction were performed to obtain respectively a complete characterization and also to reproduce an industrial extraction process with 100% water. The hydroalcoholic extractions confirmed that most of the polyphenolic compounds (72.1%) present in the seeds were retained during the mechanical oil extraction process; thus, the exhausted material could be recovered as a further possibility of exploitation of wine production waste and according to the innovative models of circular agriculture. The measured amounts of single compounds in the aqueous extract of the exhausted residue were as follows (results expressed as mg single compounds per gram of seeds): gallic acid (0.41 mg/g); catechin dimer B3 (1.52 mg/g); catechin (0.64 mg/g); catechin trimer (0.54 mg/g); catechin dimer B6 (0.77 mg/g); catechin dimer B2 (0.96 mg/g); epicatechin (0.59 mg/g); epicatechin gallate dimers I (1.06 mg/g); epicatechin gallate dimers II (5.49 mg/g); catechin tetramers (9.51 mg/g); catechin/epicatechin trimers digallated I (13.47 mg/g); catechin/epicatechin trimers digallated II (8.92 mg/g). Total polyphenols were 43.88 mg/g.

The aqueous extraction of seed waste after oil extraction allowed for a more sustainable, even though lower, recovery of polyphenolic compounds; in this case, an increased percentage of gallic acid was observed in byproducts with respect to the seeds (0.93% vs. 0.04%)—this could be due to partial hydrolysis of heavier molecules.

Recent studies have shown high antioxidant and antimicrobial properties for gallic acid in particular, and higher nematocidal activity for extracts particularly rich in free gallic acid has also been observed [88,89]; thus, it is of interest to test new agronomical formulations containing oil extraction residue from grape seeds: these formulations could slowly release condensed tannins into the ground to obtain antimicrobial and nematostatic/nematicidal effects.

In this order, a new gel formulation containing the minced grape seed residue post-oil extraction was designed, produced, and monitored for 4 months by spectrophotometric analysis repeated at regular time intervals (1 month). The preliminary analyses showed that the powder obtained from the spent residue gradually releases polyphenolic compounds into the gel matrix along with time until flavan-3-ol and procyanidin concentration, expressed as catechin equivalents per gram of gel, was 7.4 mg/g gel (0.7% p/p).

The formulations, chemically and physically stable within the time of use, are in a test phase on several crops to prevent the attack from various pathogenic species.

6. Conclusions

In Italy, the production of waste from winemaking processes is high and its use following a holistic biorefinery approach is needed. The integrated exploitation of enological byproducts represents a basis for an 'intelligent' reconversion of waste that can be attained through the use of eco-compatible 'green technologies' to ensure environmental sustainability in the supply chain. In this context, studies are needed aimed at optimizing an integrated valorization of biomass, as well as to guide producers and consumers towards virtuous and sustainable development paths.

Author Contributions: M.L., G.L.-B., and F.C. have conceived and designed the work. All authors have made a substantial contribution to the writing and revision of work, and approved it for publication. M.L. coordinated the preparation and the revisions performed by all the coauthors.

Funding: This research did not receive any specific grant from funding agencies in the public, commercial, or nonprofit sectors.

Conflicts of Interest: The authors declare that the research was conducted in the absence of any commercial or financial relationships that could be construed as a potential conflict of interest.

References

1. Gustavsson, J.; Cederberg, C.; Sonesson, U.; van Otterdijk, R.; Meybeck, A. *Global Food Losses and FW: Extent, Causes and Prevention*; FAO: Rome, Italy, 2011.
2. Xia, H.; Houghton, J.A.; Clark, J.H.; Matharu, A.S. Potential utilization of unavoidable food supply chain wastes–valorization of pea vine wastes. *ACS Sustain. Chem. Eng.* **2016**, *4*, 6002–6009. [CrossRef]
3. Waste Watcher. *V Giornata Nazionale di Prevenzione dello Spreco Alimentare 2018*; Waste Watcher: Roma, Italy, 2018.
4. Segrè, A.; Gaiani, S. *Transforming Food Waste into a Resource*; RSC Publishing: Cambridge, UK, 2012.
5. Ruggieri, L.; Cadena, E.; Martínez-Blanco, J.; Gasol, C.M.; Rieradevall, J.; Gabarrell, X.; Gea, T.; Sort, X.; Sánchez, A. Recovery of organic wastes in the Spanish wine industry. Technical, economic and environmental analyses of the composting process. *J. Clean. Prod.* **2009**, *17*, 830–838. [CrossRef]
6. Oliveira, M.; Duarte, E. Integrated approach to winery waste: Waste generation and data consolidation. *Front. Environ. Sci. Eng.* **2014**, *10*, 168–176. [CrossRef]
7. Istituto Nazionale di Statistica (ISTAT). *Atlante dell'Agricoltura Italiana, 6° Censimento Generale dell'Agricoltura*; Istituto Nazionale di Statistica: Rome, Italy, 2013.
8. OIV (Organisation Internationale de la Vigne et du Vin). *2017 Global Economic V Data*; OIV: Paris, France, 2017; pp. 1–5.
9. ASSOENOLOGI. Produzione 2016 i Dati Definitivi dell'Associazione Enologi Enotecnici Italiani Milano. 20 November 2016. Available online: http://www.assoenologi.it/main/images/pics/vendemmia_2016_dati_definitivi.pdf (accessed on 27 July 2018).
10. Mazza, G.; Miniati, E. Grapes. In *Anthocyanins in Fruits, Vegetables and Grains*; CRC Press: Boca Raton, FL, USA; Ann Harbor, MI, USA; London, UK; Tokyo, Japan, 1993; pp. 149–199.
11. Schieber, A.; Stintzing, F.C.; Carle, R. By-products of plant food processing as a source of functional compounds—Recent developments. *Trends Food Sci. Technol.* **2001**, *12*, 401–413. [CrossRef]

12. Petti, L.; Ardente, F.; Bosco, S.; De Camillis, C.; Masotti, P.; Pattara, C.; Raggi, A.; Tasselli, G. Stato dell'arte della Life Cycle Assessment (LCA) nel comparto vitivinicolo. In *La Metodologia LCA: Approccio Proattivo per le Tecnologie Ambientali. Casi Studio ed Esperienze Applicative*; Cappellaro, F., Scalbi, S., Eds.; Atti Convegno Scientifico della Rete Italiana LCA: Padova, Italy, 22 April 2010; pp. 221–228, ISBN 978-88-8286-226-8.
13. Novello, V. Filiera vitivinicola: Valorizzare residui e sottoprodotti. *Informatore Agrario* 2015, *33*, 61–63.
14. Pastrana-Bonilla, E.; Akoh, C.C.; Sellappan, S.; Krewer, G. Phenolic content and antioxidant capacity of muscadine grapes. *J. Agric. Food Chem.* 2003, *5*, 5497–5503. [CrossRef] [PubMed]
15. Chandra, H.M.; Ramalingam, S. Antioxidant potential of skin, pulp, and seed fractions of commercially important tomato cultivars. *Food Sci. Biotechnol.* 2011, *20*, 15–21. [CrossRef]
16. Dwyer, K.; Hosseinian, F.; Rod, M. The market potential of grape waste alternatives. *J. Food Res.* 2014, *3*, 91–106. [CrossRef]
17. ANPA (Agenzia Nazionale per la Protezione dell'Ambiente). *I Rifiuti del Comparto Agroalimentare*; Rapporti 11/2001; ANPA—Unità Normativa Tecnica: Roma, Italy, 2001.
18. Accardi, D.S.; Bubbico, R.; Di Palma, L.; Pietrangeli, B. Environmental and Safety Aspects of Integrated BioRefineries (IBR) in Italy. *Chem. Eng. Trans.* 2013, *32*, 169–174.
19. Ardente, F.; Beccali, G.; Cellura, M.; Marvuglia, A. A Case Study of an Italian Wine-Producing. *Environ. Manag.* 2006, *38*, 350–364. [CrossRef] [PubMed]
20. Bosco, S.; Di Bene, C.; Galli, M.; Remorini, D.; Massai, R.; Bonari, E. Greenhouse gas emissions in the agricultural phase of wine production in the Maremma rural district in Tuscany, Italy. *Ital. J. Agron.* 2011, *6*, 93–100. [CrossRef]
21. Vázquez-Rowe, I.; Rugani, B.; Benetto, E. Tapping carbon footprint variations in the European wine sector. *J. Clean. Prod.* 2013, *43*, 146–155. [CrossRef]
22. Neto, B.; Dias, A.C.; Machado, M. Life cycle assessment of the supply chain of a Portuguese wine: From viticulture to distribution. *Int. J. Life Cycle Assess.* 2013, *18*, 590–602. [CrossRef]
23. Corbo, C.; Lamastra, L.; Capri, E. From Environmental to Sustainability Programs: A Review of Sustainability Initiatives in the Italian Wine Sector. *Sustainability* 2014, *6*, 2133–2159. [CrossRef]
24. Navarro, A.; Puig, R.; Fullana-I-Palmer, P. Product vs. corporate carbon footprint: Some methodological issue. A case study and review on the wine sector. *Sci. Total Environ.* 2017, *581–582*, 722–723. [CrossRef] [PubMed]
25. ISO (International Organization for Standardization). *ISO 14040: Environmental Management—Life Cycle Assessment—Principles and Framework*; EN ISO 14040; International Organization for Standardization: Geneva, Switzerland, 2006.
26. International Wine Carbon Calculator, Developed by "Wine Institute of California". Available online: http://www.wineinstitute.org (accessed on 27 July 2018).
27. Bevilacqua, N.; Morassut, M.; Serra, M.C.; Cecchini, F. Determinazione dell'impronta carbonica dei sottoprodotti della vinificazione e loro valenza biologica. *Ingegneria dell'Ambiente* 2017, *4*, 277–285. [CrossRef]
28. UNFCCC. Kyoto Protocol to the United Nations Framework Convention on Climate Change Adopted at COP3 in Kyoto, Japan, on 11 December 1997. Available online: 20http://unfccc.int/resource/docs/cop3/07a01.pdf (accessed on 27 July 2018).
29. Ragauskas, A.J.; Williams, C.K.; Davison, B.H.; Britovsek, G.; Cairney, J.; Eckert, C.A. The path forward for biofuels and biomaterials. *Science* 2006, *311*, 484–489. [CrossRef] [PubMed]
30. Demirbas, A. *Biorefineries. For Biomass Upgrading Facilities*; Springer: London, UK, 2010.
31. Ahlgren, S.; Björklund, A.; Ekman, A.; Karlsson, H.; Berlin, J.; Börjesson, P.; Ekvall, T.; Finnveden, G.; Janssen, M.; Strid, I. Review of methodological choices in LCA of biorefinery systems—Key issues and recommendations. *Biofuels Bioprod. Bioref.* 2015, *9*, 606–619. [CrossRef]
32. ILO (International Labor Office). *Working towards Sustainable Development: Opportunities for Decent Work and Social Inclusion in a Green Economy*; ILO: Geneva, Switzerland, 2012; pp. 1–18.
33. Tuck, C.O.; Perez, E.; Horvath, I.T.; Sheldon, R.A.; Poliakoff, M. Valorization of biomass: Deriving more value from waste. *Science* 2012, *337*, 695–699. [CrossRef] [PubMed]
34. Lin, C.S.K.; Koutinas, A.A.; Stamatelatou, K.; Mubofu, E.B.; Matharu, A.S.; Kopsahelis, N.; Pfaltzgraff, L.A.; Clark, J.H.; Papanikolaou, S.; Kwan, T.H.; et al. Current and future trends in food waste valorization for the production of chemicals, materials and fuels: A global perspective. *Biofuels Bioprod. Bioref.* 2014, *8*, 686–715. [CrossRef]

35. Lin, C.S.K.; Luque, R. *Renewable Resources and Biorefineries*; Royal Society of Chemistry: Cambridge, UK, 2014.
36. Zuin, V.G.; Ramin, L.Z. Green and Sustainable Separation of Natural Products from Agro-Industrial Waste: Challenges, Potentialities, and Perspectives on Emerging Approach. *Top. Curr. Chem.* **2018**, *376*, 3. [CrossRef] [PubMed]
37. Xu, C.; Zhang, Y.; Zhang, Y.; Jun, W.; Lu, J. Extraction, distribution and characterisation of phenolic compounds and oil in grapeseeds. *Food Chem.* **2010**, *122*, 688–694. [CrossRef]
38. Garavaglia, J.; Markoski, M.M.; Oliveira, A.; Marcadenti, A. Grape Seed Oil Compounds: Biological and Chemical Actions for Health. *Nutr. Metab. Insights* **2016**, *9*, 59–64. [CrossRef] [PubMed]
39. Durante, M.; Montefusco, A.; Marrese, P.P.; Soccio, M.; Pastore, D.; Piro, G.; Mita, G.; Lenucci, M.S. Seeds of pomegranate, tomato and grapes: An underestimated source of natural bioactive molecules and antioxidants from agri-food by-products. *J. Agric. Food Chem.* **2017**, *63*, 65–72. [CrossRef]
40. Shinagawa, F.B.; de Santana, F.C.; Araujo, E.; Purgatto, E.; Mancini-Filho, J. Chemical composition of cold pressed Brazilian grape seed oil. *Food Sci. Technol.* **2017**, *38*, 164–171. [CrossRef]
41. Giannini, B.; Mulinacci, N.; Pasqua, G.; Innocenti, M.; Valletta, A.; Cecchini, F. Phenolics and antioxidant activity in different cultivars/clones of *Vitis vinifera* L. seeds over two years. *J. Plant Biosyst.* **2016**, *150*, 1408–1416. [CrossRef]
42. Romani, A.; Ieri, F.; Turchetti, B.; Mulinacci, N.; Vincieri, F.F.; Buzzini, P. Analysis of condensed and hydrolyzable tannins from commercial plant extracts. *J. Pharm. Biomed. Anal.* **2006**, *41*, 415–420. [CrossRef] [PubMed]
43. Sano, A.; Uchida, R.; Saito, M.; Shioya, N.; Komori, Y.; Tho, Y.; Hashizume, N. Beneficial effects of grape seed extract on malondialdehyde-Modified LDL. *J. Nutr. Sci. Vitaminol.* **2007**, *53*, 174–182. [CrossRef] [PubMed]
44. Kar, P.; Laight, D.; Rooprai, H.K.; Shaw, K.M.; Cummings, M. Effects of grapeseed extract in type 2 diabetic subjects: A double blind randomised placebo controlled trial looking at the effects upon inflammatory and metabolic markers. *Diabetic Med.* **2009**, *26*, 526–531. [CrossRef] [PubMed]
45. Castrillejo, V.M.; Romero, M.M.; Esteve, M.; Ardévol, A.; Blay, M.; Bladé, C.; Arola, L.; Salvadó, M.J. Antioxidant effects of a grapeseed procyanidin extract and oleoyl-estrone in obese Zucker rats. *Nutrition* **2011**, *27*, 1172–1176. [CrossRef] [PubMed]
46. Montagut, G.; Bladé, C.; Blay, M.; Fernández-Larrea, J.; Pujadas, G.; Salvadó, M.J.; Arola, L.; Pinent, M.; Ardévol, A. Effects of a grapeseed procyanidin extract (GSPE) on insulin resistance. *J. Nutr. Biochem.* **2010**, *21*, 961–967. [CrossRef] [PubMed]
47. Brito de Souza, V.; Fujita, A.; Thomazini, M.; da Silva, E.R.; Lucon, J.F., Jr.; Genovese, M.I.; Favaro-Trindade, C.S. Functional properties and stability of spray-dried pigments from Bordo grape (*Vitis labrusca*) winemaking pomace. *Food Chem.* **2014**, *164*, 380–386. [CrossRef] [PubMed]
48. Erdemli, M.E.; Akgul, H.; Ege, B.; Aksungur, Z.; Bag, H.G.; Selamoglu, Z. The effects of grapeseed extract and low level laser therapy administration on the liver in experimentally fractured mandible. *J. Turgut Ozal Med. Cent.* **2017**, *24*, 127–133. [CrossRef]
49. Agarwal, C.; Veluri, R.; Kaur, M.; Chou, S.-C.; Thompson, J.A.; Agarwal, R. Fractionation of high molecular weight tannins in grape seed extract and identification of procyanidins B2-3,3′-diO-gallate as a major active constituent causing growth inhibition and apoptotic death of DU145 Human prostate carcinoma cells. *Carcinogenesis* **2007**, *28*, 1478–1484. [CrossRef] [PubMed]
50. Chou, S.-C.; Kaur, M.; Thompson, J.A.; Agatwal, R.; Agarwal, C. Influence of gallate esterification on the activity of procyanidin B2 in Androgen-dependent prostate carcinoma LNCaP cells. *Pharm. Res.* **2010**, *27*, 619–627. [CrossRef] [PubMed]
51. Engelbrecht, A.M.; Mattheyse, M.; Ellis, B.; Loos, B.; Thomas, M.; Smith, R.; Peters, S.; Smith, C.; Myburgh, K. Proanthocyanidin from grape seeds inactivates the PI3kinase/PKB pathway and induces apoptosis in a colon cancer cell line. *Cancer Lett.* **2007**, *258*, 144–153. [CrossRef] [PubMed]
52. Kaur, M.; Mandair, R.; Agarwal, R.; Agarwal, C. Grape Seed Extract Induces Cell Cycle Arrest and Apoptosis in Human Colon Carcinoma Cells. *Nutr. Cancer* **2008**, *60*, 2–11. [CrossRef] [PubMed]
53. Keser, S.; Celik, S.; Turkoglu, S. Total phenolic contents and free-radical scavenging activities of grape (*Vitis vinifera* L.) and grape products. *Int. J. Food Sci. Nutr.* **2013**, *64*, 210–216. [CrossRef] [PubMed]
54. García-Lomillo, J.; González-SanJosé, M.L.; Del Pino-García, R.; Rivero-Pérez, M.D.; Muñiz-Rodríguez, P. Antioxidant and antimicrobial properties of wine byproducts and their potential uses in the food industry. *J. Agric. Food Chem.* **2014**, *62*, 12595–12602. [CrossRef] [PubMed]

55. Cavaliere, C.; Foglia, P.; Marini, F.; Samperi, R.; Antonacci, D.; Laganà, A. The interactive effects of irrigation, nitrogen fertilisation rate, delayed harvest and storage on the polyphenol content in red grape (*Vitis vinifera*) berries: A factorial experimental design. *Food Chem.* **2010**, *122*, 1176–1184. [CrossRef]
56. Bordiga, M.; Travaglia, F.; Locatelli, M.; Cosson, J.D.; Arlorio, M. Characterisation of polymeric skin and seed proanthocyanidins during ripening in six *Vitis vinifera* L. cv. *Food Chem.* **2011**, *127*, 180–187. [CrossRef]
57. Cecchini, F. Factors affecting antioxidant activity of grape tissues. In *Grapes*; Camara, J.S., Ed.; Nova Science Publishers, Inc.: Hauppauge, NY, USA, 2014; ISBN 978-1-63321-402-6.
58. Özcan, M.M.; Juhaimi, F.A.; Gülcü, M.; Uslu, N.; Geçgel, Ü.; Ghafoor, K.; Dursun, N. Effect of harvest time on physico-chemical properties and bioactive compounds of pulp and seeds of grape varieties. *J. Food Sci. Technol.* **2017**, *54*, 2230–2240. [CrossRef] [PubMed]
59. De Sá, M.; Justino, V.; Spranger, M.I.; Zhao, Y.Q.; Han, L.; Sun, B.S. Extraction yields and anti-oxidant activity of proanthocyanidins from different parts of grapepomace: Effect of mechanical treatments. *Phytochem. Anal.* **2014**, *25*, 134–140. [CrossRef] [PubMed]
60. Ky, I.; Lorrain, B.; Kolbas, N.; Crozier, A.; Teissedre, P.L. Wine by-products: Phenolic characterization and antioxidant activity evaluation of grapes and grape pomaces from six different French grape varieties. *Molecules* **2014**, *19*, 482–506. [CrossRef] [PubMed]
61. Yilmaz, Y.; Toledo, R.T. Oxygen radical absorbance capacities of grape/wine industry byproducts and effect of solvent type on extraction of grape seed polyphenols. *J. Food Compos. Anal.* **2006**, *19*, 41–48. [CrossRef]
62. Spigno, G.; Tramelli, L.; De Faveri, D.M. Effects of extraction time, temperature and solvent on concentration and antioxidanty activity. *J. Eng.* **2007**, *81*, 200–208.
63. Viganó, J.; da Fonseca Machado, A.P.; Martínez, J. Sub- and supercritical fluid technology applied to food waste processing. *J. Supercrit. Fluids* **2015**, *96*, 272–286. [CrossRef]
64. Casazza, A.A.; Aliakbarian, B.; Mantegna, S.; Cravotto, G.; Perego, P. Extraction of phenolics from *Vitis vinifera* wastes using non-conventional techniques. *J. Food Eng.* **2010**, *100*, 50–55. [CrossRef]
65. Chamorro, S.; Viveros, A.; Vega, E.; Brenes, A. Changes in polyphenol and polysaccharide content of grape seed extract and grape pomase after enzymatic treatment. *Food Chem.* **2012**, *133*, 308–314. [CrossRef] [PubMed]
66. Li, Y.; Skouroumounis, G.K.; Elsey, G.M.; Taylor, D. Microwave-assistance provides very rapid and efficient extraction of grape seed polyphenols. *Food Chem.* **2011**, *129*, 570–576. [CrossRef]
67. Vilkhu, K.; Mawsoa, R.; Simons, L.; Bates, D. Applications and opportunities for ultrasound assisted extraction in the food industry—A review. *Innov. Food Sci. Emerg. Technol.* **2008**, *9*, 161–169. [CrossRef]
68. Ghafoor, K.; Al-Juhaimi, F.Y.; Choi, Y.H. Supercritical fluid extraction of phenolic compounds and antioxidants from grape (Vitis labrusca B.) seeds. *Plant Foods Hum. Nutr.* **2012**, *67*, 407–414. [CrossRef] [PubMed]
69. Louli, V.; Ragoussis, N.; Magoulas, K. Recovery of phenolic antioxidants from wine industry by-products. *Bioresour. Technol.* **2004**, *92*, 201–208. [CrossRef] [PubMed]
70. Martinez, G.A.; Rebecchi, S.; Decorti, D.; Domingos, J.M.; Natolino, A.; Del Rio, D.; Bertin, L.; Da Porto, C.; Fava, F. Towards multi-purpose biorefinery platforms for the valorisation of red grape pomace: Production of polyphenols, volatile fatty acids, polyhydroxyalkanoates and biogas. *Green Chem.* **2016**, *18*, 261–270. [CrossRef]
71. Prado, J.M.; Dalmolin, I.; Carareto, N.D.D.; Basso, R.C.; Meirelles, A.J.A.; Oliveira, J.V.; Batista, E.A.C.; Meireles, M.A.A. Supercritical fluid extraction of grape seed: Process scale-up, extract chemical composition and economic evaluation. *J. Food Eng.* **2012**, *109*, 249–257. [CrossRef]
72. Prado, J.M.; Forster-Carneiro, T.; Rostagno, M.A.; Follegatti-Romero, L.A.; Maugeri Filho, F.; Meireles, M.A.A. Obtaining sugars from coconut husk, defat-ted grape seed, and pressed palm fiber by hydrolysis with subcritical water. *J. Supercrit. Fluids* **2014**, *89*, 89–98. [CrossRef]
73. Boussetta, N.; Lanoisellé, J.L.; Bedel-Cloutour, C.; Vorobiev, E. Extraction of soluble matter from grape pomace by high voltage electrical discharges for polyphenol recovery: Effect of sulphur dioxide and thermal treatments. *J. Food Eng.* **2009**, *95*, 192–198. [CrossRef]
74. Kammerer, D.; Claus, A.; Schieber, A.; Carle, R. A Novel process for the recovery of polyphenols from grape (*Vitis vinifera* L.) pomace. *J. Food Sci.* **2005**, *70*, 157–163. [CrossRef]
75. Stambuk, P.; Tomaskovic, D.; Tomaz, I.; Maslov, L.; Stupic, D. Application of pectinases for recovery of grape seeds phenolics. *3 Biotech* **2016**, *6*, 224. [CrossRef] [PubMed]

76. Canbay, H.S.; Bardakçı, B. Determination of fatty acid, C, H, N and trace element composition in grape seed by GC/MS, FTIR, elemental analyzer and ICP/OES. *SDU J. Sci.* **2011**, *6*, 140–148.
77. Hanganu, A.; Todaşcă, M.C.; Chira, N.A.; Maganu, M.; Roşca, S. The compositional characterisation of Romanian grape seed oils using spectroscopic methods. *Food Chem.* **2012**, *134*, 2453–2458. [CrossRef] [PubMed]
78. Nogales-Bueno, J.; Baca-Bocanegra, B.; Rodríguez-Pulido, F.J.; Heredia, F.J.; Hernández-Hierro, J.M. Use of near infrared hyperspectral tools for the screening of extractable polyphenols in red grape skins. *Food Chem.* **2015**, *172*, 559–564. [CrossRef] [PubMed]
79. Nogales-Bueno, J.; Baca-Bocanegra, B.; Rooney, A.; Hernández-Hierro, J.M.; Heredia, F.J.; Byrne, H.J. Linking ATR-FTIR and Raman features to phenolic extractability and other attributes in grape skin. *Talanta* **2017**, *167*, 44–50. [CrossRef] [PubMed]
80. Nogales-Bueno, J.; Baca-Bocanegra, B.; Rooney, A.; Hernández-Hierro, J.M.; Byrne, H.J.; Heredia, F.J. Study of phenolic extractability in grape seeds by means of ATR-FTIR and Raman spectroscopy. *Food Chem.* **2017**, *232*, 602–609. [CrossRef] [PubMed]
81. Gastaminza, G.; Quirce, S.; Torres, M.; Tabar, A.; Echechipía, S.; Munoz, D.; Corres, L.F. Pickled onion-induced asthma: A model of sulfite-sensitive asthma? *Clin. Exp. Allergy* **1995**, *25*, 698–703. [CrossRef] [PubMed]
82. Gruber, J.; St Clair, L. For asthma sufferers—The facts about sulphites in food. *Food Aust.* **1994**, *46*, 500.
83. García-Marino, M.; Rivas-Gonzalo, J.C.; Ibáñez, E.; García-Moreno, C. Recovery of catechins and proanthocyanidins from winery by-products using subcritical water extraction. *Anal. Chim. Acta* **2006**, *563*, 44–50. [CrossRef]
84. Nawaz, H.; Shi, J.; Mittal, G.S.; Kakuda, Y. Extraction of polyphenols from grape seeds and concentration by ultrafiltration. *Sep. Purif. Technol.* **2006**, *48*, 176–181. [CrossRef]
85. Romani, A.; Pangia, D.; Marchionni, L.; Marchionni, A. Integrated Process for Recovery of a Polyphenol Fraction and Anaerobic Digestion of Olive Mill Wastes. PCT/IT2009000246, 5 June 2009.
86. Romani, A.; Scardigli, A.; Pinelli, P. An environmentally friendly process for the production of extracts rich in phenolic antioxidants from *Olea europaea* L. and *Cynara scolymus* L. matrices. *Eur. Food Res. Technol.* **2017**, *243*, 1229–1238. [CrossRef]
87. Campo, M.; Pinelli, P.; Romani, A. Hydrolyzable Tannins from Sweet Chestnut Fractions Obtained by a Sustainable and Eco-friendly Industrial Process. *Nat. Prod. Commun.* **2016**, *11*, 409–415. [PubMed]
88. Bargiacchi, E.; Miele, S.; Romani, A.; Campo, M. Biostimulant activity of hydrolyzable tannins from sweet chestnut (*Castanea sativa* Mill.). *Acta Horticult.* **2013**, *1009*, 111–116. [CrossRef]
89. Sorrentino, E.; Succi, M.; Tipaldi, L.; Pannella, G.; Maiuro, L.; Sturchio, M.; Coppola, R.; Tremonte, P. Antimicrobial activity of gallic acid against food-related Pseudomonas strains and its use as biocontrol tool to improve the shelf life of fresh black truffles. *Int. J. Food Microbiol.* **2018**, *266*, 183–189. [CrossRef] [PubMed]

Sample Availability: Samples of the compounds are available from the authors.

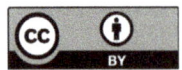

© 2018 by the authors. Licensee MDPI, Basel, Switzerland. This article is an open access article distributed under the terms and conditions of the Creative Commons Attribution (CC BY) license (http://creativecommons.org/licenses/by/4.0/).

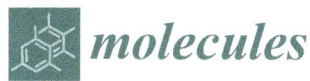

Article

Protective Effect of Cyclically Pressurized Solid–Liquid Extraction Polyphenols from *Cagnulari* Grape Pomace on Oxidative Endothelial Cell Death

Anna Maria Posadino [1,†], Grazia Biosa [2,†], Hatem Zayed [3], Haissam Abou-Saleh [4], Annalisa Cossu [1], Gheyath K. Nasrallah [3,5], Roberta Giordo [5], Daniela Pagnozzi [2], Maria Cristina Porcu [2], Luca Pretti [2,*] and Gianfranco Pintus [1,3,5,*]

1. Department of Biomedical Sciences, School of Medicine, University of Sassari, Viale San Pietro 43/B, 07100 Sassari, Italy; posadino@uniss.it (A.M.P.); cossuannalisa@libero.it (A.C.)
2. Porto Conte Ricerche S.r.l, Tramariglio, Alghero, 07041 Sassari, Italy; biosa@portocontericerche.it (G.B.); pagnozzi@portocontericerche.it (D.P.); cristina.porcu@ss.icb.cnr.it (M.C.P.)
3. Department of Biomedical Sciences, College of Health Sciences, Qatar University, P.O. Box 2713 Doha, Qatar; hatem.zayed@qu.edu.qa (H.Z.); gheyath.nasrallah@qu.edu.qa (G.K.N.)
4. Department of Biological and Environmental Sciences, College of Arts and Sciences, Qatar University, P.O. Box 2713 Doha, Qatar; hasaleh@qu.edu.qa
5. Biomedical Research Center, Qatar University, P.O. Box 2713 Doha, Qatar; roberta.giordo@qu.edu.qa
* Correspondence: pretti@portocontericerche.it (L.P.); gpintus@qu.edu.qa (G.P.); Tel.: +39-0799-98400 (L.P.); +974-4403-7558 (G.P.)
† These authors contributed equally to this work.

Received: 9 July 2018; Accepted: 17 August 2018; Published: 21 August 2018

Abstract: The aim of this work is the evaluation of a green extraction technology to exploit winery waste byproducts. Specifically, a solid–liquid extraction technology (Naviglio Extractor®) was used to obtain polyphenolic antioxidants from the *Cagnulari* grape marc. The extract was then chemically characterized by spectrophotometric analysis, high-performance liquid chromatography, and mass spectrometry, revealing a total polyphenol content of 4.00 g/L ± 0.05, and the presence of anthocyanins, one of the most representative groups among the total polyphenols in grapes. To investigate potential biological activities of the extract, its ability to counteract hydrogen peroxide-induced oxidative stress and cell death was assessed in primary human endothelial cells. The 3-(4,5-dimethylthiazol-2-yl)-2,5-diphenyltetrazolium bromide (MTT) test, used to assess potential extract cytotoxicity, failed to show any deleterious effect on cultured cells. Fluorescence measurements, attained with the intracellular reactive oxygen species (ROS) probe 2′,7′-dichlorodihydrofluorescein diacetate (H_2DCF-DA), revealed a strong antioxidant potential of the marc extract on the used cells, as indicated by the inhibition of the hydrogen peroxide-induced ROS generation and the counteraction of the oxidative-induced cell death. Our results indicate the Naviglio extraction, as a green technology process, can be used to exploit wine waste to obtain antioxidants which can be used to produce enriched foods and nutraceuticals high in antioxidants.

Keywords: *Cagnulari* marc; Naviglio Extractor®; green extraction; endothelial cell; oxidative stress; polyphenols

1. Introduction

Although wine production is one of the most important agricultural activities worldwide [1], the problems related to its waste treatment or disposal are far from being resolved [2]. Contamination problems related to winery waste byproducts have been raised [3,4]. Indeed, wine waste, such as lees and grape marc, may exert phytotoxic effects if applied to crops [4] or wetlands [5], since their content of specifc micronutrients and heavy metals is incompatible with the agricultural requirements [4–6]. Nevertheless, most of these byproducts can be used for different purposes, including the production of functional foods, dietary supplements, cosmetics, and pharmaceuticals [7,8]. The wine byproducts represent a considerable burden as industrial waste, due to the presence of variable phenolic contents in the wine, depending on the type of grape, the part of the tissue, and the processing conditions [4]. However, this burden can be significantly reduced using new or modified processing methods that aim to generate useful wine bioproducts, such as natural antioxidants. In this context, phenolic compounds with high antioxidants properties have been extracted from grape marc using new extraction techniques, such as pressurized liquid extraction and supercritical carbon dioxide [9].

Extraction methods, such as supercritical fluid extraction (SFE), pressurized liquid extraction (PLE), and assisted microwave irradiation extraction (MAE), can be employed as an alternative to conventional extraction techniques, since they have many practical aspects, including the reduction of solvent consumption and increasing the extraction rate process [9,10]. In this context, the Naviglio Extractor® is a solid–liquid extraction technology that works by generating a negative gradient pressure from the inside toward the outside of the solid matrix, which transports the extractable material outside of the matrix, by causing a suction effect. This extraction technique has been proven to be reproducible, quantitatively comparable, and affordable compared to other techniques, such as SFE and accelerated solvent extraction (ASE) [11–14]. Although the Naviglio Extractor® has been employed on several matrices [13,15–17], to our knowledge, its use on grape marc is yet to be explored. In addition, to be valuable, an extraction technology should not affect or should be able to retain the biological activities of the compounds extracted from that matrix, and therefore, its employment needs to be tested for this aspect.

Association of increased reactive oxygen species (ROS) with cardiovascular diseases (CVD) [18] suggests that counteracting oxidative stress with antioxidants could prevent disease occurrence or ameliorate their effects. For this reason, a significant amount of attention is now focusing on naturally occurring antioxidants as potential candidates for CVD prevention and/or treatment. The endothelial cell (EC) plays a crucial role in the integration and modulation of signals within the vascular wall [19], and perturbation of such homeostasis by oxidative damage is the trigger for the onset and development of CVD [18]. Therefore, we used human umbilical vein endothelial cells (HUVECs) to evaluate the potential antioxidant activity of the obtained extract. Indeed, HUVECs have been reported to be a useful model to study the vascular cells' response to natural antioxidant treatment [20–25].

Thus, the aim of the present work is to investigate whether (i) the green technology, Naviglio Extractor®, can be used to extract valuable antioxidant products from the wine waste, and (ii) the obtained products exert antioxidant activity, by protecting human endothelial cells against H_2O_2-induced oxidative stress and cell death.

2. Materials and Methods

2.1. Chemicals

Unless stated in the text, all the used reagents were from Sigma-Aldrich (St. Louis, MO, USA).

2.2. Pomace Acquisition and Preparation

The pomace of *Vitis vinifera* var. *Cagnulari* was purchased from a winery cooperative (Santa Maria La Palma, Alghero, Italy). Around 50 kg of exhausted pomace (RH% 52.6 ± 2.1) was air-dried in a cabinet tray drier with air flowing in alternate directions at 35 °C. After 72 h, the dried pomace (RH% 5.76 ± 0.2) was milled and sieved to a particle size of less than 4 mm diameter, and then vacuum stored at 4 °C until use.

2.3. Pomace Extraction Procedure

The detailed principle and procedures for the Naviglio Extractor have been previously reported [11]. Briefly, the extractor works by alternating a static phase with a dynamic one; during the static phase, the extracting solvent is brought to a pressure of about 10 atm, and is kept in this state for sufficient time to reach an equilibrium between the inside and the outside pressure of the solid matrix; at the end of the static phase, a dynamic phase begins, produced by a sudden movement of the pistons, which generates a rapid pressure decrease. The negative pressure gradient created between the inside and the outside of the solid matrix allows the extraction, due to a suction effect [11]. About 4 kg of dried pomace was recovered in a porous bag made of 50 µm filter membrane, and then introduced into the extraction chamber of the Naviglio Extractor (Mod. EXNA 1015) in 12.2 kg of water/ethanol 60:40 (v/v). To allow total polyphenols recovery, 21 extractive cycles of 1 min and 25 s each for a total of 38 min (12 min in static phase and 26 min in dynamic phase) were performed. The obtained hydro-alcoholic extract was recovered and stored at $-20\ °C$.

2.4. Chemical Characterization of the Extract

2.4.1. Folin–Ciocalteu (FC) Assay

The total polyphenol content of the extract was determined spectrophotometrically according to the classical Folin–Ciocalteau (FC) method. A 50 µL aliquot of standard solution, composed by a set of gallic acid solutions (concentrations from 50 to 500 ppm), was added to different quartz cuvettes (1 cm optical path) filled with 2350 µL of water and 150 µL of FC reagent. After 3 min, a solution of 20% sodium carbonate (450 µL) was added. Blank solution was prepared in the same way, but adding water instead of samples. All solutions were mixed in the dark for 2 h at RT, and then the absorbance was recorded at 760 nm with a Varian Cary 3E UV–vis spectrophotometer. Before analysis, 20 µL of extract were desalted and purified through a passage in a solid phase extraction C18 cartridges (Phenomenex, Torrance, California, USA, 55 µm, 70 A) equilibrated with 10% HCOOH solution. Then the extract was diluted 50 times, then treated with the same procedure used for gallic standards. The total polyphenol concentration was estimated by linear interpolation with a calibration curve made by the set of gallic acid solutions.

2.4.2. High-Performance Liquid Chromatography Analysis

Qualitative analysis of the extract was performed by high-performance liquid chromatography (HPLC) using an HP 1100/1200 instrument (Agilent Technologies, Palo Alto, CA, USA), equipped with an autosampler (100 µL sample loop), and a diode array detector [26]. About 225 µg of raw extract was loaded in 100 µL of HPLC starting conditions (6% of eluent A, composed by water/acetonitrile/formic acid, 87:3:10 $v/v/v$) on a C12 column (Synergi 4 µm Max-RP 80 A, 250 × 4.6 mm ID, Phenomenex, Torrance, California, USA), preceded by a Synergi guard column (4 × 3.00 mm, Phenomenex) with the same stationary phase, at room temperature. The flow rate was set at 0.5 mL/min with a multistep gradient of eluent B (water/acetonitrile/formic acid, 40:50:10 $v/v/v$ in A from 6% to 90%, according to the scheme provided in Table 1. Elution was followed by recording the absorbance between 190 and 700 nm. As a reference, a standard pool composed by 60 µL of a 2.5 ng/µL solution of malvidin-3-O-glucoside chloride, 60 µL of a 5 ng/µL solution of cyanidin-3-O-glucoside chloride, and 60 µL of a 2.5 ng/µL solution of peonidin-3-O-glucoside chloride (Sigma-Aldrich) was run on the same gradient.

Table 1. HPLC gradient used for the anthocyanin compounds separation.

Time (min)	Eluent B (%)
0	6
5	6
25	20
40	40
45	60
50	90
60	90

2.4.3. Mass Spectrometry Analysis

Identification of anthocyanins was confirmed by mass spectrometry (MS). Raw extract sample and selected fractions collected from HPLC run were analyzed using a MALDI-TOF Micro MX (Waters, Manchester, UK) spectrometer [27], equipped with a nitrogen laser (337 nm), and reflectron analyzer, in delayed extraction mode. Samples were mixed with an equal volume of the matrix, which was a DHB solution (2,5-dihydroxybenzoic acid, 20 mg/mL in 90% acetonitrile). Spectra were acquired in the 100–800 mass to charge ratio (m/z). The m/z range was externally calibrated by acquiring the spectrum of a mixture of compounds with known masses. The calibration was performed by air-drying on the plate 2 µL of a 1:1 mixture of standard polyphenols (resveratrol, 228.0786 g/mol, 0.14 µg/µL, peonidin-3-O-glucoside chloride, 463.1240 g/mol, 0.28 µg/µL cyanidin-3-O-glucoside chloride, 449.3848 g/mol, 0.28 µg/µL, malvidin-3-O-glucoside chloride, 493.1346 g/mol, 0.28 µg/µL), and DHB solution.

2.5. Assessment of Extract Biological Activity

2.5.1. Endothelial Cell Culture and Treatments

Human umbilical vein endothelial cells (HUVECs) were isolated from the vein of human umbilical cords and cultured as previously described [22–28]. Briefly, cells were detached from the interior of the umbilical vein of a 30 cm segment cord by treatment for 10 min at 37 °C with 0.05% (w/v) collagenase type II from *Clostridium hystolyticum* in medium M199 containing 100 U/mL of penicillin G sodium salt and 100 µg/mL streptomycin sulphate. HUVECs were harvested at 1000g for 10 min and finally resuspended in 5 mL medium M199 supplemented with 10% (v/v) fetal calf serum (FCS), 10% (v/v) newborn calf serum, 2 mM glutamine, and antibiotics. Cells were then plated in 25 cm^2 tissue culture flasks (Falcon, Oxnard, CA, USA) and cultured in an atmosphere of 5% CO_2/95% air. Cells were identified as endothelial cells by their "cobblestone" morphology and by factor VIII staining. Second passage HUVECs coming from a pool of different umbilical cords were used for experimentation. The day before each experiment, cells were plated in 48-well plates (Corning, Lowell, MA, USA) at a concentration of 10^4 cells/mL, and pretreated with the extract for 3 h, before oxidative stress was induced for 2 h by treatment with the indicated concentration of hydrogen peroxide (H_2O_2). In agreement with our previous study using a supercritical fluid extraction (SFE) extract of *Salvia desoleana* (*S. desoleana*) [25], the doses of 0.1, 1, and 10 µg/mL were tested in our human vascular model.

2.5.2. Measurements of Intracellular ROS

Intracellular ROS levels were determined by using the ROS molecular probe 2′,7′-dichlorodihydrofluorescein diacetate (H_2DCF-DA) (Molecular Probe, Eugene, OR, USA), as previously described [23,24]. Within the cell, esterases cleave the acetate groups on H_2DCF-DA, thus trapping the reduced form of the probe (H_2DCF). Intracellular ROS oxidize H_2DCF, yielding the fluorescent product, DCF. Cells were incubated for 3 h with the concentrations of extract indicated in the figure legends. After treatment, cells were incubated for 30 min with Hanks' Balanced Salt Solution

(HBSS) containing 5 µM H$_2$DCF-DA, then washed twice with HBSS and assessed for the fluorescence by using a Tecan GENios plus microplate reader (Tecan, Männedorf, CH, USA) in a light-protected condition. Treatment-induced variation of fluorescence was measured for 2 h in cell culture medium without phenol red. Excitation and emission wavelengths used for fluorescence quantification were 485 nm and 535 nm, respectively. All fluorescence measurements were corrected for background fluorescence and protein concentration. Using untreated cells as a reference, the overall anti- and pro-oxidant outcome was evaluated by comparison of five different measurements and expressed as percent of controls.

2.5.3. Assessment of Cell Viability

Potential toxicity and potential protection against oxidative cell death of the obtained extract were investigated under the different experimental conditions. To this end, cell viability was assessed in 96-well plates (BD Falcon) by using the colorimetric 3-(4,5-dimethylthiazol-2-yl)-2,5-diphenyltetrazolium bromide (MTT) assay, as previously reported [21,29]. To determinate potential toxicity, cells were treated for 20 h with the indicated concentrations of extract. To determinate potential protection against oxidative-induced cell damage, cells were pre-incubated for 3 h with the concentrations of extract indicated in the figure legends, then H$_2$O$_2$ (75 µM) was added for 20 h. After treatments, cells were added with 20 µL MTT solution (5 mg/mL) in cell culture medium and incubated at 37 °C in a cell incubator for additional 4 h; the medium was then removed, and the cell monolayer was washed twice with HBSS. The converted dye was solubilized with acidic isopropanol (0.04 N HCl in absolute isopropanol), and plates were analyzed at 570 nm using a GENios Plus microplate reader (Tecan, Männedorf, CH, USA) with background subtraction at 650 nm. All the measurements were corrected for protein concentrations and results expressed as a percentage of untreated controls.

2.6. Statistical Analysis

Data were checked for normal distribution and processed by one-way analysis of variance (ANOVA) followed by post hoc Newman–Keuls multiple comparison tests to determine the differences between mean values among treatments, with significance defined as $p < 0.05$. All the analyses were performed using the GraphPad Prism 6 software (GraphPad Software Inc., San Diego, CA, USA).

3. Results and Discussion

The treatment and disposal of waste originating from agricultural activities are important issues that are far from being resolved [2,4–6]. Fortunately, fruit and vegetable processing waste is rich in valuable compounds, such as antioxidants, and their utilization as a source of natural food additives is gaining a great deal of attention [7,8]. On the other hand, the pressing requirement to resolve food waste problems in an eco-sustainable manner necessitates the resolution of disadvantages associated with old extraction methods and promoting waste exploitation by employing green technologies. In this context, the rapid solid–liquid dynamic Naviglio® extractor represents a technology of solid–liquid extraction that possess several advantages as compared to the other currently existing extractive techniques. Contrary to many of the current methods, which aim to heat the extractive system to raise efficiency and shorten extraction times, the Naviglio® extractor carries out the extraction at room or sub-room temperature, and uses an increase of pressure of the extracting liquid on the solid matrix, thus avoiding thermal stress on thermolabile substances [11]. Moreover, the employment of higher pressures allows a reduction in the extraction time and a concomitant improvement of the extraction process [11–14].

In this study, we used the Naviglio® extractor on *Cagnulari* grape marc to isolate valuable natural antioxidants from wine waste. Indeed, while wine processing residues are unusable for agricultural purposes, its content in polyphenol antioxidants constitutes one of the higher value options for wine byproducts exploitation, since they provide many health benefits [7,8]. As revealed by the FC assay performed on the extract, the Naviglio® extractor was able to recover 4.00 g/L ± 0.05 of total polyphenol. This finding indicates that valuable polyphenolic substances are still present in the wine waste, and that the green technology employed was able to extract them from the waste matrix. As compared to other extraction technologies, our data indicate that the Naviglio® extractor recovered a number of polyphenols, characteristic of the used matrix [30,31]. Indeed, the overlap of pomace extract (blue curve) and standard (red curve) chromatograms clearly shows the correspondence between two anthocyanin standard peaks and two species present in the extract (#1 and #2, Figure 1). MS analysis of the pre-HPLC extract confirmed the presence of several anthocyanins characteristics of the exploited matrix, including malvidin, peonidin-3-O-glucoside, malvidin-3-(6-acetyl)-glucoside, and M-3-G (Figure 2A). Moreover, the MS analysis of HPLC fraction 1 (#1) and 2 (#2) further confirmed the presence of the specific anthocyanins peonidin-3-O-glucoside and M-3-G respectively (Figure 2B,C). Interestingly, the extract chromatogram (Figure 1, blue curve) showed a considerably high abundance of malvidin-3-glucoside (#2), in agreement with previous findings [30–32].

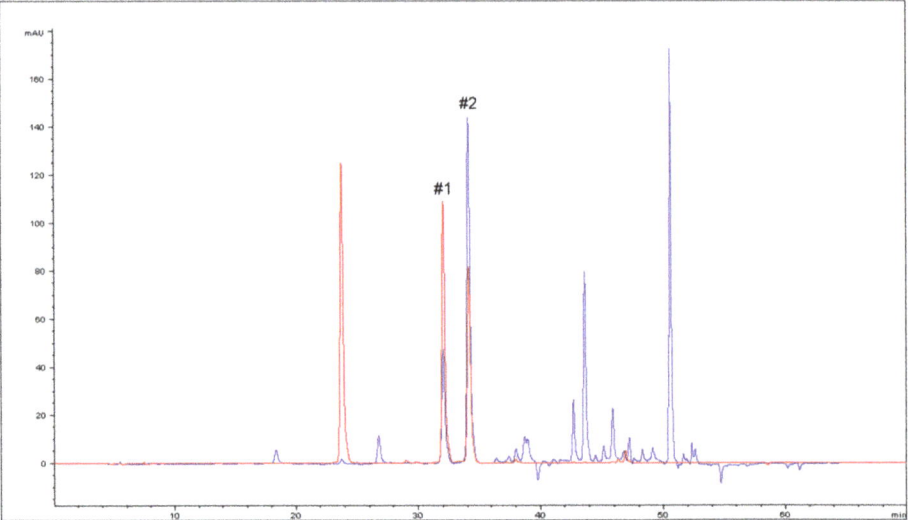

Figure 1. HPLC analysis. Overlapping of HPLC chromatograms obtained by anthocyanin standards (red curve) and pomace extract (blue curve), wavelength = 520 nm. #1 and #2 indicate the fractions collected and further analyzed by MS.

Within the different natural antioxidants, plant polyphenols are considered among the most important providers of health benefits, such as those related to the cardiovascular system [33]. In this context, red wine polyphenols are thought to be responsible for the cardiovascular benefits associated with the regular consumption of moderate amounts of wine [34,35]. M-3-G is one of the anthocyanins present in red wine responsible for the red pigmentation of red grapes and red wine [32]. While its antioxidant activity in vitro has been reported [36], as compared to the resveratrol, a natural red wine polyphenol, relatively few reports investigated its antioxidant activity and vasculoprotective effect in a vascular cell model. Indeed, although chemical tests to assess antioxidant activity are often used, the best approach to study the antioxidant activity/effect of a given compound would be directly in vivo or in a cellular model. An in vivo model, such as the cell, would provide the optimal environment for possible interaction (e.g., compound–cellular receptor, compound–cellular signal transduction) that would be missed in a chemical assay system.

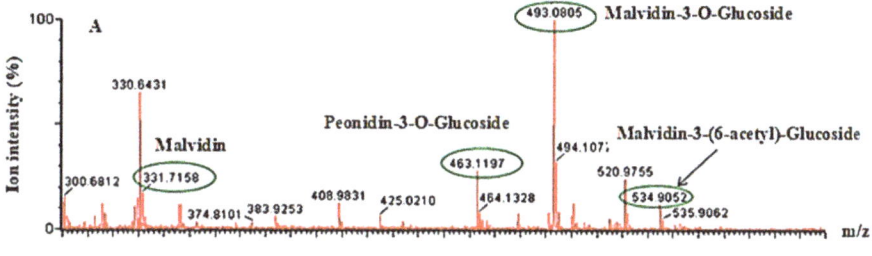
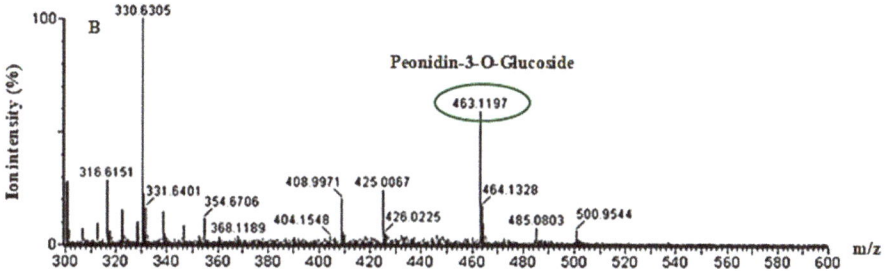
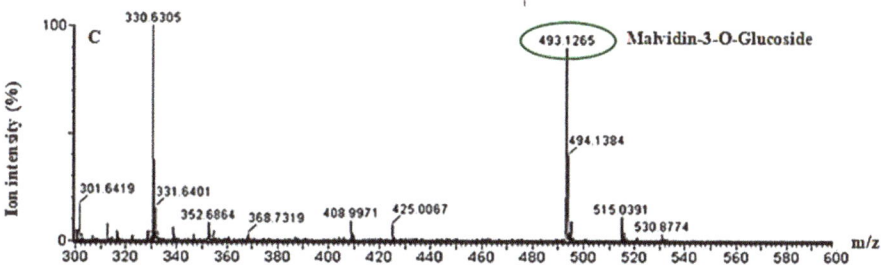

Figure 2. MALDI-TOF MS analysis. (**A**) Raw extract spectrum, confirming the presence of several anthocyanins, including malvidin, malvidin-3-O-glucoside, peodinin-3-O-glucoside, and malvidin-3-(6-acetyl)-glucoside. (**B**) Fraction 1 and (**C**) Fraction 2 spectra, confirming the presence of peodinin-3-O-glucoside and malvidin-3-O-glucoside, respectively.

The endothelium plays a pivotal role in cardiovascular homeostasis, and oxidative-induced endothelial cell (EC) injury is the key step in the onset and progression of CVD [18]. Therefore, the EC is a very useful model to investigate the potential effects of M-3-G on the vascular system. When tested on our cell vascular model, the extract obtained from the *Cagnulari* grape marc with the Naviglio Extractor® was safe. In fact, based on our previous experimentations with extracts from *Salvia desoleana* [25], we tested the pomace extract at concentrations of 0.1, 1, and 10 µg/mL without evidence of toxic effects on cultured cells (Figure 3A). Based on the high polyphenol content found in the grape marc extract, we sought to investigate whether it may counteract H_2O_2-elicited oxidative changes in our vascular models. Therefore, we pre-incubated the cells with the three different concentrations of the extract, and then we cultured them in the presence and absence of H_2O_2 to assess a potential antioxidant effect. Using the ROS fluorescent sensor H_2DCF-DA, the data derived from five pooled measurements were expressed as percentages of the untreated cells (CTRL) in Figure 3B. Exposure of the HUVEC cells to these increasing concentrations of the extract showed significant antioxidant effects with respect to the H_2O_2-treated cells (Figure 3B). Since oxidative stress is known to induce cell damage and even death, we sought to determine whether the observed antioxidant effect could be protective against the H_2O_2-induced oxidative damage. To this end, we pre-treated the cell with the indicated concentrations of extract and then we measured the cell viability by using the MTT assay both in oxidatively-stressed and -unstressed cells. Consistently with the observed antioxidant effect on H_2O_2-induced ROS generation, pre-treatment of cells with increasing doses of grape marc extract was able to significantly protect HUVECs from the oxidative cell death elicited by H_2O_2 (Figure 3C).

Due to the ever-growing production of waste by modern society, the environmental sustainability requirements related to waste treatment or disposal are becoming an issue of primary importance [3,4]. In this context, exploiting these residues to obtain valuable compounds by mean of green technologies may be the answer to this problem, both in terms of environmental sustainability and for potential profit. In some case, these residues can indeed be an alternative source for obtaining natural antioxidants, which are considered safer in comparison with synthetic antioxidants, largely used in the food industry with undesirable effects on the enzymes of human organs [7,8,37,38]. Hence, phenolic compounds can be considered added-value byproducts, which justifies their isolation from the industrial wastes [38]. Antioxidant and anti-inflammatory activities of anthocyanins have been extensively reported, therefore promoting studies concerning their extracts from different sources [4,39]. In this study, we used a green extraction technology (Naviglio®) to provide a proof of principle that wine industry wastes can be a rich resource of natural antioxidants.

As reported in the current study, the employed extraction technology was able to extract a remarkable amount (4.00 g/L ± 0.05) of phenolic compounds from the wine waste (*Cagnulari* Grape Marc). The performed chemical analysis revealed the Naviglio Extractor was able to recover specific anthocyanins, such as the malvidin, peonidin-3-O-glucoside, malvidin-3-(6-acetyl)-glucoside, and M-3-G, which are characteristic phenolic compounds of the exploited matrix. Tested on a cell vascular model, the Naviglio extract showed a strong antioxidant effect. Indeed, in H_2O_2-treated cells exposed to a low concentration of extract (1 µg/mL) the levels of ROS did not significantly differ from the one in control cells (CTRL), showing 53% more antioxidant effect as compared to cells treated with only H_2O_2 ($p = 0.0021$) (Figure 3B). At higher concentration (10 µg/mL), the extract showed an antioxidant effect that was 85% higher when compared to cells treated with only H_2O_2 ($p = 0.0001$). The observed dose-dependent antioxidant was paralleled to a protective effect of similar extent when cells were analyzed for H_2O_2-induced cell death in the presence of the different extract concentrations (Figure 3C). Noteworthy, contrary to what was observed for other natural antioxidants, such as resveratrol and coumaric acid for instance [22–24], this powerful antioxidant effect was free of any cytotoxicity or harmful effects on cells, even when treated with increasing concentrations of extract (Figure 3A), meaning that the extract does not affect the levels of intracellular ROS needed to finely control the cellular functions.

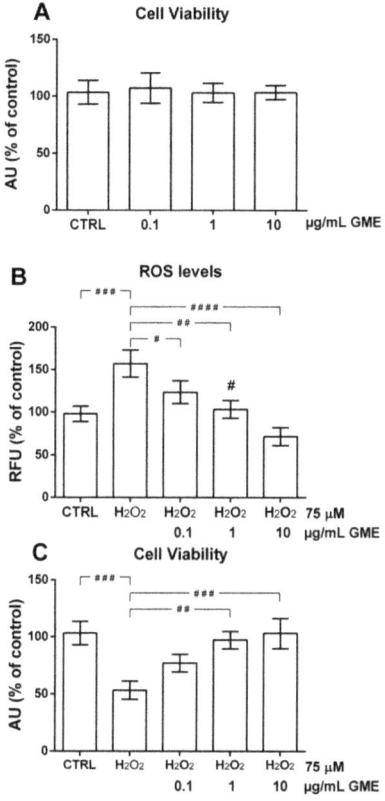

Figure 3. Effect of grape marc extracts on human umbilical vein endothelial cell (HUVEC) viability. (**A**) HUVECs were incubated for 20 h with the indicated concentrations of the extract, then cell viability was determined using the MTT assay, as reported in the materials and methods. Grape mark extract inhibits hydrogen peroxide (H_2O_2)-induced ROS generation in HUVECs. (**B**) HUVECs were exposed for 3 h to the indicated concentrations of grape marc extracts, and then incubated in the absence (CTRL) or presence of 75 µM H_2O_2. Fluorescence was measured, as reported, in the Materials and Methods. #, $p = 0.0428$; ##, $p = 0.0021$; ###, $p = 0.001$; ####, $p = 0.0001$. Grape mark extract inhibits hydrogen peroxide (H_2O_2)-induced oxidative cell death of HUVECs. (**C**) HUVECs were exposed for 3 h to the indicated concentrations of grape marc extracts and then incubate for 20 h in the absence (CTRL) or presence of 75 µM H_2O_2. Cell viability was assessed as reported in the materials and methods. Data are expressed as percentage of the control. CTRL, untreated cells; H_2O_2, hydrogen peroxide; GME, Grape marc extract. ##, $p = 0.0017$; ###, $p = 0.0006$.

4. Conclusions

Our results show that the grape pomace can be an important source of polyphenolic substances that provide antioxidant activity and vasculoprotective effect. The Naviglio® is a green extractive technology that does not make use of any solvent or thermal treatments, and is affordable compared to other conventional solvents or supercritical fluid phase extraction procedures. Our current data indicate that the green technology used to exploit the wine waste is capable of extracting antioxidants compounds that are characteristic of the employed grape pomace, namely anthocyanins. Considering that red grape is used in millions of tons in wine-producing countries, the polyphenolic compounds extracted from grape processing byproducts such as grape marc, seeds, or peels could be used as sources of natural antioxidants to be employed in different contexts. Ultimately, besides the "green aspect" related to the technology employed and the waste recycling, our proposed extraction process may be applied to other natural sources of polyphenols in various fruits, spices, and dried herbs, such as cocoa products, some berries, flaxseeds, and nuts (chestnut, hazelnut), and some vegetables, including olive and artichoke [40], which play an important role on cardiovascular protection. From this perspective, further studies need to be performed to investigate other polyphenol-rich byproducts, and to highlight their antioxidant and protective role in health and disease.

Author Contributions: Conceptualization, L.P., G.P.; Data Curation, A.M.P., A.C., R.G.; Funding Acquisition, L.P., G.P.; Investigation, A.M.P., G.B., A.C., R.G., D.P., M.C.P.; Methodology, A.C., D.P., M.C.P.; Project administration, L.P.; Resources, H.A.-S.; Supervision, H.Z., L.P., G.P.; Writing-Original Draft Preparation, A.M.P.; Writing-Review & Editing, G.B., H.Z., H.A.-S., D.P., M.C.P., L.P., G.K.N., G.P.; Authorship must be limited to those who have contributed substantially to the work reported.

Funding: This study was funded by the [Sardinia Region Government through Sardegna Ricerche Technology Park], grant number [Project Green Chemistry] and the [Qatar University], grant number [QUCG-CHS-2018\2019-1]. The article processing charge (APC) for the publication of this article was funded by the [Qatar National Library].

Conflicts of Interest: Authors declare no conflict of interest.

References

1. Arienzo, M.; Christen, E.W.; Quayle, W.C. Phytotoxicity testing of winery wastewater for constructed wetland treatment. *J. Hazard. Mater.* **2009**, *169*, 94–99. [CrossRef] [PubMed]
2. Bierhansl, L.; Conradi, L.C.; Treps, L.; Dewerchin, M.; Carmeliet, P. Central Role of Metabolism in Endothelial Cell Function and Vascular Disease. *Physiology (Bethesda)* **2017**, *32*, 126–140. [CrossRef] [PubMed]
3. Bustamante, M.A.; Moral, R.; Paredes, C.; Perez-Espinosa, A.; Moreno-Caselles, J.; Perez-Murcia, M.D. Agrochemical characterisation of the solid by-products and residues from the winery and distillery industry. *Waste Manag.* **2008**, *28*, 372–380. [CrossRef] [PubMed]
4. Cossu, A.; Posadino, A.M.; Giordo, R.; Emanueli, C.; Sanguinetti, A.M.; Piscopo, A.; Poiana, M.; Capobianco, G.; Piga, A.; Pintus, G. Apricot melanoidins prevent oxidative endothelial cell death by counteracting mitochondrial oxidation and membrane depolarization. *PLoS ONE* **2012**, *7*, e48817. [CrossRef] [PubMed]
5. Devesa-Rey, R.; Vecino, X.; Varela-Alende, J.; Barral, M.; Cruz, J.; Moldes, A. Valorization of winery waste vs. the costs of not recycling. *Waste Manag.* **2011**, *31*, 2327–2335. [CrossRef] [PubMed]
6. Faggion, H.; Beninca, C.; Naviglio, D.; Voll, F.A.P.; Zanoelo, E.F. Kinetics of Pressure Cycling Extraction of Solute from Leaves of Mate (*Ilex paraguariensis*) Dispersed in Water. *Chem. Eng. Commun.* **2017**, *204*, 406–413. [CrossRef]
7. Formato, A.; Gallo, M.; Ianniello, D.; Montesano, D.; Naviglio, D. Supercritical fluid extraction of alpha- and beta-acids from hops compared to cyclically pressurized solid-liquid extraction. *J. Supercrit. Fluids* **2013**, *84*, 113–120. [CrossRef]
8. Gallo, M.; Conte, E.; Naviglio, D. Analysis and Comparison of the Antioxidant Component of Portulaca Oleracea Leaves Obtained by Different Solid-Liquid Extraction Techniques. *Antioxidants (Basel)* **2017**, *6*, 64. [CrossRef] [PubMed]
9. Gallo, M.; Formato, A.; Ianniello, D.; Andolfi, A.; Conte, E.; Ciaravolo, M.; Varchetta, V.; Naviglio, D. Supercritical fluid extraction of pyrethrins from pyrethrum flowers (*Chrysanthemum cinerariifolium*) compared to traditional maceration and cyclic pressurization extraction. *J. Supercrit. Fluids* **2017**, *119*, 104–112. [CrossRef]
10. Gallo, M.; Vitulano, M.; Andolfi, A.; DellaGreca, M.; Conte, E.; Ciaravolo, M.; Naviglio, D. Rapid Solid-Liquid Dynamic Extraction (RSLDE): A New Rapid and Greener Method for Extracting Two Steviol Glycosides (Stevioside and Rebaudioside A) from Stevia Leaves. *Plant Foods Hum. Nutr.* **2017**, *72*, 141–148. [CrossRef] [PubMed]
11. Giordo, R.; Cossu, A.; Pasciu, V.; Hoa, P.T.; Posadino, A.M.; Pintus, G. Different redox response elicited by naturally occurring antioxidants in human endothelial cells. *Open Biochem. J.* **2013**, *7*, 44–53. [CrossRef] [PubMed]
12. Habauzit, V.; Morand, C. Evidence for a protective effect of polyphenols-containing foods on cardiovascular health: An update for clinicians. *Ther. Adv. Chronic Dis.* **2012**, *3*, 87–106. [CrossRef] [PubMed]

13. Incalza, M.A.; D'Oria, R.; Natalicchio, A.; Perrini, S.; Laviola, L.; Giorgino, F. Oxidative stress and reactive oxygen species in endothelial dysfunction associated with cardiovascular and metabolic diseases. *Vascul Pharmacol.* **2017**, *100*, 1–19. [CrossRef] [PubMed]
14. Kammerer, D.R.; Kammerer, J.; Valet, R.; Carle, R. Recovery of polyphenols from the by-products of plant food processing and application as valuable food ingredients. *Food Res. Int.* **2014**, *65*, 2–12. [CrossRef]
15. Leifert, W.R.; Abeywardena, M.Y. Cardioprotective actions of grape polyphenols. *Nutr. Res.* **2008**, *28*, 729–737. [CrossRef] [PubMed]
16. Lofrano, G.; Meric, S. A comprehensive approach to winery wastewater treatment: A review of the state-of-the-art. *Desalin. Water Treat.* **2016**, *57*, 3011–3028. [CrossRef]
17. Maddau, L.; Cabras, A.; Franceschini, A.; Linaldeddu, B.T.; Crobu, S.; Roggio, T.; Pagnozzi, D. Occurrence and characterization of peptaibols from Trichoderma citrinoviride, an endophytic fungus of cork oak, using electrospray ionization quadrupole time-of-flight mass spectrometry. *Microbiology* **2009**, *155*, 3371–3381. [CrossRef] [PubMed]
18. Manach, C.; Mazur, A.; Scalbert, A. Polyphenols and prevention of cardiovascular diseases. *Curr. Opin. Lipidol.* **2005**, *16*, 77–84. [CrossRef] [PubMed]
19. Mariani, A.; Pomarici, E.; Boatto, V. The international wine trade: Recent trends and critical issues. *Wine Econ. Policy* **2012**, *1*, 24–40. [CrossRef]
20. Mazza, G. Anthocyanins in Grapes and Grape Products. *Crit. Rev. Food Sci. Nutr.* **1995**, *35*, 341–371. [CrossRef] [PubMed]
21. Monrad, J.K.; Howard, L.R.; King, J.W.; Srinivas, K.; Mauromoustakos, A. Subcritical solvent extraction of anthocyanins from dried red grape pomace. *J. Agric. Food Chem.* **2010**, *58*, 2862–2868. [CrossRef] [PubMed]
22. Moure, A.; Cruz, J.M.; Franco, D.; Domínguez, J.M.; Sineiro, J.; Domínguez, H.; Núñez, M.A.J.; Parajó, J.C. Natural antioxidants from residual sources. *Food Chem.* **2001**, *72*, 145–171. [CrossRef]
23. Munoz-Gonzalez, C.; Rodriguez-Bencomo, J.J.; Martin-Alvarez, P.J.; Moreno-Arribas, M.V.; Pozo-Bayon, M.A. Recovery of Aromatic Aglycones from Grape Pomace Winemaking By-Products by Using Liquid-Liquid and Pressurized-Liquid Extraction. *Food Anal. Methods* **2014**, *7*, 47–57. [CrossRef]
24. Naviglio, D. Naviglio's principle and presentation of an innovative solid-liquid extraction technology: Extractor Naviglio (R). *Anal. Lett.* **2003**, *36*, 1647–1659. [CrossRef]
25. Naviglio, D.; Caruso, T.; Iannece, P.; Aragon, A.; Santini, A. Characterization of high purity lycopene from tomato wastes using a new pressurized extraction approach. *J. Agric. Food Chem.* **2008**, *56*, 6227–6231. [CrossRef] [PubMed]
26. Otero-Pareja, M.J.; Casas, L.; Fernández-Ponce, M.T.; Mantell, C.; Ossa, E.J. Green extraction of antioxidants from different varieties of red grape pomace. *Molecules* **2015**, *20*, 9686–9702. [CrossRef] [PubMed]
27. Pasciu, V.; Posadino, A.M.; Cossu, A.; Sanna, B.; Tadolini, B.; Gaspa, L.; Marchisio, A.; Dessole, S.; Capobianco, G.; Pintus, G. Akt Downregulation by Flavin Oxidase-Induced ROS Generation Mediates Dose-Dependent Endothelial Cell Damage Elicited by Natural Antioxidants. *Toxicol. Sci.* **2010**, *114*, 101–112. [CrossRef] [PubMed]
28. Pérez-Bibbins, B.; Torrado-Agrasar, A.; Salgado, J.; de Souza Oliveira, R.P.; Dominguez, J. Potential of lees from wine, beer and cider manufacturing as a source of economic nutrients: An overview. *Waste Manag.* **2015**, *40*, 72–81. [CrossRef] [PubMed]
29. Pintus, G.; Tadolini, B.; Posadino, A.M.; Sanna, B.; Debidda, M.; Carru, C.; Deiana, L.; Ventura, C. PKC/Raf/MEK/ERK signaling pathway modulates native-LDL-induced E2F-1 gene expression and endothelial cell proliferation. *Cardiovasc. Res.* **2003**, *59*, 934–944. [CrossRef]
30. Posadino, A.M.; Cossu, A.; Giordo, R.; Zinellu, A.; Sotgia, S.; Vardeu, A.; Hoa, P.T.; Deiana, L.; Carru, C.; Pintus, G. Coumaric acid induces mitochondrial damage and oxidative-mediated cell death of human endothelial cells. *Cardiovasc. Toxicol.* **2013**, *13*, 301–306. [CrossRef] [PubMed]
31. Posadino, A.M.; Cossu, A.; Giordo, R.; Zinellu, A.; Sotgia, S.; Vardeu, A.; Hoa, P.T.; Nguyen le, H.V.; Carru, C.; Pintus, G. Resveratrol alters human endothelial cells redox state and causes mitochondrial-dependent cell death. *Food Chem. Toxicol.* **2015**, *78*, 10–16. [CrossRef] [PubMed]
32. Posadino, A.M.; Phu, H.T.; Cossu, A.; Giordo, R.; Fois, M.; Thuan, D.T.B.; Piga, A.; Sotgia, S.; Zinellu, A.; Carru, C.; et al. Oxidative stress-induced Akt downregulation mediates green tea toxicity towards prostate cancer cells. *Toxicol. In Vitro* **2017**, *42*, 255–262. [CrossRef] [PubMed]

33. Posadino, A.M.; Porcu, M.C.; Marongiu, B.; Cossu, A.; Piras, A.; Porcedda, S.; Falconieri, D.; Cappuccinelli, R.; Biosa, G.; Pintus, G.; et al. Antioxidant activity of supercritical carbon dioxide extracts of Salvia desoleana on two human endothelial cell models. *Food Res. Int.* **2012**, *46*, 354–359. [CrossRef]
34. Putnik, P.; Bursać Kovačević, D.; Ježek, D.; Šustić, I.; Zorić, Z.; Dragović-Uzelac, V. High-pressure recovery of anthocyanins from grape skin pomace (*Vitis vinifera* cv. Teran) at moderate temperature. *J. Food Process. Preserv.* **2018**, *42*, e13342. [CrossRef]
35. Ruberto, G.; Renda, A.; Daquino, C.; Amico, V.; Spatafora, C.; Tringali, C.; De Tommasi, N. Polyphenol constituents and antioxidant activity of grape pomace extracts from five Sicilian red grape cultivars. *Food Chem.* **2007**, *100*, 203–210. [CrossRef]
36. Sanna, V.; Roggio, A.M.; Posadino, A.M.; Cossu, A.; Marceddu, S.; Mariani, A.; Alzari, V.; Uzzau, S.; Pintus, G.; Sechi, M. Novel docetaxel-loaded nanoparticles based on poly(lactide-co-caprolactone) and poly(lactide-co-glycolide-co-caprolactone) for prostate cancer treatment: Formulation, characterization, and cytotoxicity studies. *Nanoscale Res. Lett.* **2011**, *6*, 260. [CrossRef] [PubMed]
37. Shahidi, F. *Natural Antioxidants: Chemistry, Health Effects, and Applications*; The American Oil Chemists Society: Urbana, IL, USA, 1997.
38. Wallace, T.C. Anthocyanins in cardiovascular disease. *Adv. Nutr.* **2011**, *2*, 1–7. [CrossRef] [PubMed]
39. Wang, H.; Nair, M.G.; Strasburg, G.M.; Chang, Y.C.; Booren, A.M.; Gray, J.I.; DeWitt, D.L. Antioxidant and antiinflammatory activities of anthocyanins and their aglycon, cyanidin, from tart cherries. *J. Nat. Prod.* **1999**, *62*, 294–296. [CrossRef] [PubMed]
40. Yu, J.; Ahmedna, M. Functional components of grape pomace: Their composition, biological properties and potential applications. *Int. J. Food Sci. Technol.* **2013**, *48*, 221–237. [CrossRef]

Sample Availability: Upon specific and motivated request, samples of the extract used in this work are available from the authors.

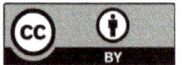 © 2018 by the authors. Licensee MDPI, Basel, Switzerland. This article is an open access article distributed under the terms and conditions of the Creative Commons Attribution (CC BY) license (http://creativecommons.org/licenses/by/4.0/).

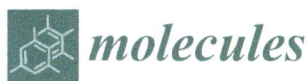

Article

Black Tea Samples Origin Discrimination Using Analytical Investigations of Secondary Metabolites, Antiradical Scavenging Activity and Chemometric Approach

Wojciech Koch [1], Wirginia Kukula-Koch [2,*] and Łukasz Komsta [3]

1   Chair and Department of Food and Nutrition, Medical University of Lublin, 4a Chodźki Str., 20-093 Lublin, Poland; kochw@interia.pl
2   Chair and Department of Pharmacognosy with Medicinal Plant Unit, Medical University of Lublin, 1 Chodźki Str., 20-093 Lublin, Poland
3   Department of Medicinal Chemistry, Medical University of Lublin, 4 Jaczewskiego str., 20-090 Lublin, Poland; lukasz.komsta@umlub.pl
*   Correspondence: virginia.kukula@gmail.com; Tel.: +48-81-448-7087

Received: 3 February 2018; Accepted: 24 February 2018; Published: 26 February 2018

Abstract: A comprehensive study on the composition and antioxidant properties of black tea samples with a chemometric approach was performed via LC-ESI-Q-TOF-MS, DPPH radical scavenging assay, and Folin–Ciocalteu assay (TPC). Marked differences between the teas from seven different countries (China, India, Iran, Japan, Kenya, Nepal, Sri Lanka) were shown. The Indian samples demonstrated the highest total catechin content (184.8 mg/100 mL), the largest TPC and DPPH scavenging potential (58.2 mg/100 mL and 84.5%, respectively). The applied principal component analysis (PCA) and ANOVA revealed several correlations between the level of catechins in tea infusions. EC (epicatechin), ECG (epicatechin gallate), EGC (epigallocatechin), and EGCG (epigallocatechin-3-gallate) content was not correlated with DPPH, gallic acid, and TPC; however, a strong correlation of EC and ECG between themselves and a negative correlation of these two catechins with EGCG and EGC was noted. Interestingly, simple catechins were not found to be responsible for antioxidant properties of the black teas. The samples collected in the higher altitudes were similar.

Keywords: *Camellia sinensis*; black teas; catechins; antioxidant activity; LC-ESI-Q-TOF-MS; principal component analysis

1. Introduction

Tea is the most widely consumed drink across the world after water [1]. Every day almost 2/3 of the world's population drinks 18–20 billion cups of tea, and its annual production is estimated to be around 2.9 million tons [2]. Tea ((*Camellia sinensis* (L.) Kuntze)) belongs to the family Theaceae and is cultivated in over 45 countries across all continents except North America and Antarctica. Naturally, the best growth of tea is observed in tropical and subtropical climate with sufficient amount of precipitation on a slightly acidic soil [3]. Tea as a food product is obtained from young leaves, immature buds, and delicate stalks of tea bush, which are then processed. Based on the type of production process, *C. sinensis*-based teas can be divided into black, green, Pu-erh, oolong, yellow, and white teas [4,5]. However, recent research demonstrated that *C. sinensis* also can be divided into seven types, namely green, yellow, white, oolong, black, aged pu-erh and ripened pu-erh [6]. Green tea is produced from freshly harvested leaves that are immediately steamed to prevent enzymatic inactivation [7]. Furthermore, white tea is a non-fermented product obtained from first, young leaves and buds harvested in spring before their maturation. It is considered as the most high quality type of tea. Only black tea is fully fermented, obtained under the influence of warm air and oxidizing enzymes [8].

The production of black tea accounts for over 75% of the whole tea production in the world; therefore, it can be considered as the most important kind of tea for general population. Although green tea is considered as the most active and rich in phenolic compounds, recent studies have shown that black tea also possesses very high biological activity [9,10]. It contains basic polyphenolic compounds called as catechins, such as (–)-gallocatechin (GC), (–)-epicatechingallate (ECG), (–)-epigallocatechin (EGC), (+)-catechin (C), (–)-epicatechin (EC), (–)-gallocatechingallate (GCG), and (–)-epigallocatechin-3-gallate (EGCG) and also complicated polymers such as theaflavins (TFs), thearubigins (TRs), and theabrownins (TBs) [11,12]. The latter complex phenolic compounds (TFs, TRs, and TBs) emerge in the fermentation process as a result of oxidation of catechins and their gallates during production of black teas [12]. Although black tea infusions are considered to have lower antioxidant activity compared to green tea, they possess a wide spectrum of biological properties because of high concentration of simple catechins as well as TFs or TBs [13]. Black tea infusions are known to have antimutagenic and anticarcinogenic properties. They accelerate cell apoptosis and prevent the occurrence of some cancer types (lungs, skin, liver, or pancreas) [10,14,15]. Furthermore, they are characterized by strong antibacterial, antiviral, and antifungal properties [9,16,17]. Recent studies suggest that black teas decrease blood pressure and cholesterol level, especially in patients with high fat intake, which can be crucial in the prevention of cardiovascular diseases [18,19].

Even though various pharmacological activities of black tea samples have been studied so far, no publications can be found, which report the actual compositional differences between the components of black tea in relation to their origin.

Black tea leaf infusions contain a large number of compounds of natural origin as well as some obtained during fermentation process; therefore, chemometric tools can complement the chromatographic analysis. The application of principal component analysis (PCA) allows treating a sample of tea as a point in a multivariate space. Furthermore, some intercorrelations between all constituents can be examined and all variability of content can be presented as several independent (orthogonal) trends. If the constituents are intercorrelated, the whole dataset can be compressed to several trends, explaining almost all information inside the results.

The majority of the studies published deal with the analysis of green tea catechins with chemometric approach helping to elucidate chromatographic analysis [11,20]. Therefore, the primary goal of this study was to quantitatively differentiate catechins' composition, which is scarcely published in the scientific literature, but also total phenolic content (TPC), and antioxidant activity of black tea infusions and classify them according to their origin. The secondary goal of this work was to find the correlations between the chemical composition of different origin tea samples using PCA-based methodology. To our knowledge, a study of this kind has not yet been performed so far, regarding the differences in catechin's concentration in the infusions, antioxidant activity of black teas from different regions and correlations between these parameters. Because the tea is not consumed as a fresh product but only as a beverage, all results were expressed per 100 mL of the infusion.

2. Results and Discussion

2.1. LC-ESI-Q-TOF-MS Determination of Catechin Content

The identification of these phenolic compounds was obtained in a tailored chromatographic method applying a gradient of two solvents: acetonitrile and water, with an addition of formic acid, which increases conductivity in the ESI (electrospray ionization) source, but also suppresses ionization of phenolic compounds during this chromatographic step and finally improves the peak shape.

The operation parameters of the applied mass spectrometer enabled the ionization of the constituents of tea infusions and the MS/MS fragmentation spectra (see Supplementary Information File, Figure S1). The selected capillary voltage and the fragmentor voltage provided a successful analysis of these compounds. The collision-induced dissociation (CID) energy values set at 10 and 20 V induced a sufficient and not excessive ions' fragmentation, which was more clear in case of the former value, because of a clearly visible deprotonated molecule in the spectrum. Negative ionization mode was found preferable for the analysis of these compounds, with the signal ca. 10 times more intensive than in the positive one.

All studied catechins were separated on the column with retention times: 4.8 min for GA, 10.9 min for EGC, 11.5 min for C, 12.3 min for EC, 12.8 for EGCG, 14.1 min for EGC. Based on that separation, we were able to do an analysis of the fragmentation patterns. The investigated gallates of catechins were found to lose the gallate group in the fragmentation process. Furthermore, the opening of the flavan-3-ol ring resulted in the presence of the following m/z value: 137 m/z.

The elaborated chromatographic method was checked for its suitability in the determination of GA and catechins. The linearity range for the studied compounds in the optimized method was within the range 0.03–12 µg/mL and the LOD and LOQ values were presented in Table 4 in the Materials and Methods chapter.

2.2. The Determination of Catechin Content in the Investigated Samples

Our study revealed the presence of four catechins (EGC, EGCG, ECG, and EC) and gallic acid (GA) in the tea infusions, which is in accordance with other investigations on tea catechins [6,21–23]. Moreover, Tao and co-workers suggest that EGCG, ECG, and EGC are the most abundant catechins in all three types of tea (green, black, and oolong), which together account for over 80% of all catechins [24]. Table 1 presents the average content of GA and catechins determined in the investigated black teas.

Only for teas cultivated in Nepal, (both regions), all catechins were determined in the extracts, however, the total concentration of all catechins and GA in these teas was not high. The sum of all five compounds was the highest in Indian teas because of a very high concentration of EGC (178 mg/100 mL of tea infusion), which was also the main catechin in all investigated teas. This is in agreement with our recent study, which proved EGC to be the main simple catechin in black tea infusions [25]. The second group of teas rich in catechins were those cultivated in Sri Lanka with a total concentration of 54.1 mg/100 mL of infusion. However, the sum of all investigated catechins in the Iranian samples was calculated as 10.5 mg/100 mL only, with an average concentration of EGC of 9.91 mg/100 mL. It was the only group of samples in which EGCG was not detected. ECG and EC were the catechins present in the lowest concentrations in all tested teas (far below 1 mg/100 mL). Furthermore, ECG was detected only in the Iranian and Nepal samples. EC was not detected in teas from China, India, and Sri Lanka.

According to Khokhar and co-workers, EGCG and EGC are the predominant catechins in black and green teas. They also suggest that the levels of (+)-catechin are below the detection limit, which is probably due to a very low concentration of (+)-catechin in the tea leaves and a strong degradation of this compound during the fermentation process of black tea [21].

Still, the application of a high-resolution mass spectrometry (HR-MS) in this study—and namely a Q-TOF-MS apparatus—resulted in the identification of catechin in the obtained extracts, although its quantity was scarce (<0.1 µg/100 mL). Therefore, catechin was not quantified in the investigated samples. The above cited findings of Khokhar and co-investigators [21] are consistent with our results; however, our data suggest that the primary catechin in black tea is not EGCG but EGC. This may be connected with the hydrolysis of EGCG during storage and the production process of black teas. In all black teas investigated in this study, the concentration of EGC was much higher compared to EGCG. These data are in agreement with previous studies suggesting that EGCG is the primary catechin in green and oolong tea, but not in the black tea [24].

Table 1. The content of gallic acid and catechins in the black teas.

Parameter	GA *	EGC *	EGCG *	ECG *	EC *	Total
		CH (China)				
Mean (mg/100 mL)	3.54	18.0	0.29	-	-	
SD	0.28	1.92	0.02			21.8
Range	3.37–4.11	15.7–20.6	0.18–0.45			
		JA (Japan)				
Mean (mg/100 mL)	2.66	14.2	0.15	-	0.04	
SD	0.43	1.77	0.04		0.01	17.1
Range	2.05–3.09	12.0–17.3	0.12–0.20		0.03–0.07	
		K (Kenya)				
Mean (mg/100 mL)	5.34	33.0	0.12	-	0.38	
SD	0.45	2.93	0.03		0.03	38.8
Range	4.69–5.94	29.9–36.5	0.08–0.15		0.35–0.41	
		I (India)				
Mean (mg/100 mL)	6.0	178.0	0.86	-	-	
SD	0.73	19.5	0.07			184.8
Range	5.28–7.11	156.8–205.2	0.64–0.96			
		S (Sri Lanka)				
Mean (mg/100 mL)	3.74	49.2	1.18	-	-	
SD	0.59	5.25	0.17			54.1
Range	3.29–4.53	41.2–58.4	0.84–1.32			
		IR (Iran)				
Mean (mg/100 mL)	0.27	9.91	-	0.08	0.28	
SD	0.01	1.16		0.007	0.05	10.5
Range	0.21–0.29	8.35–11.4		0.06–0.09	0.19–0.34	
		NH (Nepal)				
Mean (mg/100 mL)	3.68	25.5	0.05	0.36	0.51	
SD	0.35	4.18	0.009	0.04	0.08	30.1
Range	3.18–3.95	18.5–32.8	0.04–0.06	0.33–0.43	0.42–0.57	
		NM (Nepal)				
Mean (mg/100 mL)	9.42	33.9	0.06	0.12	0.57	
SD	1.74	4.01	0.02	0.022	0.08	44.1
Range	7.12–11.5	28.1–39.4	0.04–0.09	0.1–0.15	0.48–0.68	

* GA (gallic acid), EC (epicatechin), ECG (epicatechin gallate), EGC (epigallocatechin), and EGCG (epigallocatechin-3-gallate).

2.3. Antioxidant Activity Assessment and TPC in the Studied Samples

Not only green, but also black tea extracts possess strong antioxidant activity, which indicates that, not only simple catechins, but also TFs and TRs have high biological potential [23]. The review made by Wiseman and co-workers on antioxidants in tea suggests that green and black tea infusions have equally strong antioxidant activity [26]; however, according to Han and Chen, a comparison of relative inhibitory potency between simple catechins and TFs may be difficult to perform [27]. According to the previous findings, black tea infusions may be an important antioxidant-based food product in human nutrition.

Results of TPC and antiradical activity (Table 2) were in good agreement with chromatographic analysis of GA.

The teas cultivated in India were characterized by the highest phenolic content (expressed as GAE) and antioxidant activity. As it was previously described, these products contained the highest amounts of EGC, which was far above the concentrations determined in other investigated teas. High concentration of phenolics and high antiradical activity was also determined for teas from Nepal and Kenya. However, samples from China, Japan, and Iran used in this study were characterized by low antioxidant activity, which was well correlated with TPC and catechin content, which also were significantly lower compared to other teas. It should be strongly emphasized that not only simple catechins, but also condensed compounds such as TRs, TFs, and TBs, possessed a wide spectrum of biological properties, including antioxidant activity. Therefore, in this study, the Folin–Ciocalteu method was used, as a quick and simple tool for fast characterization of TPC content in black tea. Although this method is not specific, it could extend chromatographic data, especially for products with complex polyphenolic profile as black teas.

Table 2. Total phenolic content (TPC) and antiradical activity of selected black teas.

Tea	TPC * (mg/100 mL)	SD	Antiradical Activity (%)	SD	Trolox Equivalent (mM/L)	SD
CH (China)	17.5 [a]	1.73	33.6	3.19	1.74	0.18
JA (Japan)	28.4 [b]	2.62	35.6	5.28	1.85	0.16
K (Kenya)	49.9 [c]	5.12	75.6	8.80	2.55	0.22
I (India)	58.2 [c]	6.16	84.5	7.31	3.11	0.34
S (Sri Lanka)	33.8 [b]	4.28	54.8	7.70	1.97	0.21
IR (Iran)	20.2 [a]	3.11	31.8	4.20	1.51	0.14
NH (Nepal)	52.7 [c]	4.78	82.6	9.43	3.00	0.22
NM (Nepal)	44.0 [c]	5.05	73.4	8.48	2.38	0.23

* expressed as gallic acid equivalents; different letters by column are statistically significantly different at $p < 0.05$.

2.4. Chemometric Analysis of the Obtained Results

To investigate the dependences between determined compounds and sample properties, a scaled PCA was applied to the whole data matrix consisting of rows expressing the samples' type and columns containing their properties. The following seven variables were used: GA, EGC, EGCG, ECG, and EC content (all expressed in mg/100 mL), DPPH (%) and TPC (mg/100 mL).

Figure 1 presents the resulted scores and their corresponding loadings are placed in Figure 2.

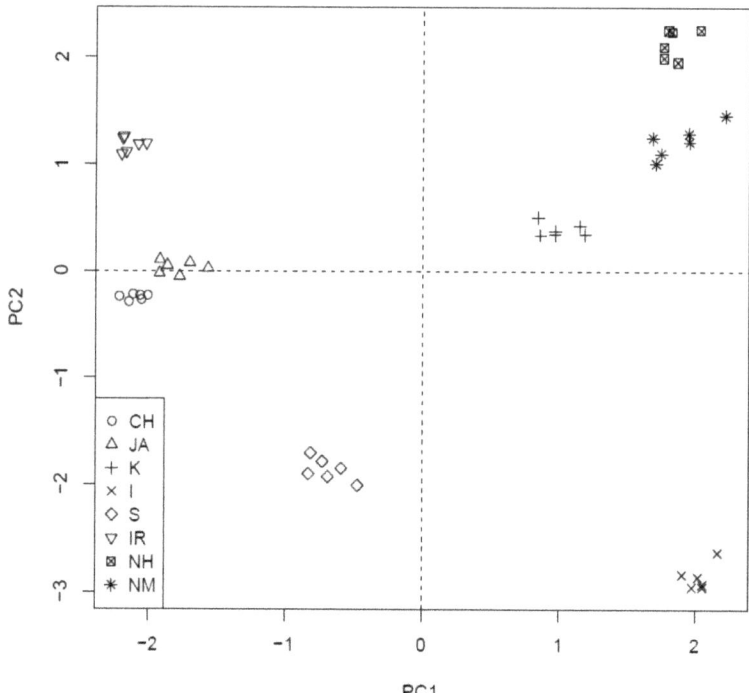

Figure 1. The scores of first two principal components of PCA analysis, explaining together 80% of information in the obtained dataset.

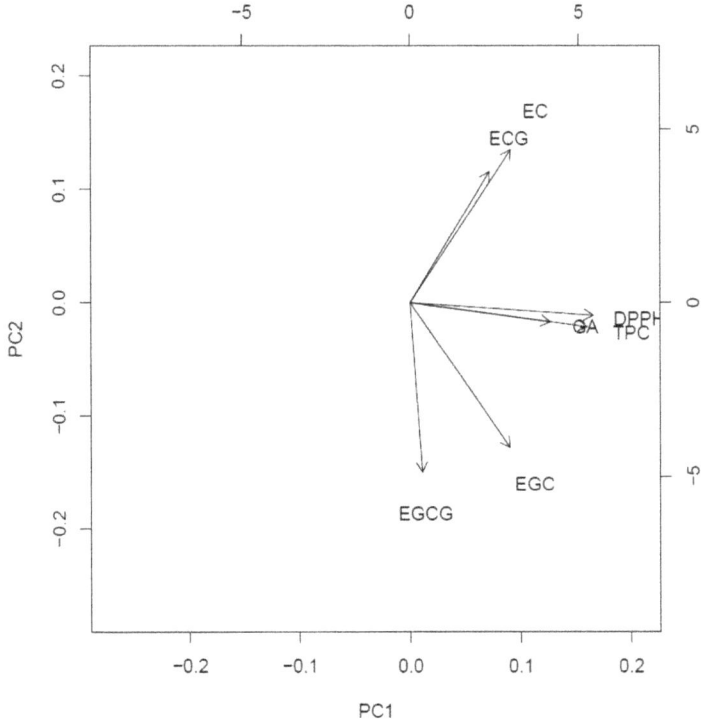

Figure 2. The loadings of first two components depicted on Figure 2. For explanations, see text.

The first principal component (PC1) explained the 45.2% of the total variance, connected with antioxidant activity. GA, TPC, and DPPH are strictly correlated with themselves; therefore, samples lying on the right side of score plot are characterized by the highest antioxidant activity (I, NM, and NH). The samples located on the left side (low PC1 value) are characterized by lowest antioxidant activity (CH, JA, and IR).

The second principal component (PC2) explains 35.3% of the samples' variance. It represents the (independent to PC1) trend, connected with changes in EC, ECG, EGC, and EGCG content. The loading vectors of these compounds are located along the vertical axis. It means that they are almost uncorrelated with DPPH, GA, and TPC. EC and ECG are strictly correlated between themselves and they are visibly negatively correlated with EGCG and EGC, which form the second intercorrelated group. Therefore, a high PC2 value means high content of ECG and EC with simultaneous low content of EGCG and EGC (for example IR, NM, and NH). The low PC2 value indicates an opposite behavior (high EGCG and EGC with low ECG and EC, for example I and S).

There is a high variability of the samples in the context of both of these trends and one can find samples representing all possible combinations of low/high PC1 and PC2 values. This fact results in the conclusion that catechins are almost not connected with antioxidant activity, whereas there is a visible correlation between their content in the investigated samples (including negative between two groups). Performed ANOVA corroborated significant differences between investigated parameters. This study confirmed that, because of the low catechin concentration in the black tea infusions (in comparison to the green tea), other compounds of phenolic nature are predominantly responsible for strong antioxidant properties of the black tea. For details, see Figures S2–S3 and Tables S1–S4 in the Supplementary Material.

The applied chemometric approach did not reveal any correlation between catechins' content, antioxidant activity, and geographical origin. Fraser and co-workers [28,29] reported potential use of secondary metabolites analysis using different chemometric tools in the origin discrimination of black teas. However, their results were based on different parameters and revealed significant differences between the tea type (black, oolong and green), rather than location. In the present study, an interesting trend was also observed—the teas cultivated in the countries or regions located on the higher altitude above the sea level (Nepal and Kenya) were characterized by different—similar to one another—catechin content and antiradical properties in comparison to other tested samples (see Figure 2). There are several studies on different groups of secondary metabolites, which shed light on the relationship between the content of natural products in the extracts and the altitude of the cultivars' occurrence [30,31]. Some of them have analyzed the levels of catechins in tea samples, but the conclusions drawn were inconclusive. Han and co-investigators [31] suggested that higher altitudes along with related lower temperatures induced the composition of Chinese green tea samples, leading to a better tea quality (based on the composition). However, Chen and co-workers [30], who investigated oolong tea samples, drew a conclusion that both the level of galloylation and the catechins' concentration were inversely correlated with the altitude of the cultivar.

Our studies preliminarily suggest the presence of a correlation between the parameters described above also in black tea samples.

3. Materials and Methods

3.1. Plant Material

The investigated tea samples were purchased in Poland in 2015–2016 from professional tea shops. In total, 48 black teas, cultivated in seven countries, were used in this study. For each tea origin, a special code was given, which was presented in Table 3. The origin of the teas was guaranteed be the seller, which specializes in the trade of high quality, premium teas. No blended products were used in this study. In general, 864 black tea samples were investigated (8 geographic regions × 6 representatives × 6 batch numbers purchased × 3 samples taken). Table 3 shows a summary of the information on the number of replicate tea samples from each sampling region.

Table 3. The geographical origin and number of samples for the investigated black teas.

Code	Sampling Region	Number (Representatives)
CH	China	6
JA	Japan	6
K	Kenya	6
IR	Iran	6
NH	Nepal (border of the Darjeeling region, altitude >2000 m)	6
NM	Nepal (altitude 1500–1700 m)	6
I	India (Assam region)	6
S	Sri Lanka	6

3.2. Reagents

Sodium carbonate (Na_2CO_3, reagent grade), citric acid and Folin–Ciocalteu reagent were obtained from Stanlab (Lublin, Poland). The solvents for liquid chromatography coupled with mass spectrometry (LC-MS) (spectrophotometric grade) such as acetonitrile, water, and formic acid were purchased from J.T. Baker (Center Valley, PA, USA). The standards of all investigated catechins (EGC, EGCG, ECG, and EC), trolox, gallic acid and 2,2-diphenyl-1-picrylhydrazyl (DPPH) radical were purchased from Sigma-Aldrich (St. Louis, MO, USA). All other reagents used for extraction were of reagent grade.

3.3. Preparation of Tea Infusions

Each tea was first milled using an electrical mill (type WZ-1, ZBPP, Poland). To prepare aqueous extracts, according to the conventional tea brewing method [32], about 1.0 g (±0.001 g) tea was weighed and transferred to a 250 mL conical flask. Then, brew was prepared using 100 mL of boiling distilled water and infused for 5 min under the watch glass cover. Because a moderate acid environment of the tea solution plays a pivotal role in the stability of the aqueous tea sample, after the extraction, pH of the extract was adjusted to 3.2 using citric acid, and it was diluted five times with distilled water (only for chromatographic determinations) [21,33]. Subsequently, the solution was filtered through 0.45 µm filter (Cronus, Gloucester, UK) prior to LC-MS analysis.

3.4. LC-MS Analysis

The LC-MS system consisted of an electrospray ionization with quadrupole time-of-flight mass spectrometer (ESI-Q-TOF-MS 6500 Series mass spectrometer, Agilent Technologies, Santa Clara, CA, USA) and an LC system (1200 Series, Agilent Technologies) composed of an autosampler, a degasser, a DAD detector, and a binary pump. The analytes were separated on a Zorbax RP 18 column from Agilent Technologies (size 150 mm × 2.1 mm, dp = 3.5 µm) at a flow rate of 0.2 mL min^{-1} and temperature of 20 °C. The mobile phase consisted of a combination of solvent A (0.1% formic acid in water) and solvent B (acetonitrile). The gradient elution was as follows: t = 0 min, 10% B; t = 10 min, 40% B; t = 12 min, 40% B; t = 17 min, 95% B; t = 20 min, 10% B; t = 22 min, 10% B and the stop time was set at 30 min. The photodiode array detector continuously recorded the absorbance from 190 to 600 nm, and later the chromatograms were analyzed at 254, 280, 320, and 365 nm. The mass spectra were simultaneously acquired using the ESI in the negative and positive ionization modes with a capillary voltage of 4.0 kV, fragmentation voltage of 130 V, skimmer voltage of 65 V, the gas and sheath gas (nitrogen) flows of 12 L/min each, and their temperatures of 350 and 400 °C, respectively. The mass spectra were recorded in the negative ionization mode, within the range of 40–1000 *m/z*, similarly to the MS/MS spectra, which were collected at two collision energy values of 10 and 20 V. Two highest signals obtained in MS1 spectra were selected for further fragmentation and after obtaining 1 spectrum of a given mass, the signal was excluded for the next 0.3 min. The nebulization pressure was 35.0 psig. The injection volume was set at 20 µL of each standard and tea infusion.

Identification of each catechin was performed based on their retention times and mass spectra (see Figure 1 and Figure S1 in the Supplementary Material). The standards of all catechins and gallic acid (GA) were used in the concentration of 2 mg/mL (stock solution) and then several dilutions (to calculate a 5-point calibration curve) were performed to plot the calibration curves for each compound and characterized the method (calculation of limit of detection (LOD), limit of quantitation (LOQ) values and linearity of the method). The LOQ was determined as a triple value of the obtained LOD, which was calculated as 3 times the signal-to-noise ratio (S/N ratio) value. Results of quantitative analysis of all obtained extracts were evaluated based on the calibration curve equations for each catechin and GA. Table 4 presents the parameters of the method and Figure 3 presents the chromatograms.

Table 4. Validation parameters obtained in the optimized LC-MS method (*n* = 5).

Compound	LOD (ng/mL)	LOQ (ng/mL)	R^2	Calibration Curve Equation	Linearity Range (µg/mL)
GA	0.52	1.56	0.9990	$y = 2.4 \times 10^7 x - 1.2 \times 10^6$	0.030–30
EGCG	0.46	1.38	0.9988	$y = 4.6 \times 10^7 x - 2.8 \times 10^6$	0.015–35
EGC	0.42	1.26	0.9987	$y = 6.0 \times 10^7 x - 1.9 \times 10^6$	0.020–40
ECG	0.42	1.26	0.9992	$y = 6.6 \times 10^7 x - 1.2 \times 10^6$	0.015–40
EC	0.42	1.26	0.9994	$y = 7.8 \times 10^8 x + 3.3 \times 10^5$	0.010–40

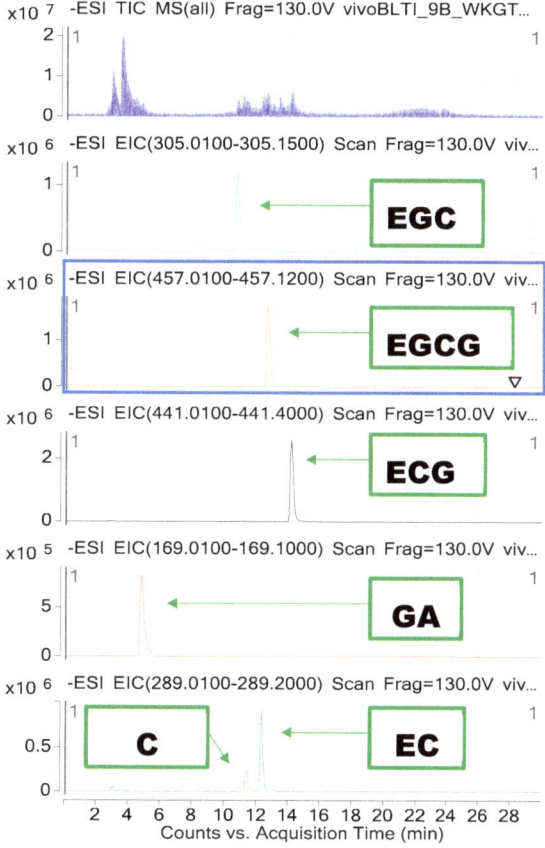

Figure 3. The EIC chromatograms of all catechins identified in the extracts in the negative mode of LC ESI-Q-TOF-MS analysis, identified based on the comparison with reference compounds.

3.5. Antioxidant Activity of Investigated Black Tea Infusions

3.5.1. TPC

The analysis was conducted according to the modified method with Folin–Ciocalteu reagent, described elsewhere [34]. Briefly, 0.5 mL of each tea infusion was mixed with 30 mL of distilled water and 2.5 mL of Folin–Ciocalteu reagent. After 1 min (but no longer than 8 min), 7.5 mL of 20% Na_2CO_3 solution was added and the mixture was filled with distilled water to a total volume of 50 mL. After 2 h, the absorbance was measured at a wavelength of 760 nm in 1-cm cuvettes using a UV-Vis spectrophotometer (Thermo Fisher Scientific Evolution, Waltham, MA, USA). The blank was prepared according to the same protocol, but, instead of a sample, 0.5 mL of distilled water was added to the reaction mixture. Moreover to avoid sample's inherent absorbance the corrections were made (absorbance of the solution of the sample, without Folin–Ciocalteu reagent). A calibration curve was performed with an aqueous solution of GA (50–500 mg/mL). For this purpose, instead of the analyte, 0.5 mL of aqueous solutions of GA was added at concentrations of 50, 100, 200, 300, and 500 mg/L. TPC in the studied samples was expressed as mg gallic acid equivalents (GAE) per 100 mL of tea infusions.

3.5.2. DPPH Test

DPPH test was performed according to a previously described procedure with minor modifications [35]. Black tea infusion (0.1 mL each) was mixed with 3.9 mL of DPPH solution (6×10^{-5} M in methanol). The absorbance at 515 nm was read at $t = 0$ (AC0) and in 5-min intervals until the reaction reached the plateu value (ACt). For all samples, it was no longer than 30 min. A control sample was prepared by replacing the addition of extract with methanol. The obtained results were expressed as a percentage of inhibition using the following equation: inhibition [%] = [($AC_0 - AC_t$)/AC_0] × 100. To express the antioxidant potential of the investigated samples, water solutions of Trolox in the concentration range 0–15 mM/L were prepared and used according to the same protocol.

3.5.3. Statistical Analysis

The statistical evaluation of data, including the principal component analysis (PCA), one-way Anova and post hoc tests, was performed in Statistica 12 program (StatSoft, Tulsa, OR, USA). The statistical significance of all obtained results was determined at $p < 0.05$.

4. Conclusions

This study shows a detailed analysis of catechins content, TPC analysis, and radical scavenging activity assessment of black tea samples from different cultivation areas: China, Japan, Kenya, Iran, Nepal, India, and Sri Lanka. EGC was the dominant catechin in the studied samples, followed by EGCG. The obtained results recorded by LC-ESI-Q-TOF-MS indicated the highest catechin content in black tea samples from India because of the presence of highest EGC concentration. These products were also characterized by the highest TPC and antiradical activity. However, the tea extracts from Iran were found to be the weakest source of catechins and the mildest antioxidant agent.

PCA revealed that the EC, ECG, EGC, and EGCG content was not correlated with DPPH, GA, and TPC content; however, a strong correlation of EC and ECG between themselves was noted and a negative correlation of these two catechins and EGCG and EGC was revealed. Despite the above findings, the chemometric analysis revealed that the level of simple catechins in the black tea infusions still did not influence the antioxidant potential of the samples. In case of black teas, the antioxidant properties must be strongly influenced by other compounds of phenolic nature, possibly the condensed phenolics, which occur in the fermentation process of *C. sinensis* leaves [13].

Finally, the chemometric approach did not reveal any correlation between the black tea composition and the place of origin. However, the influence of the altitude of the cultivar on the tea quality was observed in case of tea samples from Kenya and Nepal, whose composition and antioxidant potential were very similar.

Supplementary Materials: Supplementary materials are available online.

Acknowledgments: This study was supported from statutory funds of Medical University of Lublin No. DS 07/2017.

Author Contributions: W.K. designed the research, collected the samples, conducted the analysis and wrote the manuscript. W.K.-K. designed, optimized and conducted high-resolution mass spectrometry method for tea catechins and wrote some parts of the manuscript. Statistical elaboration of results was performed by Ł.K.

Conflicts of Interest: The authors declare no conflict of interest. The founding sponsors had no role in the design of the study; in the collection, analyses, or interpretation of data; in the writing of the manuscript, and in the decision to publish the results.

References

1. Mejia, E.G.; Ramirez-Mares, M.V.; Puangpraphant, S. Bioactive components of tea: Cancer, inflammation and behavior. *Brain Behav. Immun.* **2009**, *23*, 721–731. [CrossRef] [PubMed]
2. Marcos, A.; Fischer, A.; Rea, G.; Hill, S.J. Preliminary study using trace element concentrations and a chemometrics approach to determine geographical origin of tea. *J. Anal. Atom. Spectrom.* **1998**, *13*, 521–525. [CrossRef]
3. Barua, A. Romancing the Camellia assamica (Assam and the story of tea). *Assam Rev. Tea News.* **2008**, 18–27.
4. Almajano, P.; Carbo, R.; Lopez Jimenez, J.A.; Gordon, M.H. Antioxidant and antimicrobial activities of tea infusions. *Food Chem.* **2008**, *108*, 55–63. [CrossRef]
5. Zhang, H.F.; Shi, Y.P. Magnetic retrieval of chitosan: Extraction of bioactive constituents from green tea beverage samples. *Analyst* **2012**, *137*, 910–916. [CrossRef] [PubMed]
6. Yi, T.; Zhu, L.; Peng, W.-L.; He, X.-C.; Chen, H.-L.; Li, J.; Yu, T.; Liang, Z.-T.; Zhao, Z.-Z.; Chen, H.-B. Comparison of ten major constituents in seven types of processed tea using HPLC-DAD-MS followed by principal component and hierarchical cluster analysis. *LWT-Food Sci. Technol.* **2015**, *62*, 194–201. [CrossRef]
7. Chacko, S.M.; Thambi, P.T.; Kuttan, R.; Nishigaki, I. Beneficial effects of green tea: A literature review. *Chin. Med.* **2010**, *5*, 1–9. [CrossRef] [PubMed]
8. Hilal, Y.; Engelhardt, U. Characterisation of white tea—Comparison to green and black tea. *Journal für Verbraucherschutz und Lebensmittelsicherheit* **2007**, *2*, 414–421. [CrossRef]
9. Cantatore, A.; Randall, S.D.; Traum, D.; Adams, S.D. Effect of black tea extract on herpes simplex virus-1 infection of cultured cells. *BMC Complement. Altern. Med.* **2013**, *13*, 139–148. [CrossRef] [PubMed]
10. Pan, M.-H.; Lai, C.-S.; Wang, H.; Lo, C.-Y.; Ho, C.-T.; Li, S. Black tea in chemo-prevention of cancer and other human diseases. *Food Sci. Hum. Wellness* **2013**, *2*, 12–21. [CrossRef]
11. Pauli, E.D.; Scarminio, I.S.; Tauler, R. Analytical investigation of secondary metabolites extracted from *Camellia sinensis* L. leaves using a HPLC-DAD-ESI/MS data fusion strategy and chemometric methods. *J. Chemom.* **2016**, *30*, 75–85. [CrossRef]
12. Yao, L.H.; Jiang, Y.M.; Caffin, N.; D'Arcy, B.; Datta, N.; Liu, X.; Singanusong, R.; Xu, Y. Phenolic compounds in tea from Australian supermarkets. *Food Chem.* **2006**, *96*, 614–620. [CrossRef]
13. Halder, J.; Bhaduri, A.N. Protective role of black tea against oxidative damage of human red blood cells. *Biochem. Biophys. Res. Commun.* **1998**, *244*, 903–907. [CrossRef] [PubMed]
14. Lung, H.L.; Ip, W.Q.; Chen, Z.Y.; Mak, N.K.; Leung, K.N. Comparative study of the growth-inhibitory and apoptosis-inducing activities of black tea theaflavins and green tea catechin on murine myeloid leukemia cells. *Int. J. Mol. Med.* **2004**, *13*, 465–471. [CrossRef] [PubMed]
15. Yang, C.S.; Wang, X.; Lu, G.L.; Picinisch, S.C. Cancer prevention by tea: Animal studies, molecular mechanisms and human relevance. *Nat. Rev. Cancer* **2009**, *9*, 429–439. [CrossRef] [PubMed]
16. Ferrazzano, G.F.; Amatoa, I.; Ingenitoa, A.; De Natale, A.; Pollio, A. Anti-cariogenic effects of polyphenols from plant stimulant beverages (cocoa, coffee, tea). *Fitoterapia* **2009**, *80*, 255–262. [CrossRef] [PubMed]
17. Friedman, M. Overview of antibacterial, antitoxin, antiviral, and antifungal activities of tea flavonoids and teas. *Mol. Nutr. Food Res.* **2007**, *51*, 116–134. [CrossRef] [PubMed]
18. Bahorun, T.; Luximon-Ramma, A.; Neergheen-Bhujun, V.S.; Gunness, T.K.; Googoolye, K.; Auger, C.; Crozier, A.; Aruoma, O.I. The effect of black tea on risk factors of cardiovascular disease in a normal population. *Am. J. Prev. Med.* **2012**, *54*, 98–102. [CrossRef] [PubMed]
19. Grassi, D.; Draijer, R.; Desideri, G.; Mulder, T.; Ferri, C. Black tea lowers blood pressure and wave reflections in fasted and postprandial conditions in hypertensive patients: A randomised study. *Nutrients* **2015**, *7*, 1037–1051. [CrossRef] [PubMed]
20. Masoum, S.; Heshamt, S. Photoluminescence quantitative analysis of gallic acid and caffeine in green tea using multi-way chemometric approaches. *Iran. J. Math. Chem.* **2015**, *6*, 109–119.
21. Khokhar, S.; Venema, D.; Hollmann, P.C.H.; Dekker, M.; Jongen, W. A RP-HPLC method for the determination of tea catechins. *Cancer Lett.* **1997**, *114*, 171–172. [CrossRef]
22. Horie, H.; Kohata, K. Application of capillary electrophoresis to tea quality estimation. *J. Chromatogr. A* **1998**, *802*, 219–223. [CrossRef]
23. Wang, H.; Provan, G.J.; Helliwell, K. Tea flavonoids: Their functions, utilisation and analysis. *Trends Food Sci. Technol.* **2000**, *11*, 152–160. [CrossRef]

24. Tao, W.; Zhou, Z.; Zhao, B.; Wei, T. Simultaneous determination of eight catechins and four theaflavins in green, black and oolong tea using new HPLC–MS–MS method. *J. Pharm. Biomed. Anal.* **2016**, *131*, 140–145. [CrossRef] [PubMed]
25. Koch, W.; Kukula-Koch, W.; Głowniak, K. Catechin composition and antioxidant activity of black teas in relation to brewing time. *J. AOAC Int.* **2017**, *100*, 1694–1699. [CrossRef] [PubMed]
26. Wiseman, S.A.; Balentine, D.A.; Frei, B. Antioxidants in tea. *Crit. Rev. Food Sci. Nutr.* **1997**, *37*, 705–718. [CrossRef] [PubMed]
27. Han, C.; Chen, J. The screening of active anticarcinogenic ingredients' in tea. In Proceedings of the 95 International Tea-Quality-Human Health Symposium, Shanghai, China, 7–10 November 1995; pp. 39–41.
28. Fraser, K.; Harrison, S.J.; Lane, G.A.; Otter, D.E.; Hemar, Y.; Quek, S.-Y.; Rasmussen, S. Non-targeted analysis of tea by hydrophilic interaction liquid chromatography and high-resolution mass spectrometry. *Food Chem.* **2012**, *134*, 1616–1623. [CrossRef] [PubMed]
29. Fraser, K.; Lane, G.A.; Otter, D.E.; Hemar, Y.; Quek, S.-Y.; Harrison, S.J.; Rasmussen, S. Analysis of metabolic markers of tea origin by UHPLC and high-resolution mass spectrometry. *Food Res. Int.* **2013**, *53*, 827–853. [CrossRef]
30. Chen, G.H.; Yang, C.Y.; Lee, S.J.; Wu, C.C.; Tzen, J.T.C. Catechin content and the degree of its galloylation in oolong tea are inversely correlated with cultivation altitude. *J. Food Drug Anal.* **2014**, *22*, 303–309. [CrossRef] [PubMed]
31. Han, W.Y.; Huang, J.G.; Li, X.; Li, Z.X.; Ahhamed, G.J.; Yan, P.; Stepp, J.R. Altitudinal effects on the quality of green tea in east China: A climate change perspective. *Eur. Food Res. Technol.* **2017**, *243*, 323–330. [CrossRef]
32. Wang, H.; Helliwell, K. Determination of flavonols in green and black tea leaves and green tea infusions by high-performance liquid chromatography. *Food Res. Int.* **2001**, *34*, 223–227. [CrossRef]
33. Su, Y.L.; Leung, L.K.; Huang, Y.; Chen, Z.Y. Stability of tea theaflavins and catechins. *Food Chem.* **2003**, *83*, 183–195. [CrossRef]
34. Singleton, V.L.; Orthofer, R.; Lamuela-Raventos, R.M. Analysis of total phenols and other oxidation substrates and antioxidant by means of Folin–Ciocalteu reagent. *Methods Enzymol.* **1999**, *299*, 152–178. [CrossRef]
35. Koch, W.; Baj, T.; Kukula-Koch, W.; Marzec, Z. Dietary intake of specific phenolic compounds and their effect on the antioxidant activity of daily food rations. *Open Chem.* **2015**, *13*, 869–876. [CrossRef]

Sample Availability: Samples of the compounds are available from the authors.

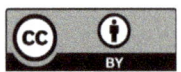

© 2018 by the authors. Licensee MDPI, Basel, Switzerland. This article is an open access article distributed under the terms and conditions of the Creative Commons Attribution (CC BY) license (http://creativecommons.org/licenses/by/4.0/).

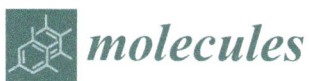

Article

Antioxidant Activity and Spectroscopic Characteristics of Extractable and Non-Extractable Phenolics from *Terminalia sericea* Burch. ex DC.

Chinedu Anokwuru [1], Muendi Sigidi [2], Marlaine Boukandou [2], Peter Tshisikhawe [3], Afsatou Traore [2,*] and Natasha Potgieter [4]

1. Chemistry Department, University of Venda, Private Bag X5050, 0950 Thohoyandou, South Africa; anokwuruchi@gmail.com
2. Microbiology Department, University of Venda, Private Bag X5050, 0950 Thohoyandou, South Africa; Muedi.sigidi@univen.ac.za (M.S.); bouk_marlaine@yahoo.fr (M.B.)
3. Botany Department, University of Venda, Private Bag X5050, 0950 Thohoyandou, South Africa; peter.tshisikhawe@univen.ac.za
4. School of Mathematical and Natural Sciences, University of Venda, Private Bag X5050, 0950 Thohoyandou, South Africa; natasha.potgieter@univen.ac.za
* Correspondence: afsatou.traore@univen.ac.za; Tel.: +27-15-962-8474; Fax: +27-15-962-8002

Received: 30 April 2018; Accepted: 24 May 2018; Published: 29 May 2018

Abstract: The aim of this study was to determine the antioxidant activity of the extractable and non-extractable phenolics of *Terminalia. Sericea* Burch. Ex DC. Free, ester bound, ether or glycoside bound and insoluble phenolics were extracted from the fruit, leaves, stem, and root samples. Follin Ciocalteu was used to estimate the phenolic content while DPPH (2,2-diphenyl-1-picrylhydrazyl) assay was used to determine the antioxidant activity. The data obtained were subjected to multivariate analysis for relationships. The result indicated that the highest average total phenolic contents and antioxidant activities were found in the free (14.8 mgGAE/g; IC_{50} 6.8 µg/mL) and ester bound (15.1 mgGAE/g; IC_{50} 6.4 µg/mL) extractable phenolics. There was a strong negative correlation between TPC and DPPH ($r = -0.828$). Agglomerative hierarchical clustering revealed three clusters. Cluster one contained the insoluble and glycoside phenolics while cluster 2 contained only free phenolic acid of the root. The third cluster was predominantly free and ester bound phenolic extracts. The principal component analysis score plot indicated two major clusters with factor 1 (F1) explaining 61% of the variation. The nuclear magnetic resonance spectroscopy spectra indicated that gallic acid and resveratrol are the major phenolic compounds present in the root. This study has demonstrated that extractable phenolics contributed more to the antioxidant activities compared to the non-extractables.

Keywords: extractable; non-extractable; antioxidant activity; agglomerative hierarchical clustering; principal component analysis; multivariate analysis; nuclear magnetic spectroscopy

1. Introduction

Accumulation of reactive oxygen and nitrogen species during oxidative metabolic processes can result in diseases such as diabetes, aging, inflammation, cardiovascular, neurodegenerative, and brain dysfunction [1–3]. Antioxidants are molecules that prevent oxidative damage caused by reactive species through scavenging free radicals, inhibiting lipid perodixation, and metal chelation [1,4]. Synthetic antioxidants such as butylatedhydroxytoluene (BHT), butylatedhydroxyanisole (BHA), and propylgallate (PG) are commercially used to preserve food by increasing the shelf-life through the inhibition of lipid peroxidation [4–6]. However, studies have revealed that synthetic antioxidants are toxic and carcinogenic, leading to the search for alternative sources of antioxidants from the natural origin [7].

Food and medicinal plants have been identified as rich natural sources of antioxidants [8]. Phenolics are secondary metabolites in plants and are known as major sources of antioxidants [9,10]. They protect plants against UV radiation, oxidative stress, and microbial infections [11–14]. The health benefits of phenolics have been ascribed to their pharmacological potentials such as anti-carcinogenic, anti-inflammatory, and anti-microbial [15]. Phenolics are good antioxidants because of their ability to scavenge free radicals, reactive oxygen and nitrogen species, and metal chelation [16]. They are generally classified as phenols, polyphenols, stilbenes, xanthones, and coumarins [17]. Phenolic acids are further classified as hydroxybenzoic acid and hydroxycinnamic acid while flavonoids are classified as flavones and their glycosides, catechins, flavonones, isoflavonoids, flavonols, anthocyanins, flavan-3-ols and proanthocyanidins flavonols, anthocyanins, flavan-3-ols, and proanthocyanidins. Tannins are either hydrolyzable or condensed [13,18].

Phenolics exist as free, soluble conjugates and in insoluble forms [19]. Conjugated soluble phenolics are bound to soluble low molecular mass molecules (carbohydrates, proteins, lipids) by either esterification at the carboxylic moiety or etherification at the hydroxyl group [20–22]. Insoluble phenolics are usually covalently bound to polymers such as polysaccharides and lignins through an ester linkage and are only released from the matrix through acid, alkaline, or enzyme hydrolysis [23,24]. In humans, insoluble phenolics are released from the matrix in the colon during the fermentation of the ingested material. The release of these phenolics has been identified as beneficial against colon cancer [25]. Free and conjugated phenolics are known as extractable phenolics while bound or insoluble phenolics are known as non-extractable [26]. Non-extractable or insoluble phenolics usually remain in the matrix of the residue after the extraction of soluble phenolics with aqueous alcohol [27,28]. Quantification of phenolics using only extractable phenolics results in the underestimation of the total phenolic content and antioxidant activity of the plant material [29]. It is therefore important to consider the contribution of the insoluble phenolics to the antioxidant activities of a plant material.

Terminalia sericea Burch. ex DC. (Combretaceae) is a medicinal plant commonly found in the savannah woodlands of eastern, central, and southern Africa. [30]. The fruit, leaf, stem, or root have been used for the treatment of diabetes, diarrhea, venereal disease, and tuberculosis [31]. Decoction and infusion are common methods of herbal preparation for oral administration [32]. The Vhavenda people mix the root infusion in preparation of the baby's soft porridge which helps in preventing diarrhea and dysentery [33,34]. Infusion or decoction prepared from *T. sericea* fruit, leaf, stem, or root is used to treat infectious wounds, diarrhea, eye infection, hypertension, fever, pneumonia, infertility, menorrhagia, stomach ache, cough, and gonorrhea [33,35]. Aqueous or organic extracts of *T. sericea* root, stem or leaf have been reported to possess antibacterial, antidiabetic, anti-HIV, anti-inflammatory, and anti-mycobacterial activities [31]. The crude extract of the root has been reported to be toxic to Monkey kidneys or Vero cells [36]. Previous studies [37–39] on the antioxidant activities of *T. sericea* have been limited to extractable antioxidants. Lupeol, inseparable mixtures of epicatechin-catechin and epigallocatechin-gallocatechin have been identified as antioxidant constituents of the acetone extract of stem bark [38]. There is, however, no available report on the estimation of the antioxidant activities of the non-extractable phenolics. It is therefore important to evaluate the antioxidant activities of the non-extractable phenolics to avoid underestimation of the antioxidant capacity. Several studies have been conducted on the quantification and antioxidant properties of extractable and non-extractable phenolics in fruits, vegetables, and cereals [40,41] compared to non-food medicinal plants. The aim of this study, therefore, is to evaluate the antioxidant activities of the extractable and non-extractable phenolics of *T. sericea*.

2. Results and Discussion

2.1. Extraction Yield

The result of the extraction yield is illustrated in Figure 1. Aqueous ethanol was used as the extracting solvent for extractable phenolic, so as to increase the extraction of very polar phenolics [42]. In general, the highest yield was found in the free phenolic root extract while the least yield was found in the insoluble phenolic root extract. Other studies have indicated that extractable (soluble) phenolics contain higher yields compared to non-extractable or bound phenolics [21,43], soluble or extractable phenolics have higher yields than bound or non-extractable phenolics. The root had the highest free and ester bound phenolic extract yield while the leaves had the highest ether bound phenolic extract yield and the stem had the highest insoluble bound phenolic extract yield. This result has indicated that there are more extractable phenolics in the root and leaf compared to the fruit and stem. However, the stem contained more non-extractable phenolics compared to the fruit, leaf, and root. While free phenolic acids contributed more to the extractable phenolics in the root, ether bound phenolics contributed more to the extractable phenolics in the leaf.

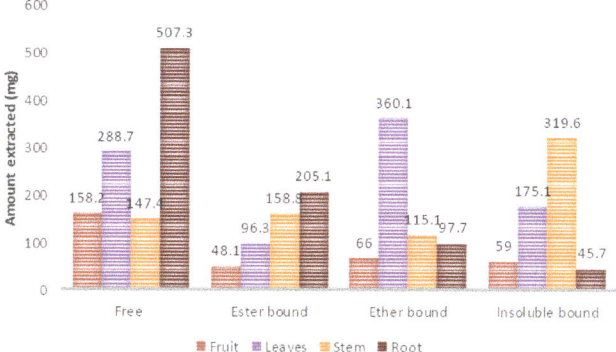

Figure 1. The extraction yield of extractable and non-extractable phenolics in the organs of *T. sericea*.

2.2. Total Phenolic Content

The result of the total phenolic content of the extractable and non-extractable phenolics is presented in Table 1. The highest TPC was found in the ester bound phenolic extract of the leaves (15.69 ± 0.04 mg GAE/g) and the root (15.62 ± 0.04 mg GAE/g) while the least TPC was found in the insoluble bound phenolic extract of the fruit (5.34 ± 0.02 mg GAE/g). In the fruit, the free and ether bound phenolics displayed the highest TPC, while the ester bound phenolics contained the highest TPC in the leaves. The free and ester bound phenolics contained the highest TPC in both stem and root. Considering the distribution of the TPC in the organs, the stem and the root displayed the highest free phenolics while the root and leaves displayed the highest ester bound phenolics.

Table 1. The total phenolic contents (mg GAE/g) of extractable and non-extractable pehnolics in *T. sericea*.

Organs	Free	Ester Bound	Ether Bound	Insoluble Bound	Average
Fruit	14.30 ± 0.02 [a]	13.87 ± 0.13 [c]	14.25 ± 0.05 [a]	5.34 ± 0.02 [g]	11.94
Leaves	14.81 ± 0.13 [a]	15.69 ± 0.04 [b]	11.17 ± 0.12 [e]	11.60 ± 0.12 [e]	13.32
Stem	15.12 ± 0.01 [b]	15.24 ± 0.05 [b]	14.03 ± 0.08 [a]	11.62 ± 0.02 [e]	14.00
Root	15.12 ± 0.07 [b]	15.62 ± 0.04 [b]	12.12 ± 0.14 [d]	10.38 ± 0.04 [f]	13.31
Average	14.84	15.11	12.89	9.74	

The values in each column or row with different alphabetical letters are significantly different at $p < 0.05$.

In the ether bound phenolics, the fruit and stem contained the highest total phenolic content while the leaves and the stem displayed the highest total phenolic content in the insoluble bound phenolics. The ester bound phenolics contained the highest average TPC (15.11 mgGAE/g) while the least average TPC was found in the insoluble bound (9.74 mgGAE/g). Although the stem contained the highest TPC (14 mgGAE/g), the actual difference between the TPC of the organs was 1–2 mgGAE/g. This study has demonstrated that the total phenolic content in the extractable phenolics was higher than non-extractable phenolics. Furthermore, the stem contained the highest average total phenolic content (14 mgGAE/g). It also demonstrated that free and ester bound phenolics contained more total phenolic content compared to the ether and insoluble bound phenolics. This study correlates to the study done by Nayaka et al. [44], which indicated that swallow root free phenolics contained higher phenolic compounds compared to the insoluble phenolic extract. The study by Kumar et al. [45] also indicated higher free phenolic content than the bound phenolics in *Emlica officinalis* and *Curcuma longa*. Gallic acid and tannic acid were found to be the major phenolics in both free and bound phenolics of *E. officinalis*. Curcumin was the major phenolic found in the free phenolics of *C. longa* while proto-catechuic acid and ferulic acid were the main phenolics in the bound phenolics. However, the study by Singh et al. [21] indicated that insoluble phenolics contained more total phenolic content in *Moringa oleifera* seed flour compared to the soluble phenolics. Gallic acid was found to be the main phenolic in the soluble phenolics while catechin and epicatechin were found to be the major phenolics in the insoluble phenolics in *M. oleifera*. In another study [46], the TPC of non-extractable phenolics was higher than the extractable phenolics of Cashew apple. The non-extractable phenolic of Mandrin waste has been reported to contain higher TPC compared to the extractable phenolics [47].

2.3. Antioxidant Activities

The result of the antioxidant activities of the soluble and insoluble extracts is presented in Table 2. The free and insoluble phenolics of the fruit displayed the highest (3.13 ± 0.75 µg/mL) and the lowest (235 ± 6.69 µg/mL) antioxidant activities, respectively. In the fruit, the free phenolics displayed the highest antioxidant activity while the ester bound phenolics (4.58 ± 0.71 µg/mL) displayed the highest antioxidant activity in the leaves. The free phenolics (8.78 ± 0.57 µg/mL) displayed the highest antioxidant activity in the stem but was not significantly different ($p > 0.05$) from the ester bound phenolics (9.32 ± 0.42 µg/mL). In the root, the ester bound phenolics displayed the highest antioxidant activities (4.89 ± 0.34 µg/mL). Considering the distribution of the antioxidants in the organs, the free phenolics of the fruit and leaves displayed higher antioxidant activity ($p < 0.05$) compared to the stem and root. The ester bound phenolics of the fruit, leaves, and root displayed higher antioxidant activities ($p < 0.05$) compared to the stem. In the glycoside or ether bound phenolics, the stem displayed the highest antioxidant while the leaves displayed the highest antioxidant activity in the insoluble phenolics. The ester bound phenolics displayed the best antioxidant activity with an average IC_{50} value of 6.4 µg/mL while the stem displayed the best antioxidant activity with the IC_{50} value of 13.2 µg/mL.

Table 2. The antioxidant activity (IC_{50} µg/mL) of free and bound phenolics in the organs of *T. sericea*.

Organs	Free	Ester Bound	Glycoside Bound	Insoluble Bound	Average
Fruit	3.13 ± 0.75 [a]	6.91 ± 0.75 [a]	12.6 ± 0.2 [c]	235 ± 7 [g]	64.4
Leaves	6.44 ± 0.81 [a]	4.58 ± 0.71 [a]	34.2 ± 1.6 [d]	15.4 ± 1.3 [e]	15.2
Stem	8.78 ± 0.57 [b]	9.32 ± 0.42 [b]	17 ± 0.7 [e]	17.8 ± 0.8 [e]	13.2
Root	8.99 ± 0.53 [b]	4.89 ± 0.34 [a]	25.3 ± 0.6 [f]	23.1 ± 0.5 [f]	15.6
Average	6.8	6.4	22.2	72.8	
Gallic acid					5.5 ± 0.1

The values in each column or row with different alphabetical letters are significantly different at $p < 0.05$.

This study has indicated that extractable phenolics, especially free and ester bound phenolics, possess higher antioxidant activities compared to the insoluble phenolics. This study also demonstrated that the stem contained more antioxidant compounds compared to the fruit, leaves, and root. In a previous study [39], the crude extracts of *T. sericea* stem displayed higher antioxidant activity compared to the leaves and the root. The ester bound extractable phenolics displayed the highest average antioxidant activity compared to the free, glycoside bound extractable phenolics and non-extractable (insoluble) phenolics. In general, the extractable phenolics (free, ester, and glycoside) displayed higher antioxidant activities compared to the non-extractable phenolics. The higher antioxidant activity in the extractable phenolics could be due to the higher total phenolics compared to the non-extractable (insoluble) phenolics. This result corresponds to the findings of Nayaka et al. [44], in which the conjugated phenolics of *Decalepis hamiltonii* root displayed higher antioxidant activities compared to the insoluble phenolic extract. However, other studies have indicated that insoluble bound phenolics display higher antioxidant activities in fruits, vegetables, and cereals [19]. There is no available literature of any report of antioxidant activities of extractable and non-extractable phenolics from genus *Terminalia*.

2.4. Multivariate Analysis

2.4.1. Agglomerative Hierarchical Clustering (AHC) Analysis

Agglomerative hierarchical clustering is a multivariate analytical tool used to cluster samples based on dissimilar characteristics and then displayed as a dendrogram [48,49]. The dendrogram (Figure 2) was constructed by Euclidean Pythagorean distance dissimilarities with Ward's Method of linkage [50,51]. Dotted lines represent automatic (entropy) truncation [49].

In this study, extractable phenolics include free, ester bound, and ether or glycoside bound phenolic acids while non-extractable phenolics are also known as insoluble phenolic acids. Ether bound extractable phenolics are also designated glycoside phenolics.

The dendrogram constructed indicated three clusters, indicating the dissimilarities in the extractable and non-extractable phenolics in the fruit, leaf, stem, and root of *T. sericea*. Cluster 1 consists of Leaf insoluble phenolic acid (LIPA), stem insoluble phenolic acid (SIPA), root insoluble phenolic acid (RIPA), leaf glycoside phenolic acid (LGPA), and root glycoside phenolic acid (RGPA). The second cluster consists only of root free phenolic acids (RFPA). The third cluster consists of fruit ester phenolic acid (FEPA), leaf ester phenolic acid (LEPA), stem ester phenolic acid (SEPA), root ester phenolic acid (REPA), fruit free phenolic acid (FFPA), leaf free phenolic acid (LFPA), stem free phenolic acid (SFPA), fruit glycoside phenolic acid (FGPA), and stem glycoside phenolic acid (SGPA). The sample FIPA (fruit insoluble phenolic acid) was removed from the plot due to the high IC_{50} value (235 µg/mL), making it an outlier compared to the values of the other samples. The dendogram clearly indicates that the glycoside bound extractable and non-extractable (insoluble) phenolics are similar and different from the phenolics found in the free and ester bound phenolic extracts. The widest variety was observed between LGPA in cluster 1 and SEPA in cluster 3. Although FGPA and SGPA are found in cluster 3, they are also found in the same sub-cluster, indicating similarities in their phenolics. The clustering of RFPA alone in cluster 2 may be due to the high extract yield and total phenolic content. This result has indicated similarities between glycoside bound extractables and non-extractable phenolics, and dissimilarities with free and ester bound extractable phenolics.

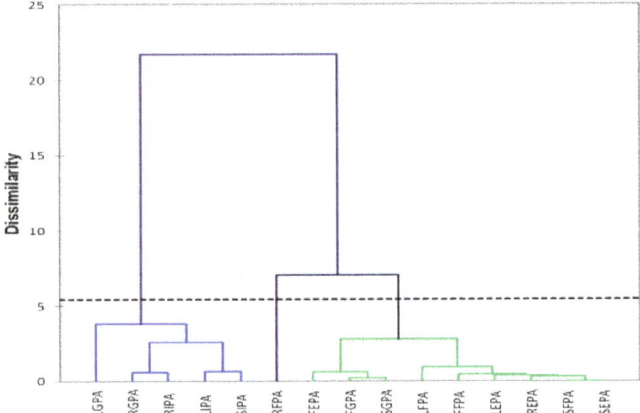

Figure 2. The dendrogram of extractable and non-extractable phenolics in the fruit, leaves, stem, and root of *T. sericea*.

2.4.2. Principal Component Analysis

The Principal Component Analysis is an unsupervised method used to identify the patterns and grouping within a data set based on the highest variation within the data [52]. The scree plot (Figure 3) presented 3 factors, however, only F1 and F2 were significant to explain 96% of the variations. A biplot illustrating the PCA correlation and score scatter plot is presented in Figure 4.

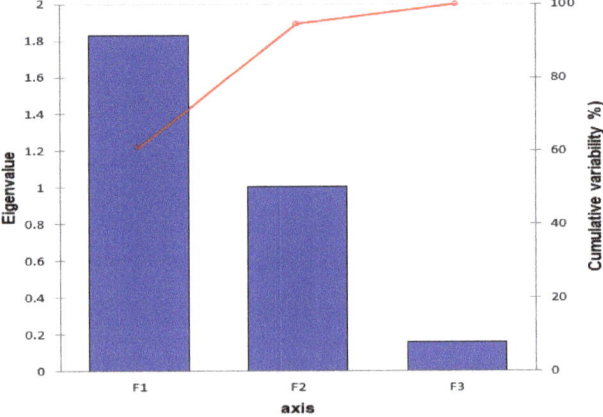

Figure 3. The scree plot indicating the number of significant factors explaining the variations. F1–3: factors 1–3.

There was no correlation (Table 3) between extraction yield and TPC ($r = 0.034$), and between extraction yield and DPPH ($r = 0.097$). However, there was a strong negative correlation between TPC and DPPH ($r = -0.828$).

Table 3. The correlation analysis between parameters and *T. sericea* phenolic acid extracts.

Parameters	YIELD	TPC	DPPH
YIELD	1	0.034	0.097
TPC	0.034	1	−0.828
DPPH	0.097	−0.828	1

TPC: total phenolic content; DPPH: 2,2-diphenyl-1-picrylhydrazyl.

About 61% of the variation in the samples was explained by factor 1 (principal component PC1) while 34% of the variation was explained by factor 2. The scatter plot revealed that the insoluble phenolics and glycosides are found in positive F1 (cluster 1) free and ester bound phenolics are found in the negative F1 (cluster 2). The samples found along the positive F1 have high IC_{50} indicating low antioxidant activities. Although FGPA is found in negative F1, it is closer to the center. This further suggests that glycosides have lower antioxidant activities. This indicates that glycosides and insoluble phenolics are poor antioxidants. The result of the antioxidant activities (Table 2) indicated that all the insoluble and glycoside (ether bound) phenolics had higher IC_{50} values (lower antioxidant activity) compared to the free and ester bound phenolic extracts.

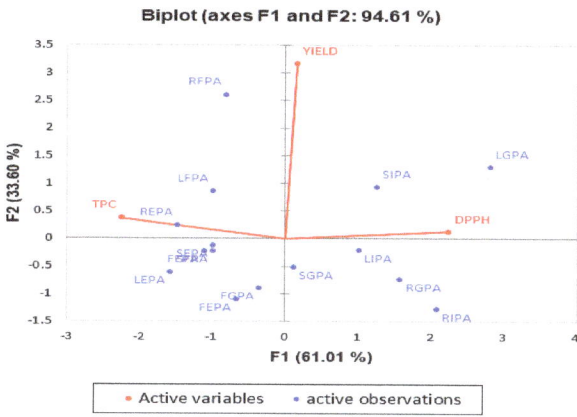

Figure 4. The principal component analysis biplot indicating the correlation circle of the active variables and the scatter plot of the active observations. F1: the first factor or principal component 1 (PC1). F2: the second factor or principal component 2 (PC2).

Along negative F1, REPA, and LEPA were the farthest samples from the center. The highest total phenolic contents (Table 1) were found in both samples. Free and ester bound phenolics contained higher phenolics and exhibited higher antioxidant activities compared to the glycosides and the insoluble phenolics. This trend explains the negative relationship between TPC and DPPH (r = −0.828). Previous studies have reported on the correlation between TPC and DPPH antioxidant activities [53,54]. The variation in the extraction yield is explained along F2. Positive F2 consists of RFPA, LFPA, SIPA, LGPA, and REPA. The highest extractable phenolics were found in leaves and root while the highest non-extractable phenolics were found in the stem. Although LGPA had a high extraction yield, it displayed a poor antioxidant activity. The same trend was found with SIPA. On the other hand, the extraction yield and antioxidant activity (low IC_{50} values) of RFPA, REPA, and LFPA were high. This trend explains why there was no correlation between DPPH and extraction yield. Although FIPA was not included in the constructing the PCA model, it contained the least phenolic content and antioxidant activity.

2.5. Nuclear Magnetic Resonance (NMR) Spectroscopy

The advantage of NMR metabolomics is its ability to detect a wider range of metabolites compared to GC/MS and LC/MS. It is also highly reproducible and non-destructive [55,56]. NMR was used in this study to identify the variation in metabolites responsible for the activity and grouping in the multivariate analysis. The results of the one-dimensional proton NMR analysis of the extractable and non-extractable phenolics are presented in Figures 5 and 6. The samples were selected for the NMR analysis based on their clustering in the AHC and PCA analysis. In the two statistical tools, free and ester bound phenolics were clustered in group 2 (or 2 and 3 in the case of AHC) while the glycosides and insoluble phenolics were clustered in group 1. All the free phenolics were selected to represent the cluster 2 (or 2 and 3, in the case of AHC) while LIPA, RGPA, and SIPA were selected to represent cluster 1. Multiplet signals (Figure 5) at aromatic region δ_H 7.7 and 7.5 ppm (A), δ_H 4.2 ppm (B), δ_H 1.7–1.27 ppm (C), and δ_H 0.92 ppm (D) are characteristics of phthalates, which are contaminants from the solvents used for the extraction [57]. The solvent peaks are indicated at δ_H 5 ppm and δ_H 3.2 ppm.

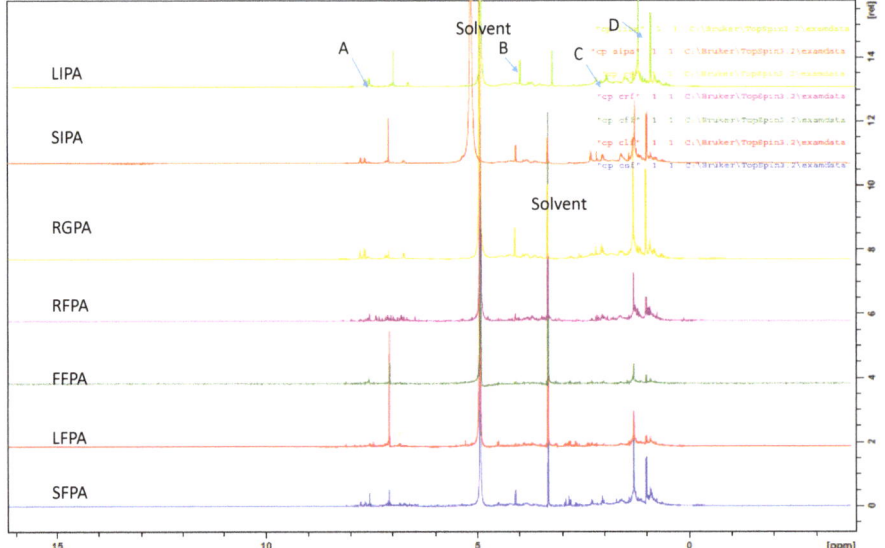

Figure 5. The ^{1}H-NMR spectra indicating the chemical shifts identical to Pthalates.

In the proton NMR spectra, δ_H 0.5–3.0 ppm are the aliphatic or organic, amino acid region while the chemical shift ranges δ_H 3.0–5.5 ppm and 5.5–10 ppm are predominantly the carbohydrate and aromatic regions, respectively [58,59]. Signals with chemical shifts characteristics of carbohydrates were not visible in any of the spectra. The result of the aromatic region of the extractable and non-extractable phenolics is presented in Figure 6.

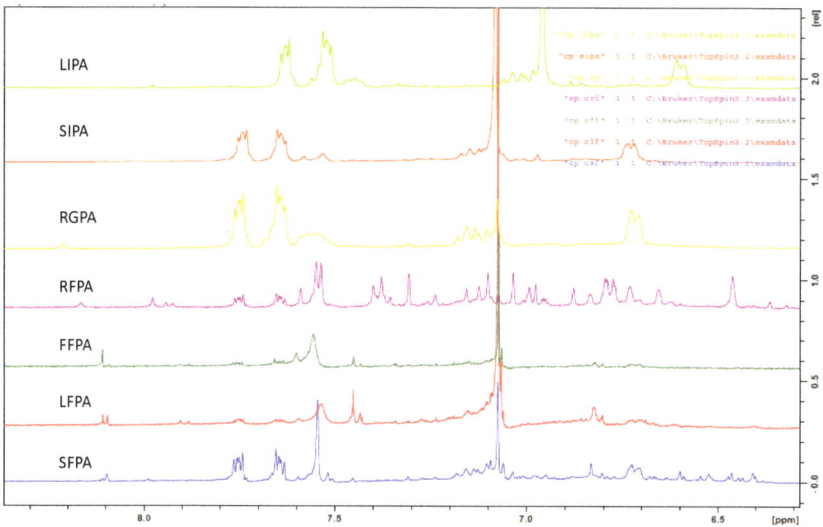

Figure 6. The ^{1}H-NMR spectra indicating the chemical shift (δ ppm) of the phenolic acid extracts at the aromatic region.

The fruit free phenolic acid (FFPA) displayed four singlet signals at $δ_H$ 8.11, 7.60, 7.45, and 7.07 ppm. The leaf free phenolic acid (LFPA) displayed a doublet signal at $δ_H$ 8.10 ppm (J = 4.8 Hz), two singlet signals at $δ_H$ 7.54 and 7.07 ppm, and two doublets at $δ_H$ 7.43 (J = 2 Hz) and 6.81 (J = 8.8 Hz). The stem free phenolic acid (SFPA) displayed singlet signals at $δ_H$ 8.09, 7.54, 7.07, 6.83 ppm and a doublet signal at $δ_H$ 6.72 ppm (J = 9.6 Hz). The root free phenolic acid (RFPA) displayed seventeen singlet signals at $δ_H$ 8.17, 7.98, 7.59, 7.31, 7.24, 7.16, 7.12, 7.10, 7.07, 7.03, 6.88, 6.84, 6.73, 6.65, 6.46, 6.36, and 6.32 ppm and six doublets signals at $δ_H$ 7.94 ppm (J = 8.0 Hz), 7.54 ppm (J = 5.2 Hz), 7.39 ppm (J = 8.8 Hz), 6.98 ppm (J = 6.0 Hz), 6.78 ppm (J = 8.8 Hz), and 6.19 ppm (J = 12 Hz). The glycoside (ether) bound phenolic acid (RGPA) displayed two singlet signals at $δ_H$ 8.21, 7.08 ppm and one doublet signal at $δ_H$ 6.72 ppm (J = 6.8 Hz). The leave insoluble phenolic acid (LIPA) displayed a singlet signal at $δ_H$ 6.96 ppm and a doublet signal at $δ_H$ 6.6 ppm (J = 8.8 Hz). The stem insoluble phenolic acid (SIPA) displayed a singlet signal at $δ_H$ 7.08 ppm and a doublet signal at $δ_H$ 6.73 ppm (J = 7.2 Hz).

All the extractable phenolics (FFPA, LFPA, SFPA, RFPA, and RGPA) displayed a singlet signal around $δ_H$ 8.0 ppm. This signal was not found in the insoluble phenolics (LIPA and SIPA). This could be a major reason for the clear separation in the three classes illustrated in the dendrogram (Figure 2) and the scatter plot (Figure 3). Additionally, included in the PCA score plot class two with the insoluble phenolics were the glycosides (SGPA, RGPA, and LGPA). The clustering of RGPA in cluster 1 may be due to the absence of the singlet signal range $δ_H$ 7.60–7.31 ppm compared to the other extractable phenolics. The absence of these signals could be responsible for the poor antioxidant activity of all the extracts found in cluster 1 of the PCA score plot.

Comparing the spectra within the extractable phenolics, LFPA was the only extract with a doublet around $δ_H$ 8.0 ppm. This may be a distinguishing feature of the leaf compared to the other organs. Another unique feature in the leaf is the similarities in the doublet signals around $δ_H$ 6 ppm (J = 8.8 Hz) in both LFPA and LIPA. The RFPA displayed the highest number of signals (Figure 6), indicating the presence of more phenolics compared to other extracts. The highest extract yield found in RFPA (Figure 1) could be due to the presence of more phenolics as indicated by the ^{1}H-NMR spectra. All the extracts, except LIPA, displayed a singlet at $δ_H$ 7.07 ppm. This chemical shift is consistent with the characteristic signal for gallic acid, a hydroxybenzoic acid [60–62]. Doublets at $δ_H$ 7.94 ppm (J = 8 Hz) and δ_H 7.39 ppm (J = 8.8) in the RFPA spectra are characteristic signals for hydroxybenzoic acid derivatives [63]. The singlet signal range δ_H 6.73–6.32 ppm in the RFPA spectra is consistent with the signals of the aromatic rings of resveratrol-3-O-β-rutinoside, a hydroxystilbene glycoside [64], which has been previously isolated from the root of *T. sericea* [65,66]. The chemical shifts in the spectra of the selected samples suggest that hydroxybenzoic acid and stilbenes are the major phenolics of *T. sericea*.

The presence of gallic acid (Figure 7) in RFPA was confirmed by comparing the 1D and 2D spectra of the gallic acid standard and RFPA. The cross peak between δ_H 7.07 ppm and δ_C 108.9 ppm in the heteronuclear single quantum correlation (HSQC) of the gallic acid (Supplementary Figure S1) corresponds with the cross peak in RFPA (Supplementary Figure S2). The proton δ_H 7.07 ppm was identified as the methine proton of C-2 or 6 (δ_C 108.9 ppm) in gallic acid. The carbon δ_C 139.6 ppm (Supplementary Figure S2) was assigned to C-3 or 5 while carbon δ_C 145.0 ppm was assigned to C-4 [63]. The chemical shifts δ_C 120.6 ppm and δ_C 169.0 ppm were assigned to C-1 and the carbonyl functional group (C = O), respectively. The cross peaks between δ_C 108.9 ppm and singlet protons δ_H 7.03, 7.10, 7.12, and 7.16 ppm suggest the presence of gallic acid derivatives or other hydroxybenzoic acid derivatives. In the heteronuclear multiple bond correlation (HMBC) spectrum of RFPA (Supplementary Figure S3), the cross peaks of δ_H 7.03 and 7.07 with δ_C 139.6 ppm further confirm that δ_H 7.03 ppm is characteristics of a hydroxybenxoic acid, probably a derivative of gallic acid. Gallic acid has been isolated from the fruit of *T. bellerica* [67], the fruit pulp of *T. chebula* [68], and the leaf of *T. arjuna* [69]. However, this is the first report of gallic acid in *T. sericea*. This study has demonstrated that gallic acid is a major phenolic compound in *T. sericea*. According to Ajila and Prasada Rao [70], gallic acid was a major phenolic acid in both raw and ripe badami and raspusi mango peel. Gallic acid and its derivative (gallic hexoside) were the major phenolic acid in berry seed meals [71].

Resveratrol consists of two aromatic rings (A and B) linked by an olefin (Figure 8). The A ring is characterized by two doublets while the B ring is characterized by two singlets. In the HSQC spectrum (Supplementary Figure S2) of RFPA, the cross peak between the doublet at δ_H 7.39 ppm (J = 8.4 Hz) and δ_C 128.5 ppm corresponds to the carbons C-2 or C-6 in the A ring. The cross peak between the doublet at δ_H 6.79 ppm (J = 8.8 Hz) and δ_C 115.1 ppm corresponds to the carbons C-3 or C-5. The identification of these cross peaks in RFPA confirms the A ring. In the HMBC spectrum (Supplementary Figure S3) of RFPA, the cross peaks of δ_H 7.39 and 6.79 with δ_C 128.5 further confirmed that both doublet protons are in ring A. Both doublets also displayed cross peak with δ_C 158.1 ppm. In the B ring, the cross peak between the singlet proton δ_H 6.73 ppm and δ_C 106 ppm corresponds to the carbon C-2' or C-6'.

In the ^{13}C spectrum (Supplementary Figure S4), the chemical shift δ_C 102.5 ppm was assigned to C-4' due to the cross peak between δ_C 102.5 ppm and the singlet proton δ_H 6.46 ppm in the HSQC. The chemical shift δ_C 160.1 ppm was assigned to C-3' or C-5' while δ_C 158.1 ppm was assigned to C-4 in the A ring [64] due to the cross peak between both δ_H 7.39 and 6.79 and δ_C 158.1 ppm in the HMBC spectrum.

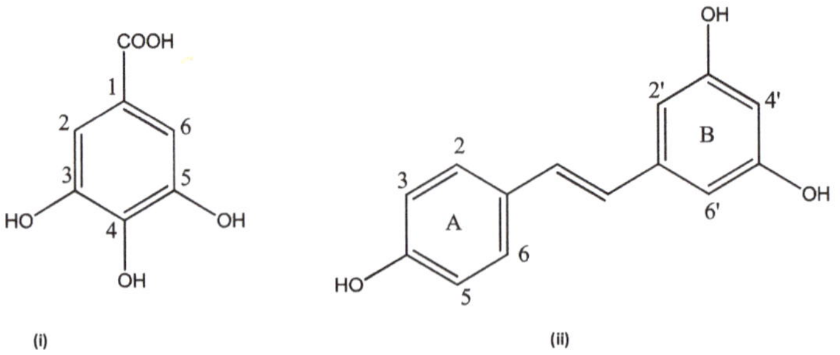

Figure 7. The structure of identified compounds (i) Gallic acid (ii) resveratrol from RFPA.

The NMR data (one and two-dimensional) have revealed that gallic acid and resveratrol are major phenolics in the root free phenolic acid. It also revealed that gallic acid is present in both extractable and non-extractable extracts of all organs. In other studies [21,43,72,73], gallic acid has been reported to be present in both extractable and non-extractable phenolics. The absence of the chemical shifts δ_H 7.39, 6.79, 6.73, and 6.65 ppm in the fruit, leaf, and stem suggests that resveratrol is not present or in very little amount.

3. Materials and Methods

3.1. Materials

Solvents were purchased at Rochelle Chemicals, South Africa, while the reagents were purchased from Merck (Darmstadt, Germany). The fruit, leaf, stem, bark, and root samples of *T. sericea* were collected from Vuwani, Limpopo province in June 2014 and identified by Prof Tshisikhawe MP (Department of Botany, University of Venda). The collected voucher specimen (MPT00114) was identified and deposited at the University of Venda Herbarium.

3.2. Extraction

The samples were washed to remove debris and air dried for two weeks. The dried materials were ground to a powder using an industrial grinder (Dietz-motoren KG, Dettingen unter Teck, Germany). The free, conjugated and bound phenolics were extracted as described by Chandrasekara and Shahidi [20]. Four grams of each dried sample was macerated with 40 mL of 50% ethanol for 24 h at room temperature. The supernatant was filtered and the residue was re-extracted with the same volume of the extracting solvent on an orbital shaker for 1 h. This process was repeated three times and all the filtrate were combined to obtain extractable or soluble phenolics. The leaf and fruit samples were previously defatted with hexane to remove the fat content before extraction [21]. The summary of the extraction of the extractable and non-extractable phenolics is illustrated in Figure 8.

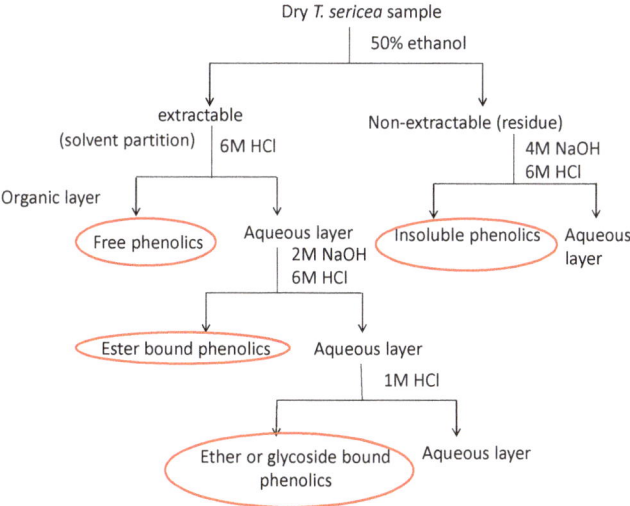

Figure 8. The flowchart indicating the extraction of free, ester, ether, and insoluble-bound phenolics.

3.2.1. Free Phenolics

The soluble phenolic aqueous solution was acidified with HCl (6 M; pH 2) and was partitioned with diethyl ether:ethyl acetate (1:1) in a separating funnel. The organic layer containing the free phenolics was collected. The aqueous layer was further partitioned (4×) with a mixture of diethyl ether and ethyl acetate to extract the free phenolics. The organic layers were combined and evaporated to dryness using a rotar vapour (Buchi, Flawil, Switzerland).

3.2.2. Ester Bound Phenolics

The aqueous fraction (10 mL) obtained after the extraction of the free phenolics was hydrolysed with 40 mL of 2 M NaOH for 4 h at room temperature. The alkaline solution was made acidic with 6 M HCl and the ester bound phenolics were extracted with diethyl ether: the ethyl acetate mixture as described previously.

3.2.3. Glycoside Bound Phenolics

The aqueous fraction (20 mL) obtained after the extraction of the ester bound phenolics was subjected to acid hydrolysis with HCl (1 M; 30 mL) by incubating in a water bath at 95 °C for 45 min. The glycoside bound phenolics were extracted with the organic mixture and dried as described earlier.

3.2.4. Insoluble Phenolics

The residue after the extraction of the soluble phenolics was hydrolysed with NaOH (4 M; 40 mL) for 1 h at room temperature. The solution was acidified with HCl (6 M; pH 2) and the insoluble phenolics were extracted with the organic mixture and dried as described earlier.

3.3. Total Phenolic Content

The total phenolic contents of the free, conjugated and insoluble phenolic extracts were determined using a method described by Anokwuru et al. [74]. Briefly, the extracts (1 mg/mL; 20 µL) were transferred to 96 well plates containing 80 µL of distilled water. Follin Ciocalteu reagent (10%; 20 µL) was added to each well containing the diluted extracts. The mixture was allowed to stand for 1 min at room temperature before Na_2CO_3 (7%; 60 µL) was added to each well. The mixture was further diluted with 120 µL of distilled water and incubated for 30 min at room temperature before measuring the absorbance with a microplate reader (Versa Max, Shanghai, China) at 760 nm. The total phenolic content was extrapolated from a gallic acid (10–80 µg/mL) calibration curve (y = 0.0009x + 0.049; R^2 = 1) and was expressed as mg Gallic Acid Equivalent per gram of the dry extract (mgGAE/g) using Equation (1) [68].

$$C = cV/m \tag{1}$$

C = the total phenolic content (mgGAE/g)
c = the concentration of Gallic acid obtained from the calibration curve
V = the volume of extract (mL)
m = the mass of the extract (g)

3.4. Antioxidant Activity

The antioxidant activity was determined using a DPPH (2,2-diphenyl-1-picrylhydrazyl) assay as described by Anokwuru et al. [74]. Briefly, 100 µL of the extracts (1 mg/mL) or gallic acid (0.10 mg/mL;) were serially diluted in a 96 well plate and DPPH solution (0.3 mM; 200 µL) was added to each well containing the diluted samples. The mixtures were left in the dark at room temperature for 30 min and the absorbance was read at 517 nm using a microplate reader (Versa Max, Shanghai, China). The blank contained only distilled water and the DPPH solution without any sample or gallic acid.

The following equation was used to calculate the percentage antioxidant activity (AA)

$$\%AA = [Ab - As/Ab] \times 100 \tag{2}$$

where Ab is the absorbance of the blank and As is the absorbance of the sample or gallic acid. The concentration required for 50% inhibition (IC_{50}) of the DPPH free radical [75,76] was derived from a plot of % AA against concentration.

3.5. Nuclear Magnetic Resonance (NMR) Spectroscopy

The proton spectra of selected extractable and non-extractable phenolic extracts were recorded on Bruker Ultra Shield™ Plus 400 MHZ (Biospin) (Bruker, Bellericea, MA, USA). The obtained spectra were processed using Bruker Topspin 3.2 on the AVIII 400 software. The extracts (10 mg) were dissolved in 1 mL deuterated methanol (Methanol-*d*4) and 700 µL was transferred into an NMR tube for analysis. Gallic acid and resveratrol were identified in the crude extract by comparing the 2D experiment (heteronuclear single quantum correlation, HSQC; heteronuclear multiple bond correlation, HMBC) of gallic acid standard and resveratrol-3-*O*-β-rutinoside (previously isolated).

3.6. Statistical Analysis

The total phenolic content and antioxidant activity were analysed in triplicates and the values were expressed as the mean ± standard error. A one-way ANOVA was used to determine the significant difference in the TPC and the antioxidant activities using SPSS 23. Fisher's least significant difference (LSD) method was used for post hoc analysis. Multivariate analysis (Agglomerative hierarchical clustering and principal component analysis) were performed on the data obtained (percentage yield, total phenolic content, and antioxidant activity) using the software XLSTAT (2017). Agglomerative hierarchical clustering (AHC) analysis was used to determine the dissimilarities between the extractable and non-extractable phenolics [48]. Principal component analysis used was Pearson correlation [26]. The scree plot was used to determine the number of significant PCA factor [77].

4. Conclusions

This study demonstrated that free and ester bound extractable phenolics contained higher total phenolic content and antioxidant activity compared to the ether bound or glycoside and insoluble phenolics of *T. sericea*. Furthermore, the use of aqueous alcohol does not underestimate the amount of phenolic compounds and antioxidant in the organs. The dendrogram constructed from the agglomerative hierarchical clustering (AHC) indicated three clusters based on the type of phenolics extracted. The insoluble and glycosides were found in cluster 1 while the free and ester bound extractable phenolics were found in cluster 3. Cluster 2 contained free phenolic acids from the root alone. The three clusters from the dendrogram were further confirmed with the principal component analysis (PCA) score plot. There was a significant ($p < 0.05$) correlation between the total phenolic acid and the DPPH antioxidant activity. One-dimensional ^{1}H-NMR spectra of the selected extracts revealed that hydroxybenzoic acids and stilbenes are major phenolics in the plant. The difference in the antioxidant activity of cluster 1 compared to cluster 2 (or 2 and 3 in the case of AHC) could be due to the variation in the chemical shift between δ_H 8.1 and 7.07 ppm. In the 2D experiment, the heteronuclear single quantum correlation (HSQC) and heteronuclear multiple bond correlation (HMBC) of RFPA revealed that Gallic acid and resveratrol are major phenolic constituents of *T. sericea* root. Further study is required for the identification of phenolics responsible for the antioxidant activities in *T. sericea*.

Supplementary Materials: Supplementary materials are available online.

Author Contributions: Muendi Sigidi and Peter Tshisikhawe collected and prepared the plant materials. Chinedu Anokwuru conducted the analysis and drafted the paper. Afsatou Traore was the project leader administration the funds. Marlaine Boukandou helped with the analysis of samples and Natasha Potgieter edited the manuscript. All authors reviewed the articles and added inputs from the 1st draft to the last version.

Acknowledgments: The authors would like to thank the University of Venda Research and Innovation Directorate for funding of this study.

Conflicts of Interest: The authors declare no conflict of interest.

References

1. Sharma, S.; Kori, S.; Parmar, A. Surfactant mediated extraction of total phenolic contents (TPC) and antioxidants from fruits juices. *Food Chem.* **2015**, *185*, 284–288. [CrossRef] [PubMed]
2. Ismail, H.F.; Hashim, Z.; Soon, W.T.; Rahman, N.S.A.; Zainudin, A.N.; Majid, F.A.A. Comparative study of herbal plants on the phenolic and flavonoid content, antioxidant activities and toxicity on cells and zebrafish embryo. *J. Tradit. Complement. Med.* **2017**, *7*, 452–465. [CrossRef] [PubMed]
3. Mirończuk-Chodakowska, I.; Witkowska, A.M.; Zujko, M.E. Endogenous non-enzymatic antioxidants in the human body. *Adv. Med. Sci.* **2018**, *63*, 68–78. [CrossRef] [PubMed]
4. Agregán, R.; Munekata, P.E.; Domínguez, R.; Carballo, J.; Franco, D.; Lorenzo, J.M. Proximate composition, phenolic content and in vitro antioxidant activity of aqueous extracts of the seaweeds *Ascophyllum nodosum*, *Bifurcaria bifurcata* and *Fucus vesiculosus*. Effect of addition of the extracts on the oxidative stability of canola oil under accelerated storage conditions. *Food Res. Int.* **2017**, *99*, 986–994. [PubMed]
5. Lee, J.H.; Park, M.J.; Ryu, H.W.; Yuk, H.J.; Choi, S.; Lee, K.; Kim, S.; Seo, W.D. Elucidation of phenolic antioxidants in barley seedlings (*Hordeum vulgare* L.) by UPLC-PDA-ESI/MS and screening for their contents at different harvest times. *J. Funct. Foods* **2016**, *26*, 667–680. [CrossRef]
6. Azima, A.S.; Noriham, A.; Manshoor, N. Phenolics, antioxidants and color properties of aqueous pigmented plant extracts: *Ardisia colorata* var. elliptica, *Clitoria ternatea*, *Garcinia mangostana* and *Syzygium cumini*. *J. Funct. Foods* **2017**, *38*, 232–241. [CrossRef]
7. Salar, R.K.; Purewal, S.S.; Sandhu, K.S. Relationships between DNA damage protection activity, total phenolic content, condensed tannin content and antioxidant potential among Indian barley cultivars. *Biocatal. Agric. Biotechnol.* **2017**, *11*, 201–206. [CrossRef]
8. Chen, C.; Wang, L.; Wang, R.; Luo, X.; Li, Y.; Li, J.; Li, Y.; Chen, Z. Phenolic contents, cellular antioxidant activity and antiproliferative capacity of different varieties of oats. *Food Chem.* **2018**, *239*, 260–267. [CrossRef] [PubMed]
9. Bergantin, C.; Maietti, A.; Cavazzini, A.; Pasti, L.; Tedeschi, P.; Brandolini, V.; Marchetti, N. Bioaccessibility and HPLC-MS/MS chemical characterization of phenolic antioxidants in Red Chicory (*Cichorium intybus*). *J. Funct. Foods* **2017**, *33*, 94–102. [CrossRef]
10. Rahman, M.J.; de Camargo, A.C.; Shahidi, F. Phenolic profiles and antioxidant activity of defatted Camelina and Sophia seeds. *Food Chem.* **2018**, *240*, 917–925. [CrossRef] [PubMed]
11. De Ascensao, A.R.; Dubery, I.A. Soluble and wall-bound phenolics and phenolic polymers in Musa acuminata roots exposed to elicitors from *Fusarium oxysporum* f. sp. cubense. *Phytochemistry* **2003**, *63*, 679–686. [CrossRef]
12. Alrahmany, R.; Avis, T.J.; Tsopmo, A. Treatment of oat bran with carbohydrases increases soluble phenolic acid content and influences antioxidant and antimicrobial activities. *Food Res. Int.* **2013**, *52*, 568–574. [CrossRef]
13. Chen, P.X.; Bozzo, G.G.; Freixas-Coutin, J.A.; Marcone, M.F.; Pauls, P.K.; Tang, Y.; Zhang, B.; Liu, R.; Tsao, R. Free and conjugated phenolic compounds and their antioxidant activities in regular and non-darkening cranberry bean (*Phaseolus vulgaris* L.) seed coats. *J. Funct. Foods* **2015**, *18*, 1047–1056. [CrossRef]
14. Coyago-Cruz, E.; Corell, M.; Moriana, A.; Hernanz, D.; Benítez-González, A.M.; Stinco, C.M.; Meléndez-Martínez, A.J. Antioxidants (carotenoids and phenolics) profile of cherry tomatoes as influenced by deficit irrigation, ripening and cluster. *Food Chem.* **2018**, *240*, 870–884. [CrossRef] [PubMed]
15. Yuan, B.; Lu, M.; Eskridge, K.M.; Isom, L.D.; Hanna, M.A. Extraction, identification, and quantification of antioxidant phenolics from hazelnut (*Corylus avellana* L.) shells. *Food Chem.* **2018**, *244*, 7–15. [CrossRef] [PubMed]
16. Hemalatha, P.; Bomzan, D.P.; Rao, B.S.; Sreerama, Y.N. Distribution of phenolic antioxidants in whole and milled fractions of quinoa and their inhibitory effects on α-amylase and α-glucosidase activities. *Food Chem.* **2016**, *199*, 330–338. [CrossRef] [PubMed]
17. Luo, C.; Wang, X.; Gao, G.; Wang, L.; Li, Y.; Sun, C. Identification and quantification of free, conjugate and total phenolic compounds in leaves of 20 sweet potato cultivars by HPLC–DAD and HPLC–ESI–MS/MS. *Food Chem.* **2013**, *141*, 2697–2706. [CrossRef] [PubMed]
18. Daniel, M. *Medicinal Plants: Chemistry and Properties*; Science Publisher: Enfield, NH, USA, 2006; pp. 140–191, ISBN 1-57808395-8.
19. Acosta-Estrada, B.A.; Gutiérrez-Uribe, J.A.; Serna-Saldívar, S.O. Bound phenolics in foods, a review. *Food Chem.* **2014**, *152*, 46–55. [CrossRef] [PubMed]

20. Chandrasekara, A.; Shahidi, F. Determination of antioxidant activity in free and hydrolyzed fractions of millet grains and characterization of their phenolic profiles by HPLC-DAD-ESI-MS n. *J. Funct. Foods* **2011**, *3*, 144–158. [CrossRef]
21. Singh, R.G.; Negi, P.S.; Radha, C. Phenolic composition, antioxidant and antimicrobial activities of free and bound phenolic extracts of *Moringa oleifera* seed flour. *J. Funct. Foods* **2013**, *5*, 1883–1891. [CrossRef]
22. Wang, W.; Guo, J.; Zhang, J.; Peng, J.; Liu, T.; Xin, Z. Isolation, identification and antioxidant activity of bound phenolic compounds present in rice bran. *Food Chem.* **2015**, *171*, 40–49. [CrossRef] [PubMed]
23. Irakli, M.N.; Samanidou, V.F.; Biliaderis, C.G.; Papadoyannis, I.N. Development and validation of an HPLC-method for determination of free and bound phenolic acids in cereals after solid-phase extraction. *Food Chem.* **2012**, *134*, 1624–1632. [CrossRef] [PubMed]
24. Pihlava, J.; Nordlund, E.; Heiniö, R.; Hietaniemi, V.; Lehtinen, P.; Poutanen, K. Phenolic compounds in wholegrain rye and its fractions. *J. Food Comp. Anal.* **2015**, *38*, 89–97. [CrossRef]
25. Verma, B.; Hucl, P.; Chibbar, R. Phenolic acid composition and antioxidant capacity of acid and alkali hydrolysed wheat bran fractions. *Food Chem.* **2009**, *116*, 947–954. [CrossRef]
26. Scaglioni, P.T.; de Souza, T.D.; Schmidt, C.G.; Badiale-Furlong, E. Availability of free and bound phenolic compounds in rice after hydrothermal treatment. *J. Cereal Sci.* **2014**, *60*, 526–532. [CrossRef]
27. Pérez-Jiménez, J.; Díaz-Rubio, M.E.; Saura-Calixto, F. Non-extractable polyphenols, a major dietary antioxidant: Occurrence, metabolic fate and health effects. *Nutr. Res. Rev.* **2013**, *26*, 118–129. [CrossRef] [PubMed]
28. Chen, P.X.; Tang, Y.; Marcone, M.F.; Pauls, P.K.; Zhang, B.; Liu, R.; Tsao, R. Characterization of free, conjugated and bound phenolics and lipophilic antioxidants in regular-and non-darkening cranberry beans (*Phaseolus vulgaris* L.). *Food Chem.* **2015**, *185*, 298–308. [CrossRef] [PubMed]
29. Ti, H.; Zhang, R.; Zhang, M.; Li, Q.; Wei, Z.; Zhang, Y.; Tang, X.; Deng, Y.; Liu, L.; Ma, Y. Dynamic changes in the free and bound phenolic compounds and antioxidant activity of brown rice at different germination stages. *Food Chem.* **2014**, *161*, 337–344. [CrossRef] [PubMed]
30. Palgrave, K.C. *Trees of Southern Africa*, 5th ed.; Struik Publishers: Cape Town, South Africa, 1988; Volume 684, ISBN 0869770810.
31. Eldeen, I.M.; Elgorashi, E.E.; Mulholland, D.A.; van Staden, J. Anolignan B: A bioactive compound from the roots of *Terminalia sericea*. *J. Ethnopharmacol.* **2006**, *103*, 135–138. [CrossRef] [PubMed]
32. Lall, N.; Kishore, N. Are plants used for skin care in South Africa fully explored? *J. Ethnopharmacol.* **2014**, *153*, 61–84. [CrossRef] [PubMed]
33. Moshi, M.; Mbwambo, Z. Some pharmacological properties of extracts of Terminalia sericea roots. *J. Ethnopharmacol.* **2005**, *97*, 43–47. [CrossRef] [PubMed]
34. Mabogo, D. The Ethnobotany of the Vhavenda. Master's Thesis, University of Pretoria, Pretoria, South Africa, 1990.
35. Fyhrquist, P.; Mwasumbi, L.; Haeggstrom, C.A.; Vuorela, H.; Hiltumen, R.; Vuorela, P. Ethnobotanical and antimicrobial investigation on some species of *Terminalia* and *Combretum* (Combretaceae) growing in Tanzania. *J. Ethnopharmacol.* **2002**, *79*, 169–177. [CrossRef]
36. Tshikalange, T.E.; Meyer, J.J.M.; Hussein, A.A. Antimicrobial activity, toxicity, and isolation of bioactive compounds from plants used to treat sexually transmitted disease. *J. Ethnopharmacol.* **2005**, *96*, 515–519. [CrossRef] [PubMed]
37. Adewusi, E.A.; Steenkamp, V. In vitro screening for acetylcholinesterase inhibition and antioxidant activity of medicinal plants from southern Africa. *Asian Pac. J. Trop. Med.* **2011**, *4*, 829–835. [CrossRef]
38. Nkobole, N. Antidiabetic activity of *Terminalia sericea* Burch. Ex DC constituents. *Nat. Prod. Commun.* **2011**, *6*, 1–4.
39. Anokwuru, C.P.; Ramaite, I.D.; Bessong, P. Phenolic content distribution and antioxidant activities of *Terminalia sericea* Burch. *Afr. J. Trad. Complement. Altern. Med.* **2015**, *12*, 21–27. [CrossRef]
40. Zhang, R.; Zeng, Q.; Deng, Y.; Zhang, M.; Wei, Z.; Zhang, Y.; Tang, X. Phenolic profiles and antioxidant activity of litchi pulp of different cultivars cultivated in Southern China. *Food Chem.* **2013**, *136*, 1169–1176. [CrossRef] [PubMed]
41. Lou, S.; Lin, Y.; Hsu, Y.; Chiu, E.; Ho, C. Soluble and insoluble phenolic compounds and antioxidant activity of immature calamondin affected by solvents and heat treatment. *Food Chem.* **2014**, *161*, 246–253. [CrossRef] [PubMed]

42. Waksmundzka-Hajnos, M.; Sharma, J. (Eds.) High Performance Liquid Chromatography in Phytochemical Analysis; CRC press: Boca Raton, FL, USA, 2010; Volume 483, ISBN 9781420092608.
43. Pradeep, P.; Sreerama, Y.N. Soluble and bound phenolics of two different millet genera and their milled fractions: Comparative evaluation of antioxidant properties and inhibitory effects on starch hydrolysing enzyme activities. *J. Funct. Foods* **2017**, *35*, 682–693. [CrossRef]
44. Nayaka, M.H.; Sathisha, U.; Dharmesh, S.M. Cytoprotective and antioxidant activity of free, conjugated and insoluble-bound phenolic acids from swallow root (*Decalepis hamiltonii*). *Food Chem.* **2010**, *119*, 1307–1312. [CrossRef]
45. Kumar, G.S.; Nayaka, H.; Dharmesh, S.M.; Salimath, P. Free and bound phenolic antioxidants in amla (*Emblica officinalis*) and turmeric (*Curcuma longa*). *J. Food Comp. Anal.* **2006**, *19*, 446–452. [CrossRef]
46. Rufino, M.D.S.M.; Pérez-Jiménez, J.; Tabernero, M.; Alves, R.E.; De Brito, E.S.; Saura-Calixto, F. Acerola and cashew apple as sources of antioxidants and dietary fibre. *Int. J. Food Sci. Tech.* **2010**, *45*, 2227–2233. [CrossRef]
47. Esparza-Martínez, F.J.; Miranda-López, R.; Mata-Sánchez, S.M.; Guzmán-Maldonado, S.H. Extractable and non-extractable phenolics and antioxidant capacity of mandarin waste dried at different temperatures. *Plant Foods Hum. Nutr.* **2016**, *71*, 294–300. [CrossRef] [PubMed]
48. Konczak, I.; Maillot, F.; Dalar, A. Phytochemical divergence in 45 accessions of *Terminalia ferdinandiana* (Kakadu plum). *Food Chem.* **2014**, *151*, 248–256. [CrossRef] [PubMed]
49. AbouZid, S.F.; Chen, S.; Pauli, G.F. Silymarin content in *Silybum marianum* populations growing in Egypt. *Ind. Crops Prod.* **2016**, *83*, 729–737. [CrossRef] [PubMed]
50. Marcial, G.; de Lampasona, M.P.; Vega, M.I.; Lizarraga, E.; Viturro, C.I.; Slanis, A.; Juárez, M.A.; Elechosa, M.A.; Catalán, C.A. Intraspecific variation in essential oil composition of the medicinal plant *Lippia integrifolia* (Verbenaceae). Evidence for five chemotypes. *Phytochemistry* **2016**, *122*, 203–212. [CrossRef] [PubMed]
51. Elechosa, M.A.; Lira, P.D.L.; Juárez, M.A.; Viturro, C.I.; Heit, C.I.; Molina, A.C.; Martínez, A.J.; López, S.; Molina, A.M.; van Baren, C.M. Essential oil chemotypes of *Aloysia citrodora* (Verbenaceae) in Northwestern Argentina. *Biochem. Syst. Ecol.* **2017**, *74*, 19–29. [CrossRef]
52. Sandasi, M.; Kamatou, G.P.; Viljoen, A.M. An untargeted metabolomic approach in the chemotaxonomic assessment of two Salvia species as a potential source of α-bisabolol. *Phytochemistry* **2012**, *84*, 94–101. [CrossRef] [PubMed]
53. Colak, N.; Primetta, A.K.; Riihinen, K.R.; Jaakola, L.; Grúze, J.; Strnad, M.; Torun, H.; Faik Ahmet Ayaz, F.A. Phenolic compounds and antioxidant capacity in different-colored and non-pigmented berries of bilberry (*Vaccinium myrtillus* L.). *Food Biosci.* **2017**, *20*, 67–78. [CrossRef]
54. Shao, Y.; Hu, Z.; Yu, Y.; Mou, R.; Zhu, Z.; Beta, T. Phenolic acids, anthocyanins, proanthocyanidins, antioxidant activity, minerals and their correlations in non-pigmented, red, and black rice. *Food Chem.* **2018**, *239*, 733–741. [CrossRef] [PubMed]
55. Kim, H.K.; Khan, S.; Wilson, E.G.; Kricun, S.D.P.; Meissner, A.; Goraler, S.; Deelder, A.M.; Choi, Y.H.; Verpoorte, R. Metabolic classification of South American Ilex species by NMR-based metabolomics. *Phytochemistry* **2010**, *71*, 773–784. [CrossRef] [PubMed]
56. Deborde, C.; Moing, A.; Roch, L.; Jacob, D.; Rolin, D.; Giraudeau, P. Plant metabolism as studied by NMR spectroscopy. *Prog. Nucl. Magn. Reson. Spectrosc.* **2017**, *102–103*, 61–97. [CrossRef] [PubMed]
57. Cohen, H.; Charrier, C.; Sarfaty, J. Extraction and identification of a plasticizer, di-(2-ethylhexyl) phthalate, from a plastic bag containing contaminated corn. *Arch. Environ. Contam. Toxicol.* **1991**, *20*, 437–440. [CrossRef]
58. Mediani, A.; Abas, F.; Khatib, A.; Maulidiani, H.; Shaari, K.; Choi, Y.H.; Lajis, N. ^{1}H-NMR-based metabolomics approach to understanding the drying effects on the phytochemicals in *Cosmos caudatus*. *Food Res. Int.* **2012**, *49*, 763–770. [CrossRef]
59. Li, Z.; Li, J.; Zhang, Z.; Mi, X.; Du, G.; Qin, X. NMR-based metabolomic analyses for the componential differences and the corresponding metabolic responses of three batches of *Farfarae Flos*. *Chemom. Intell. Lab. Syst.* **2017**, *165*, 1–10. [CrossRef]
60. Khoo, L.W.; Mediani, A.; Zolkeflee, N.K.Z.; Leong, S.W.; Ismail, I.S.; Khatib, A.; Shaari, K.; Abas, F. Phytochemical diversity of *Clinacanthus nutans* extracts and their bioactivity correlations elucidated by NMR based metabolomics. *Phytochem. Lett.* **2015**, *14*, 123–133. [CrossRef]

61. Mediani, A.; Abas, F.; Khatib, A.; Tan, C.P.; Ismail, I.S.; Shaari, K.; Ismail, A.; Lajis, N. Phytochemical and biological features of *Phyllanthus niruri* and *Phyllanthus urinaria* harvested at different growth stages revealed by 1 H NMR-based metabolomics. *Ind. Crops Prod.* **2015**, *77*, 602–613. [CrossRef]
62. Lee, S.Y.; Abas, F.; Khatib, A.; Ismail, I.S.; Shaari, K.; Zawawi, N. Metabolite profiling of *Neptunia oleracea* and correlation with antioxidant and α-glucosidase inhibitory activities using 1 H NMR-based metabolomics. *Phytochem. Lett.* **2016**, *16*, 23–33. [CrossRef]
63. Wang, P.; Rong, Z.; Ma, C.; Zhao, X.; Xiao, C.; Zheng, X. Distribution of metabolites in root barks of seven tree peony cultivars for quality assessment using nmr-based metabolomics. *Chin. Herb. Med.* **2017**, *9*, 31–41. [CrossRef]
64. Wanjala, C.C.; Majinda, R.R. A new stilbene glycoside from *Elephantorrhiza goetzei*. *Fitoterapia* **2001**, *72*, 649–655. [CrossRef]
65. Bombardelli, E. Plants of Mozambique IX. A new hydroxystilbene glycoside from *Terminalia sericea*. *Fitoterapia* **1975**, *5*, 199–200.
66. Joseph, C.C.; Moshi, M.; Innocent, E.; Nkunya, M. Isolation of a stilbene glycoside and other constituents of *Terminalia sericeae*. *Afr. J. Tradit. Complement. Altern. Med.* **2007**, *4*, 383–386. [CrossRef] [PubMed]
67. Gangadhar, M.; Bhavana, P.; Sunil, Y.; Datta, S. Isolation and characterization of gallic acid from *Terminalia bellerica* and its effect on carbohydrate regulatory system In vitro. *Int. J. Res. Ayurveda Pharm.* **2011**, *2*, 559–562.
68. Genwali, G.R.; Acharya, P.P.; Rajbhandari, M. Isolation of gallic acid and estimation of total phenolic content in some medicinal plants and their antioxidant activity. *Nepal J. Sci. Technol.* **2013**, *14*, 95–102. [CrossRef]
69. Singh, A.P.P.; Chauhan, S.M.S. Activity-guided isolation of antioxidants from the leaves of Terminalia arjuna. *Nat. Prod. Res.* **2014**, *28*, 760–763. [CrossRef] [PubMed]
70. Ajila, C.M.; Prasada Rao, U.J.S. Mango peel dietary fibre: Composition and associated bound phenolics. *J. Funct. Foods.* **2013**, *5*, 444–450. [CrossRef]
71. Ayoub, M.; de Camargo, A.C.; Shahidi, F. Antioxidants and bioactivities of free, esterified and insoluble-bound phenolics from berry seed meals. *Food Chem.* **2016**, *197*, 221–232. [CrossRef] [PubMed]
72. Peng, H.; Li, W.; Li, H.; Deng, Z.; Zhang, B. Extractable and non-extractable bound phenolic compositions and their antioxidant properties in the seed coat and cotyledon of black soybean (*Glycinemax (L.) merr*). *J. Funct. Food.* **2017**, *32*, 296–312. [CrossRef]
73. Esparza-Martínez, F.J.; Miranda-López, R.; Guzman-Maldonado, S.H. Effect of air-drying temperature on extractable and non-extractable phenolics and antioxidant capacity of lime wastes. *Ind. Crops Prod.* **2016**, *84*, 1–6. [CrossRef]
74. Anokwuru, C.; Sigidi, M.; Zininga, T.; Tshisikhawe, M.; Shonhai, A.; Ramaite, I.; Traoré, A.; Potgieter, N. Phenolic contents, antioxidant activity and spectroscopic characteristics of *Pterocarpus angolensis* DC. stem bark fractions. *NISCAIR* **2017**, *16*, 400–406.
75. Žilić, S.; Šukalović, V.H.; Dodig, D.; Maksimović, V.; Maksimović, M.; Basić, Z. Antioxidant activity of small grain cereals caused by phenolics and lipid soluble antioxidants. *J. Cereal Sci.* **2011**, *54*, 417–424. [CrossRef]
76. Lu, Y.; Wu, N.; Fang, Y.; Shaheen, N.; Wei, Y. An automatic on-line 2,2-diphenyl-1-picrylhydrazyl-high performance liquid chromatography method for high-throughput screening of antioxidants from natural products. *J. Chromatogr. A* **2017**, *1521*, 100–109. [CrossRef] [PubMed]
77. Skrzypczak-Pietraszek, E.; Pietraszek, J. Chemical profile and seasonal variation of phenolic acid content in bastard balm (*Melittis melissophyllum* L., Lamiaceae). *J. Pharm. Biomed. Anal.* **2012**, *66*, 154–161. [CrossRef] [PubMed]

Sample Availability: Not available

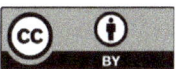

© 2018 by the authors. Licensee MDPI, Basel, Switzerland. This article is an open access article distributed under the terms and conditions of the Creative Commons Attribution (CC BY) license (http://creativecommons.org/licenses/by/4.0/).

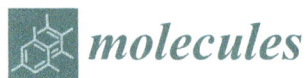

Article

The Effects of Different Degrees of Procyanidin Polymerization on the Nutrient Absorption and Digestive Enzyme Activity in Mice

Huairong Zhong [1,2], Yong Xue [3], Xiaoyuan Lu [1,2], Qiang Shao [1,2], Yuelei Cao [1,2], Zhaoxia Wu [4,*] and Gao Chen [1,2,*]

1. Biotechnology Research Center, Shandong Academy of Agricultural Sciences, Ji'nan 250100, China; zh.hr12@163.com (H.Z.); luxiaoyuan1225@163.com (X.L.); shaoqiang12345@126.com (Q.S.); caoyuelei0733@163.com (Y.C.)
2. Shandong Provincial Key Laboratory of Genetic Improvement, Ecology and Physiology of Crops, Ji'nan 250100, China
3. Department of Synthetic Biology and Bioenergy, J. Craig Venter Institute, Rockville, MD 20850, USA; yongxue@gmail.com
4. College of Food Science, Shenyang Agricultural University, Shenyang 110866, China
* Correspondence: wuzxsau@163.com (Z.W.); gxchen001@hotmail.com (G.C.); Tel.: +86-024-8848-7161 (Z.W.); +86-531-6665-7793 (G.C.)

Academic Editors: Alessandra Durazzo and Massimo Lucarini
Received: 16 October 2018; Accepted: 6 November 2018; Published: 8 November 2018

Abstract: Proanthocyanidins, including polymers with both low and high degrees of polymerization, are the focus of intensive research worldwide due to their high antioxidant activity, medicinal applications, and pharmacological properties. However, the nutritional value of these compounds is limited because they readily form complexes with proteins, polysaccharides, and metal ions when consumed. In this study, we examined the effects of proanthocyanidins with different degrees of polymerization on white mice. Twenty-four male white mice were randomly divided into three groups of eight mice each and fed proanthocyanidins with a low degree of polymerization or a high degree of polymerization or a distilled water control via oral gavage over a 56-day period. We examined the effects of these proanthocyanidins on digestive enzyme activity and nutrient absorption. Compared to the control group, the group fed high-polymer proanthocyanidins exhibited a significant reduction in net body mass, total food intake, food utility rate, amylase activity, protease activity, and major nutrient digestibility ($p < 0.05$), while the group fed low-polymerization proanthocyanidins only exhibited significant reductions in total food intake, α-amylase activity, and apparent digestibility of calcium and zinc ($p < 0.05$). Therefore, proanthocyanidins with a high degree of polymerization had a greater effect on digestive enzyme activity and nutrient absorption than did those with a low degree of polymerization. This study lays the foundation for elucidating the relationship between procyanidin polymerization and nutrient uptake, with the aim of reducing or eliminating the antinutritional effects of polyphenols.

Keywords: antioxidant properties; digestive enzyme; nutrient; polymerization; proanthocyanidins

1. Introduction

Proanthocyanidins are a large class of polyphenolic compounds produced by a wide range of plants. These compounds are composed of a mixture of molecules with different degrees of polymerization, including catechins, epicatechins, and epicatechin gallates linked by C4-C6 or C4-C8 bonds. Polymers composed of two to four monomer units are classified as oligomers while those composed of five or more monomers are high polymers [1]. Proanthocyanidins are the most potent antioxidants and free radical scavengers identified to date; the antioxidant capacity of proanthocyanidins is 20-times that of vitamin C and 50-times that of vitamin E [2]. Most pharmacological functions of proanthocyanidins, such as their anti-cancer, anti-aging, and anti-inflammatory properties and their ability to lower blood pressure, blood fat levels, and blood sugar levels, are closely related to their strong antioxidant activity.

Numerous studies conducted worldwide have examined the physiological activity and medicinal value of proanthocyanidins [3–5], and these compounds have increasingly been used to prevent and treat disease. However, due to their polyhydroxy structure, proanthocyanidins readily undergo complexation reactions with proteins, polysaccharides, and metal ions, reducing the nutritional value of these compounds [6,7]. Polyphenols are widely distributed in nature and are present in plant-derived foods, teas, medicines, and animal feed. However, when polyphenols are consumed, they combine with other compounds, which reduces their nutritional value and limits their development as human health and animal husbandry products [8]. The molecular weight of polyphenols affects their ability to bind to proteins; polyphenols with a molecular weight of less than 500 kD rarely precipitate with proteins in vitro [9].

Several recent studies have examined the effects of the degree of proanthocyanidin polymerization on food functional properties, such as foaming and foam stability. Proanthocyanidins with a higher degree of polymerization have a stabilizing effect on the foaming properties of proteins and are better able to bind to proteins than are those with a low degree of polymerization. The polyhydroxyl properties of proanthocyanidins enable them to bind to multiple protein sites simultaneously [10]. A study of apple juice turbidity revealed that juice proteins aggregated with catechin polymers but not with catechin or epicatechin monomers, suggesting that low-molecular-weight proanthocyanidins do not effectively crosslink proteins [11].

To date, most studies examining the effects of polyphenols with different molecular weights on the digestion and absorption of nutrients have been performed in vitro. Stojadinovic et al. [12] simulated the gastrointestinal digestive environment to study the mechanism by which polyphenols and β-proteins interact, and found that non-covalent bonding between polyphenols and proteins inhibits the digestion of β-lactoglobulin by pepsin and trypsin; the higher the binding strength, the slower the rate of protein digestion. Gonçalves et al. [13] confirmed that t high-polymer proanthocyanidins inhibit α-amylase activity to a greater extent than do oligomeric proanthocyanidins in vitro, due to the broader interaction between α-amylase and homomeric proanthocyanidins. Furthermore, Baxter et al. [14] showed that insoluble aggregates resulting from an interaction between polyphenols and proline-rich proteins contributed to sputum formation. Sarni-Manchadoy et al. [15] confirmed that the precipitate mainly forms in vitro via the interaction between high-polymer polyphenols and salivary proteins, perhaps because the higher hydroxyl content of high-polymer polyphenols enables them to interact with salivary proteins more extensively than with low-polymer polyphenols.

Although the results of in vitro simulation experiments are somewhat correlated with the results of in vivo tests, these experiments do not fully account for the actual digestion and absorption processes of the body. Therefore, in the current study, we explored the relationship between the degree of procyanidin polymerization and nutrient uptake in mice. The results of this study lay the foundation for reducing or eliminating the antinutritional effects of polyphenols.

2. Results

2.1. Effects of Proanthocyanidins with Different Degrees of Polymerization on Body Weight in Mice

The initial body weights of mice in the experimental groups were not significantly different from those of the control group, However, after a 56-day treatment with high- or low-polymer proanthocyanidins or a distilled water control, the body weight of mice in the high-polymer group was significantly lower than that of the control group ($p < 0.05$), whereas that of mice in the low-polymer group was not ($p > 0.05$; Table 1). These results indicate that proanthocyanidins with a high degree of polymerization affect the normal growth and development of mice.

The total food intake of the high-polymer group was significantly lower than that of the control group ($p < 0.05$), indicating that the proanthocyanidin solution inhibited food intake by the mice. Perhaps the activity of digestive enzymes secreted by the mice and of enzymes produced by microorganisms in their digestive tracts was reduced through their interaction with the polyphenols, and this affected satiety and levels of fiber and insoluble compounds, resulting in a reduction in food intake [16].

We calculated the net mass gain of the mice based on their initial and final body masses and the food utility rate of the mice using formula (1) (Table 1). The food utility rate was significantly lower for mice in the high-polymer group vs. the control group ($p < 0.05$). Although the food utility rate of mice in the low-polymer group was lower than that of the control group, the difference was not significant ($p > 0.05$). These results indicate that high-polymer proanthocyanidins reduce the food utilization rate of mice. These results suggest that high-polymer proanthocyanidins have a stronger tendency than low-polymer proanthocyanidins to form complexes with enzymes and biological macromolecules such as proteins, fats, and sugars, resulting in a lower nutrient utilization rate.

Table 1. Effects of procyanidins with different degrees of polymerization on body weight gain, food consumption, and the feed conversion ratio in mice.

Group	Initial Weight (g)	Final Weight (g)	Weight Increase (g)	Total Feed Intake (g)	Food Utility Rate (%)
Control	28.92 ± 2.04 [a]	40.81 ± 2.45 [a]	11.89 ± 1.45 [a]	276.26 ± 10.43 [a]	4.30 ± 0.45 [a]
Low polymer	29.01 ± 1.78 [a]	39.19 ± 2.78 [a]	10.18 ± 0.98 [a]	244.26 ± 7.45 [b]	4.17 ± 0.39 [a]
Highpolymer	29.41 ± 1.56 [a]	37.94 ± 3.12 [b]	8.53 ± 1.01 [b]	242.22 ± 9.09 [b]	3.52 ± 0.52 [b]

[a, b] Differentsuperscripts in the same line indicate significant differences ($p < 0.05$).

2.2. Effects of Proanthocyanidins with Different Degrees of Polymerization on Digestive Enzyme Activity

We calculated the inhibitory effects of proanthocyanidins with different degrees of polymerization on digestive enzyme activity using Formula (2). The effects of these treatments on the activities of various digestive enzymes are described below.

2.2.1. α-Amylase Activity

The α-amylase activity in the small intestine and pancreas was significantly lower in the experimental groups than the control group ($p < 0.05$; Table 2). This enzyme activity was also significantly lower in mice in the high- vs. low-polymer group ($p < 0.05$). In the small intestine, α-amylase activity was inhibited at a rate of 21% in the low-polymer group and 41% in the high-polymer group. In the pancreas, α-amylase activity was inhibited at a rate of 26% in the low-polymer group and 45% in the high-polymer group. The α-amylase digestive enzyme activity was significantly lower in the experimental groups than in the control group, likely because the large number of phenolic hydroxyl groups in the polyphenols interacted with the peptidyl-NH-CO-, amino-NH$_2$-, and carboxyl-COOH groups of the enzymes in the form of hydrogen bonds, forming a non-digestible complex that caused the catalytic activity of the enzymes to be reduced or lost. α-amylase activity was significantly lower in mice in the high- vs. low-polymer group, likely because the proanthocyanidins with high degrees of polymerization had more sites that bind with α-amylase, increasing the number of interactions between these molecules.

2.2.2. Trypsin and Pepsin Activity

The trypsin and pepsin activity in the small intestine, pancreas, and stomach was significantly lower in the high-polymer group compared to the control ($p < 0.05$; Table 2). Although this activity was lower in the low-polymer group than in the control, the difference was not significant ($p > 0.05$).

Perhaps proanthocyanidins with a high degree of polymerization were more susceptible to binding by proteases than were the other proanthocyanidins. In the small intestine, trypsin activity was inhibited at a rate of 15% in the low-polymer group and 32% in the high-polymer group. In the pancreas, trypsin activity was inhibited at a rate of 21% in the low-polymer group and 39% in the high-polymer group. In the stomach, pepsin activity was inhibited at a rate of 13% in the low-polymer group and 38% in the high-polymer group.

2.2.3. Pancreatic Lipase Activity

Pancreatic lipase activity in the small intestine and pancreas was lower in the experimental groups than in the control group, but the difference was not significant ($p > 0.05$; Table 2), suggesting that both groups of proanthocyanidins had a small inhibitory effect on lipase activity. In the small intestine, pancreatic lipase activity was inhibited at a rate of 7% in the low-polymer group and 10% in the high-polymer group. In the pancreas, pancreatic lipase activity was inhibited at a rate of 10% in the low-polymer group and 13% in the high-polymer group. Compared to amylase and protease activity, proanthocyanidins had a smaller effect on pancreatic lipase activity, perhaps because pancreatic lipase has a weaker affinity for these compounds than the other digestive enzymes.

Table 2. Effects of procyanidins with different degrees of polymerization on digestive enzyme activity in mice [1].

Relative Enzyme Activity	Control Group	Low-Polymer Group	Rate of Inhibition of Digestive Enzyme Activity in the Low-Polymer Group	High-Polymer Group	Degree of Digestive Enzyme Activity Inhibition in the High-Polymer Group
α-amylase activity in small intestine	0.34 ± 0.05 [a]	0.27 ± 0.06 [b]	21%	0.20 ± 0.03 [c]	41%
α-amylase activity in the pancreas	0.47 ± 0.05 [a]	0.35 ± 0.04 [b]	26%	0.26 ± 0.04 [c]	45%
Pancrelipase activity in the small intestine	2.21 ± 0.08 [a]	2.05 ± 0.2 [a]	7%	1.99 ± 0.16 [a]	10%
Pancrelipase activity in the pancreas	3.28 ± 0.21 [a]	2.95 ± 0.25 [a]	10%	2.84 ± 0.39 [a]	13%

[a,b] Different superscripts in the same line indicate significant differences ($p < 0.05$); digestive enzyme activity unit (U mg prot^{-1}). [1] The rate of inhibition by proanthocyanidins with different degrees of polymerization on digestive enzyme activity = (Digestive enzyme activity of control group—Digestive enzyme activity of experimental group)/Digestive enzyme activity of control group.

2.3. Effects of Proanthocyanidins with Different Degrees of Polymerization on Nutrient Digestibility

Proanthocyanidins with different degrees of polymerization had different effects on the apparent digestibility of proteins. The apparent digestibility of proteins was significantly lower in the high-polymer group than in the control group ($p < 0.05$; Table 3), but there was no significant difference in this value between the low-polymer and control group ($p > 0.05$). The decrease in apparent protein digestibility in the high-polymer group might have been due to the binding of polyphenols to proteases in mice, resulting in the inhibition of enzyme activity, a reduction in protein digestion, and, ultimately, a decrease in protein digestibility in vivo. In addition, polyphenols can directly combine with macromolecular proteins to form molecular complexes that are not easily digested and absorbed by the human body, reducing the effective utilization of nitrogen by intestinal microbes and ultimately reducing the utilization of proteins in food. Proteins are also major components of the cell membrane. Polyphenols can reduce the permeability of the plant cell membrane by binding to macromolecular substances on the cell surface, reducing the solubility of nutrients in the cell and ultimately decreasing the digestibility of proteins in feed. The apparent digestibility of protein was significantly lower in the high- vs. low-polymer group, perhaps because polyphenols containing more hydroxyl groups or with a higher molecular weight react more readily with proteins. Although polyphenols bind to proteins, this binding is selective. The molecular mass, spatial configuration, and other aspects of polyphenols affect their reaction with proteins.

Table 3. Effects of procyanidins with different degrees of polymerization on nutrient absorption in mice.

Apparent Digestibility	Control Group	Low-Polymer Group	High-Polymer Group
Apparent digestibility of protein (%)	86.33 ± 0.67 [a]	84.89 ± 1.36 [a]	78.53 ± 1.91 [b]
Apparent digestibility of fat (%)	87.41 ± 0.98 [a]	86.08 ± 0.51 [a]	82.65 ± 1.91 [b]
Apparent digestibility of calcium (%)	33.01 ± 2.12 [a]	29.06 ± 3.08 [b]	27.97 ± 1.85 [b]
Apparent digestibility of zinc (%)	28.86 ± 0.80 [a]	24.45 ± 1.47 [b]	23.38 ± 1.50 [b]

[a, b] Different superscripts in the same line indicate significant differences ($p < 0.05$).

2.4. Effects of Proanthocyanidins with Different Degrees of Polymerization on Fat Digestibility

The apparent digestibility of fat was significantly lower in the high polymerization group than the control group ($p < 0.05$; Table 3), but there was no significant difference between these values in the low-polymer group vs. the control ($p > 0.05$). The decrease in lipid digestibility in the high-polymer group might have been due to the strong complexation of polyphenols with lipid macromolecules, which hindered the biodegradation of lipids and ultimately led to a decrease in fat digestibility. In addition, polyphenols could bind to phospholipids, proteins, and polysaccharides on the surfaces of cell membranes, thereby reducing the permeability of the membrane and affecting the discharge of nutrients, ultimately leading to a decrease in fat digestibility. The combination of polyphenols with digestive enzymes in animals and enzymes secreted by microorganisms might also result in a decrease in fat digestibility.

2.5. Effects of Proanthocyanidins with Different Degrees of Polymerization on Ca and Zn Digestibility

The apparent digestibility of calcium and zinc was lower in the experimental groups than the control group ($p < 0.05$; Table 3). These values were lower in the high-polymer group than the low-polymer group, but the difference was not significant ($p > 0.05$). The decrease in apparent digestibility of calcium and zinc in the experimental groups might have been due to the formation of chelates of polyphenols and metal ions that are poorly digested and absorbed by the body [17]. In addition, polyphenols may damage the intestinal mucosa by binding to proteins on the mucosa of the small intestine, thus reducing the bioavailability of mineral elements. Under our experimental conditions, both low- and high-polymer proanthocyanidins reduced the digestibility of Ca and Zn in mice, with no significant differences between these values.

3. Discussion

Energy and protein are the core factors affecting the metabolism and growth performance of animals. A deficiency or imbalance in dietary protein and energy can affect lean tissue deposition and protein turnover, resulting in low weight gain and feed conversion rates [18].

Proteins are a basic component of living cells and tissues that play key roles in numerous life activities. Protein digestion and absorption disorders affect human growth and development. In the current study, the apparent digestibility of proteins in the high-polymer group was significantly reduced, which was likely detrimental to the growth of mice. The apparent digestibility of proteins was significantly lower in mice in the high- vs. low-polymer group. Perhaps high-molecular-weight proanthocyanidins substantially alter the conformation of proteins, thereby affecting their digestibility and absorption.

The combination of polyphenols and amino acids can affect the quantity and proportion of certain essential amino acids, and the reduced nutritional value of the protein will inevitably affect normal growth and development [19]. Indeed, the reaction of polyphenols with soy proteins blocks the absorption of lysine, tryptophan, and cysteine, thereby reducing the bioavailability of essential amino acids, as revealed by Rawel et al. [20]. Moreover, since the enzyme protease is a protein, the inhibition of protease activity also affects protein digestion.

In the current study, high-polymer proanthocyanidins had a strong effect on proteases and to some extent also affected the biodegradation of proteins. Because the weak binding forces within these molecules have little effect on the conformation of proteins and proteases, they do not substantially alter the biological activity or physiological functions of proteins. Therefore, oligomeric proanthocyanidins are less likely to interfere with the absorption and utilization of proteins by the organism than are high-polymer proanthocyanidins. The diverse structures of proanthocyanidins make their interactions with proteins stereospecific. The degree of binding between these molecules is not only affected by the degree of polymerization of proanthocyanidins, but also by factors such as the molecular shape, hydrodynamic radius, phenolic hydroxyl position, degree of acylation, and steric hindrance. Although the number of active sites on polyphenols available for protein binding increases proportionally with the number of structural units of flavonols, this number is not proportional to the amount of precipitate obtained. In vitro, the affinity of catechin for proline is stronger than that of epicatechin. According to De et al. [21], the affinity of proanthocyanidin B3 and B4 (C4-C8) for proline is greater than that of their analogs B6 and B8 (C4-C6), respectively, whereas the degrees of specific binding of proanthocyanidin C1 (trimer) to proline, proanthocyanidins B2 (dimer), and epicatechin (monomer) are similar. A similar experiment using proanthocyanidins with different degrees of polymerization could be performed in the future.

The combination of polyphenols and the active sites of digestive enzymes (the phenolic hydroxyl groups present in polyphenols bind to the peptidyl groups of the enzymes (-NH-CO-, amino-NH_2-, and carboxyl-COOH) via hydrogen bonds) alters the molecular structure of the enzyme, for instance by reducing the number of free amino acids and altering the structure of the amino acid side chain, resulting in a decrease or loss of biological activity, and thereby affecting the digestion and absorption of carbohydrates. Goncalves et al. [13] confirmed the wider interaction between α-amylase and high-polymer proanthocyanidins through fluorescence quenching, dynamic light scattering analysis, and turbidimetry. In the current study, the rate of inhibition of α-amylase activity in the high polymer group was close to 50%, which would reduce the biodegradation of carbohydrates, and thus limit growth and development. As shown in the above table, the affinity between polyphenols and various enzymes differed. The rate of α-amylase inhibition was greater than that of other digestive enzymes, which may be related to the stereostructure of the enzyme, the molecular weight, and/or the number of specific amino acids on the surface of the enzyme molecule.

Compared to other digestive enzymes, amylase was more strongly affected by proanthocyanidin solution, likely because many amino acid residues on its surface bind to proanthocyanidins. The digestion and absorption of carbohydrates are also closely related to the presence of a glucose transporter. Johnston et al. [22] found that proanthocyanidins can inhibit the transport of glucose by inhibiting the activity of glucose transporter II, thereby reducing the rate of glucose release and absorption in the small intestine.

Polyphenols can alter the emulsifying properties of fat by binding to the lipid layer or the hydrophilic head of lecithin outside the emulsion droplets [23]. In the current study, fat digestibility in mice was lower in the high-polymer group than the low-polymer group. Perhaps the high-molecular-weight polyphenols function as connectors between the complexes, thereby increasing the droplet size and inhibiting the digestion and absorption of fat. According to Haslam [24], the mechanism of polyphenol–lipid complex formation is similar to the polyphenol–protein binding mechanism, which is based on hydrogen bonds and hydrophobic bonds. The high-polymer group of mice had lower fat digestibility, possibly due to the stronger binding between the high-polymer proanthocyanidins and lipids, which would limit the biodegradation of pancreatic lipase. Compared to pancreatic amylase and trypsin activity, the inhibitory effect of proanthocyanidins on pancreatic lipase activity is generally small, perhaps because this enzyme has fewer amino acid residues that bind to proanthocyanidins due to its spatial configuration and smaller molecular weight. Recent studies on the effects of polyphenols on pancreatic lipase activity have yielded mixed results. Sugiyama et al. performed in vitro simulated digestion experiments that showed that catechin and epicatechin have no inhibitory effect on pancreatic lipase activity. As the degree of polymerization (dimer–pentamer) increased, the inhibitory effects of proanthocyanidins on pancreatic lipase activity increased. The inhibition of pancreatic lipase activity by proanthocyanidins above the polymer is not much different [25]. Griffiths et al. [26] demonstrated that polyphenols inhibit murine α-amylase and trypsin activity and promote pancreatic lipase activity. Longstaff et al. [27] found that polyphenols inhibited α-amylase, trypsin, and pancreatic lipase activity in chickens, but when the protein content in the feed increased to a certain level, polyphenols increased pancreatic lipase activity, perhaps due to the stronger binding of protein molecules to polyphenols, which weakened the effects of polyphenols on lipase. The results of experiments investigating the effects of polyphenols on pancreatic lipase activity may be affected by factors such as experimental methods, experimental subjects, and polyphenol types.

4. Materials and Methods

4.1. Separation and Measurement of Proanthocyanidins with Different Degrees of Polymerization

Proanthocyanidins were isolated from grape (*Vitis vinifera*) seeds by the methanol-chloroform solvent two-phase precipitation method [28]. Proanthocyanidin levels and quality were determined by the vanillin-glacial acetic acid method, and the average degree of polymerization of the samples was calculated by combining the average molecular weights of the compounds [29]. Animal feeding experiments were performed using fragments with degrees of polymerization of 2–4 units and >10 units for the low- and high-polymer group, respectively.

4.2. Feed Management and Sample Collection

Twenty-four adult male-specific pathogen-free Wistar rats (Chinese Academy of Medical Sciences Animal Breeding Center, Beijing, China) were used in the experiments. Animal experiments were performed according to ethical standard issued by the National Institutes of Health Guide for the Care and Use of Laboratory Animals and approved by Institutional Animal Care and Use Committee.

The conditions of the animal breeding room were 20–25 °C, 55–60% humidity, and a 12 h:12 h light/dark cycle. The mice were free to eat and drink for one week. After 7 days of laboratory conditioning, the mice were randomly divided into three groups of eight animals per group. The mice were fed intragastrically once per day at 3 pm for 8 weeks. The first group of mice was fed with distilled water as a blank control. The second group was fed with an oligomeric proanthocyanidin solution at a dose of 150 mg/kg. The third group was fed with a high-polymer proanthocyanidin solution at a dose of 150 mg/kg. The mice ate basal feed freely, and weight gain and feed consumption were recorded weekly. The mouse feces were collected and weighed for 6–8 weeks. After the experiment, all experimental mice were sacrificed in the morning on an empty stomach, the rats were euthanized by lethal intraperitoneal injection of pentobarbital (150 mg/kg; <200 mg/mL) and quickly dissected. Subsequently, the contents of the small intestine and stomach were collected, and the pancreas was collected, weighted and homogenized in 1: 9 (w/v) physiological saline for 30 s by using the FJ-200 type high-speed tissue homogenizer, then centrifuged at 4 °C for 10 min and placed in liquid nitrogen, and transferred to a -80 °C freezer for further assays [30].

4.3. Determination of Food Utility Rate

Food utility rate was calculated as follows:

$$\text{Food utility rate (\%)} = \text{weight gain (g)}/\text{feed intake (g)} \tag{1}$$

4.4. Determination of Enzyme Activity

The activities of alpha-amylase, pancreatic lipase, trypsin, and pepsin were determined using commercial kits purchased from Nanjing Jiancheng Institute of Bioengineering (Nanjing, China) according to the manufacturer's instructions.

Digestive enzyme activity was calculated as follows:

$$\text{Digestive enzyme activity} = (\text{digestive enzyme activity in the control group} - \text{digestive enzyme activity in the experimental group})/\text{digestive enzyme activity in the control group} \quad (2)$$

4.5. Determination of Protein Digestibility

The content of crude protein in feed and feces was determined by the Kjeldahl method. Each feed or feces sample was weighed, sequentially combined with copper sulfate, potassium sulfate, and concentrated sulfuric acid, gently shaken, and heated with a small flame in an electric furnace. After the contents were completely carbonized and foam generation had stopped, the flame intensity increased. After the liquid turned blue-green, the sample was heated for a bit longer, removed from the furnace, and cooled to a constant volume. The reaction was carried out using NaOH solution in a Auto-Kjeldahl Apparatus (KDY–9820, China). NH_3 was released by distillation and collected in H_3BO_3 solution. Titration was carried out using a known concentration of a sulfuric acid standard solution, and the nitrogen content was calculated based on the consumption of H_2SO_4. The nitrogen content was multiplied by 6.25, and the protein content was calculated as follows:

$$\text{Apparent protein digestibility (\%)} = (\text{intake of nitrogen} - \text{fecal nitrogen})/\text{intake of nitrogen} \times 100 \quad (3)$$

4.6. Determination of Fat Digestibility

Soxhlet extraction techniques were used to determine the crude fat content of feed and feces. A 2 g sample of ground feed or feces was transferred to a tube of filter paper, which was placed into a Soxhlet extraction tube. Anhydrous ether was added to the upper end of the extraction tube, and the sample was heated in a water bath for reflux extraction until the extraction was complete. After removing the fat receiving bottle, the remaining ether in the water bath was evaporated, and the fat receiving bottle was placed in a desiccator and dried. The operation was repeated until a constant weight was achieved, and the increase in weight of the receiving bottle was used to calculate the crude fat content in the sample.

$$\text{Apparent digestibility of fat (\%)} = (\text{intake of fat} - \text{fat in feces})/\text{intake of fat} \times 100 \quad (4)$$

4.7. Determination of Minerals Digestibility

The calcium and zinc contents in animal feed and feces were determined by atomic absorption spectrometry. After placing 1 g of ground feed or feces into a crucible, the samples were placed on an electric heating plate for low-temperature carbonization. The sample was completely carbonized, and the crucible was transferred to a muffle furnace at 550 °C for high-temperature ashing. After adding HCl to dissolve all inorganic elements in the ash, the sample was diluted to a constant volume. The sample was introduced into the air-acetylene flame of the atomic absorption spectrophotometer (Perkin-Elmer Corp., Shelton, CT, USA), and the Ca and Zn contents were quantitatively determined using the standard curve method. The apparent digestibility of calcium and zinc was calculated according to the following formulas:

$$\text{Apparent absorption rate of calcium and zinc (\%)} = (\text{intake of calcium and zinc} - \text{amount of calcium and zinc in the feces})/\text{intake of calcium and zinc} \times 100 \quad (5)$$

$$\text{Intake of calcium and zinc (mg/day)} = \text{contents of calcium and zinc in feed}/\% \text{ amount of feed consumption (mg/day)} \quad (6)$$

Amount of fecal calcium and zinc (mg/day) = contents of calcium and zinc in feces/% × amount of fecal output (mg/day) (7)

4.8. Statistical Analysis

The experimental data for each treatment group were expressed as the average ± standard deviation. The Duncan new repolarization difference method to analyze differences amongst multiple samples. Correlation analysis was performed using SPSS 17.0 software (SPSS Inc., Chicago, IL, USA). Differences between samples were considered to be significant at $p < 0.05$.

5. Conclusions

Our 56-day intragastric experiment suggested that treatment with high-polymer proanthocyanidins had a significant effect on digestive enzyme activity and the digestion and absorption of nutrients in mice. The anti-nutritional properties of polyphenols depend on their content [31]. The current study confirmed that the high degree of polymerization of proanthocyanidins is a major reason for their antinutritional properties. Therefore, during the process of food production, the anti-nutritional properties of polyphenols could be minimized by reducing the degree of polymerization of proanthocyanidins. However, in this study, we only explored the effects of proanthocyanidins with different degrees of polymerization on nutrient digestion and digestive enzyme activities in vivo from a macroscopic perspective. The specific reaction patterns were not studied in depth. We plan to conduct a follow-up investigation on this metabolic mechanism at the cellular or molecular level, by analyzing the amino acid sequences, secondary structures, and conformational changes of the complexed proteins. Such studies should provide scientific guidelines for including proanthocyanidin use in the food, chemical, pharmaceutical, and other industries, thereby improving the comprehensive utilization rate of these beneficial compounds.

Author Contributions: H.Z., Z.W., and G.C. conceived and designed the experiments; H.Z., Y.X., X.L., Q.S., and Y.C. performed the experiments; Z.W. and G.C. contributed reagents/materials/analysis tools; H.Z, Z.W., and G.C. wrote the paper.

Funding: This research was funded by Natural Science Foundation of Shandong Province, China (ZR2016CM48), National Key Research and Development Program of Shandong (2018GSF121019), Young Talents Training Program of Shandong Academy of Agricultural Sciences (2016), and China Postdoctoral Science Foundation (2014M551942).

Conflicts of Interest: The authors declare no conflict of interest.

References

1. Ibars, M.; Ardidruiz, A.; Suárez, M.; Muguerza, B.; Bladé, C.; Aragonès, G. Proanthocyanidins potentiate hypothalamic leptin/STAT3 signalling and *Pomc* gene expression in rats with diet-induced obesity. *Int. J. Obes.* **2017**, *41*, 129–136. [CrossRef] [PubMed]
2. Bagchi, D.; Garg, A.; Krohn, R.L.; Bagchi, M.; Tran, M.X.; Stohs, S.J. Oxygen free radical scavenging abilities of vitamins C and E, and a grape seed proanthocyanidin extract in vitro. *Res. Commun. Mol. Pathol. Pharmacol.* **1997**, *95*, 179–189. [PubMed]
3. Casanova-Martí, À.; Serrano, J.; Blay, M.T.; Terra, X.; Ardévol, A.; Pinent, M. Acute selective bioactivity of grape seed proanthocyanidins on enteroendocrine secretions in the gastrointestinal tract. *Food Nutr. Res.* **2017**, *61*. [CrossRef] [PubMed]
4. Chung, S.W.; Yao, H.W.; Caito, S.; Hwang, J.W.; Arunachalam, G.; Rahman, I. Regulation of SIRT1 in cellular functions: role of polyphenols. *Arch. Biochem. Biophys.* **2010**, *501*, 79–90. [CrossRef] [PubMed]
5. Ramosromero, S.; Hereu, M.; Molinartoribio, E.; Almajano, M.P.; Méndez, L.; Medina, I.; Taltavull, N.; Romeu, M.; Nogués, M.R.; Torres, J.L. Effects of the combination of ω-3 PUFAs and proanthocyanidins on the gut microbiota of healthy rats. *Food Res. Int.* **2017**, *97*, 364–371. [CrossRef] [PubMed]
6. Rodrigo, R.; Miranda, A.; Vergara, L. Modulation of endogenous antioxidant system by wine polyphenols in human disease. *Clin. Chim. Acta* **2011**, *412*, 410–424. [CrossRef] [PubMed]

7. Smeriglio, A.; Barreca, D.; Bellocco, E.; Trombetta, D. Proanthocyanidins and hydrolysable tannins: Occurrence, dietary intake and pharmacological effects. *Br. J. Pharmacol.* **2017**, *174*, 1244–1262. [CrossRef] [PubMed]
8. Casanova-Martí, À.; Serrano, J.; Portune, K.J.; Sanz, Y.; Blay, M.T.; Terra, X.; Ardévol, A.; Pinent, M. Grape seed proanthocyanidins influence gut microbiota and enteroendocrine secretions in female rats. *Food Funct.* **2018**, *9*, 1672–7682. [CrossRef] [PubMed]
9. Lu, Y.P.; Yao, K.; Jia, D.Y. Antinutrition and Biodegradation of Vegetable Tannins in Forage. *J. Anim. Sci.* **2003**, *2*, 42–43.
10. Prigent, S.V.; Voragen, A.G.; Koningsveld, G.A.V.; Baron, A.; Renard, C.M.G.C.; Gruppen, H. Interactions between globular proteins and procyanidins of different degrees of polymerization. *J. Dairy Sci.* **2009**, *92*, 5843–5853. [CrossRef] [PubMed]
11. Eastmond, R.; Gardner, R.J. Effect of various polyphenols on the rate of haze formation in beer. *J. Inst. Brew.* **1974**, *80*, 192–200. [CrossRef]
12. Stojadinovic, M.; Radosavljevic, J.; Ognjenovic, J.; Vesic, J.; Prodic, I.; Stanic-Vucinic, D.; Velickovic, T.C. Binding affinity between dietary polyphenols and β-lactoglobulin negatively correlates with the protein susceptibility to digestion and total antioxidant activity of complexes formed. *Food Chem.* **2013**, *136*, 1263–1271. [CrossRef] [PubMed]
13. Gonçalves, R.; Mateus, N.; De Freitas, V. Inhibition of α-amylase activity by condensed tannins. *Food Chem.* **2011**, *125*, 665–672. [CrossRef]
14. Baxter, N.J.; Lilley, T.H.; Haslam, E.; Williamson, M.P. Multiple interactions between polyphenols and a salivary proline-rich protein repeat result in complexation and precipitation. *Biochemistry* **1997**, *36*, 5566–5577. [CrossRef] [PubMed]
15. Sarni-Manchado, P.; Canals-Bosch, J.M.; Mazerolles, G.; Cheynier, V. Influence of the glycosylation of human salivary proline-rich proteins on their interactions with condensed tannins. *J. Agric. Food Chem.* **2008**, *56*, 9563–9569. [CrossRef] [PubMed]
16. Rasoamanana, R.; Even, P.C.; Darcel, N.; Tomé, D.; Fromentin, G. Dietary fibers reduce food intake by satiation without conditioned taste aversion in mice. *Physiol. Behav.* **2013**, *110*, 13–19. [CrossRef] [PubMed]
17. De Oliveira, D.R.; Schaffer, L.F.; Busanello, A.; Barbosa, C.P.; Peroza, L.R.; de Freitas, C.M.; Krum, B.N.; Bressan, N.G.; Boligon, A.A.; Athayde, M.L.; et al. Silymarin has antioxidant potential and changes the activity of Na+/K+-ATPase and monoamine oxidase in vitro. *Ind. Crops Prod.* **2015**, *70*, 347–355. [CrossRef]
18. Chiba, L.I.; Lewis, A.J.; Peo, E.R. Amino acid and energy interrelationships in pigs weighing 20 to 50 kilograms: I. Rate and efficiency of weight gain. *J. Anim. Sci.* **1991**, *69*, 694–707. [CrossRef] [PubMed]
19. Jakobek, L. Interactions of polyphenols with carbohydrates, lipids and proteins. *Food Chem.* **2015**, *175*, 556–567. [CrossRef] [PubMed]
20. Rawel, H.M.; Czajka, D.; Rohn, S.; Kroll, J. Interactions of different phenolic acids and flavonoids with soy proteins. *Int. J. Biol. Macromol.* **2002**, *30*, 137–150. [CrossRef]
21. De, F.V.; Mateus, N. Structural features of procyanidin interactions with salivary proteins. *J. Agric. Food Chem.* **2001**, *49*, 940–945.
22. Johnston, K.; Sharp, P.; Clifford, M.; Morgan, L. Dietary polyphenols decrease glucose uptake by human intestinal Caco-2 cells. *FEBS Lett.* **2005**, *579*, 1653–1657. [CrossRef] [PubMed]
23. Shishikura, Y.; Khokhar, S.; Murray, B.S. Effects of tea polyphenols on emulsification of olive oil in a small intestine model system. *J. Agric. Food Chem.* **2006**, *54*, 1906–1913. [CrossRef] [PubMed]
24. Haslam, E. Tannins, polyphenols and molecular complexation. *Chem. Ind. For. Prod.* **1992**, *12*, 1–24.
25. Sugiyama, H.; Akazome, Y.; Shoji, T.; Yamaguchi, A.; Yasue, M.; Kanda, T.; Ohtake, Y. Oligomeric procyanidins in apple polyphenol are main active components for inhibition of pancreatic lipase and triglyceride absorption. *J. Agric. Food Chem.* **2007**, *55*, 4604–4609. [CrossRef] [PubMed]
26. Griffiths, D.W.; Moseley, G. The effect of diets containing field beans of high and lob polyphenolic content on the activity of digestive enzymes in the intestine of rats. *J. Sci. Food Agric.* **1980**, *31*, 225–259. [CrossRef]
27. Longstaff, M.A.; Feuerstein, D.; McNab, J.M.; Mccorquodale, C. The influence of proanthocyanidin-rich bean hulls and level of dietary protein on energy metabolizability and nutrient digestibility by adult cockerels. *Br. J. Nutr.* **1993**, *70*, 355–367. [CrossRef] [PubMed]
28. Saucier, C.; Mirabel, M.; Daviaud, F.; Longieras, A.; Glories, Y. Rapid fractionation of grape seed proanthocyanidins. *J. Agric. Food Chem.* **2001**, *49*, 5732–5735. [CrossRef] [PubMed]

29. Butler, L.G.; Price, M.L.; Brotherton, J.E. Vanillin assay for proanthocyanidins (condensed tannins): Modification of the solvent for estimation of the degree of polymerization. *J. Agric. Food Chem.* **1982**, *30*, 1087–1089. [CrossRef]
30. Zhao, Z.G.; Zhu, H.X.; Zhang, L.M.; Zhang, Y.P.; Niu, C.Y. Mesenteric lymph drainage alleviates acute kidney injury induced by hemorrhagic shock without resuscitation. *Sci. World J.* **2014**, *1*. [CrossRef] [PubMed]
31. Burns, J.C. Antiquality factors as related to forage quality. *J. Dairy Sci.* **1978**, *61*, 1809–1820. [CrossRef]

Sample Availability: Samples of the compounds are not available from the authors.

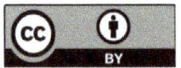

© 2018 by the authors. Licensee MDPI, Basel, Switzerland. This article is an open access article distributed under the terms and conditions of the Creative Commons Attribution (CC BY) license (http://creativecommons.org/licenses/by/4.0/).

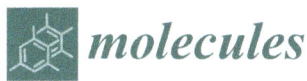

Article

Time-Dependent Degradation of Polyphenols from Thermally-Processed Berries and Their In Vitro Antiproliferative Effects against Melanoma

Zorița Diaconeasa

Faculty of Food Science and Technology, University of Agricultural Science and Veterinary Medicine Cluj-Napoca, Calea Mănăștur 3-5, 400372 Cluj-Napoca, Romania; zorita.sconta@usamvcluj.ro; Tel.: +40-751-033-871

Received: 3 September 2018; Accepted: 30 September 2018; Published: 4 October 2018

Abstract: Polyphenols are natural occurring micronutrients that can protect plants from natural weathering and are also helpful to humans. These compounds are abundantly found in fruits or berries. Because of berry seasonal availability and also due to their rapid degradation, people have found multiple ways to preserve them. The most common options are freezing or making jams. Polyphenol stability, during processing is a continuous challenge for the food industry. There are also multiple published data providing that they are sensitive to light, pH or high temperature, vectors which are all present during jam preparation. In this context the aim of this study was to assess phytochemical composition and bioactive compounds degradation after jam preparation. We also monitored their degradation during storage time and their in vitro antiproliferative potential when tested on melanoma cells. The obtained results revealed that when processed and stored in time, the bioactive compounds from berries jams are degrading, but they still exert antioxidant and antiproliferative potential. Prior to LC-MS analysis, polyphenolic compounds were identified as: flavonoids (anthocyanins (ANT), flavonols (FLA)) and non-flavonoid (hydroxycinnamic acids (HCA) and hydroxybenzoic acids (HBA)). The most significant decrease was observed for HCA compared to other classes of compounds. This variation is expected due to differences in constituents and phenolic types among different analyzed berries.

Keywords: berries jam; phenolic acids; flavonols glycosides; degradation; HPLC-ESI/MS

---

1. Introduction

Fruits and vegetables are important sources of bioactive compounds which were shown to have positive health benefits [1,2]. In recent years, food and nutrition sciences aimed to improve health through intelligent foods containing bioactive plant-based molecules that were proven to have positive health benefits, such as the prevention of cardiovascular diseases or cancer [3,4]. The demand for innovative and functional food products had increased lately due to the fact that consumers are more aware of their bodies and mental health. Diets rich in vegetables or fruits were proven to provide essential bioactive molecules which can play important roles in human health. These plant-based bioactive molecules include polyphenols (phenolic acids, flavonoids, anthocyanins, catechins), enzymes, amino acids, vitamins (vitamin C, folate, and provitamin A), minerals (potassium, calcium, and magnesium), and fibers (inulin, pectin, lignan). The related body of literature indicates a strong correlation between diet and degenerative diseases, and due to this fact, the use of natural compounds as ingredients in food has become a major concern for food technologists [5,6]. Berries and fruits are the main sources of bioactive compounds with many applications in the food, pharmaceutical, nutraceutical and cosmetic industries [7–10]. These bioactive compounds are mainly polyphenols, and among them, anthocyanins which have proved to have high nutritional and potential health value [11]. In vivo studies have shown that anthocyanins have many positive effects on the prevention of cardiovascular diseases, diabetes, and cancers (lung, colon, breast, and skin). Red berries, including the chokeberry, blueberry, blackcurrant, elderberry, raspberry, and cranberry, are widely consumed fresh or in processed forms, such as jams, juices, syrups, and various types of jellies. These fruits have been extensively investigated from the chemical point of view, particularly in fresh, juice, or dried forms [12]. Due to the fact that fresh berry consumption is not always possible, jam production is a good option for the food industry. In order to obtain high quality berry jams, the technological process must use low temperatures, environmentally-friendly and non-destructive methods. In this way, bioactive compounds can be protected from degradation, and the colour of the products can also be preserved. In order to influence consumers' acceptance, the product—jam in this case—must still have an attractive colour. This colour is related to the anthocyanin content and has a strong association with the antioxidant capacity. However, the temperature and time of processing must be chosen properly to ensure the stability of the anthocyanins and the conservation of the antioxidant activity [13–15]. Moreover, several other factors can affect the colour of berry jams, including the storage temperature, amount of light exposure, and pH [16–18]. The antioxidant capacity can decrease, remain unchanged, or even increase during processing or storage. Previous studies have revealed that the optimum storage temperature for jam is 4 °C, and the brief storage of raspberry jam at 4 °C has been associated with a lower rate of anthocyanin degradation compared to jam stored at a higher temperature (15 °C) [19]. The thermal treatment of anthocyanins is related to both anthocyanin and antioxidant capacity degradation [20]. In this context, the aim of present study is to prepare homemade jams using chokeberry, elderberry, blackcurrant, or blackthorn and to evaluate phenolic compounds degradation during storage time. Moreover the in vitro antiproliferative potential of the rich polyphenolic extracts will be tested on melanoma cell line. However, to the best of our knowledge, no previous studies have investigated the effect of food compounds processing on the phenolic compound content and the antioxidant capacity of homemade jams prepared using chokeberry (*Aronia melanocarpa*), elderberry (*Sambucus nigra*), blackcurrant (*Ribes nigrum*) or blackthorn (*Prunus spinosa*).

2. Results

2.1. LC-PDA-ESI/MS Identification and Quantification of Phenolic Compounds

2.1.1. Chokeberry Jam

The obtained jams and fresh berries were characterized by the presence of 11 compounds: five anthocyanins, four flavonols, one HCA and one HBA (Table 1). The identified anthocyanins were only glycosylated cyanidin, whereas, in the case of flavonols, we identified glycosylated quercetin as well as caffeic and ellagic acids which are forms of HCA and HBA, respectively. Cyanidin-3-O-galactoside was found to be the main compound among all the identified anthocyanins (Figure 1). It was identified by the m/z 449 molecular ion, which was confirmed by the fragment ion m/z 287, which corresponds to aglycone cyanidin (Figure 2).

The ESI-MS analysis of peaks 8, 9, and 10 showed the presence of molecular ions at m/z 419, corresponding to cyanidin-3-O-arabinoside; m/z 449, corresponding to cyanidin-3-O-glucoside; and m/z 419, corresponding to cyanidin-3-O-xyloside. Regarding the quantitative analysis, the flavonol profiles were consistent with those reported previously, except that quercetin-3-O-rutinoside was found to be present in a higher amount [21,22]. In addition to the flavonols identified in our study, Mikulic-Petkovsek et al. identified four more quercetin glycosides: glucuronide, xyloside, arabinopyranoside, and robinobioside [21,23]. At peak 1, the MS parent ion m/z 163 was identified as caffeic acid which is in agreement with the available literature [24].

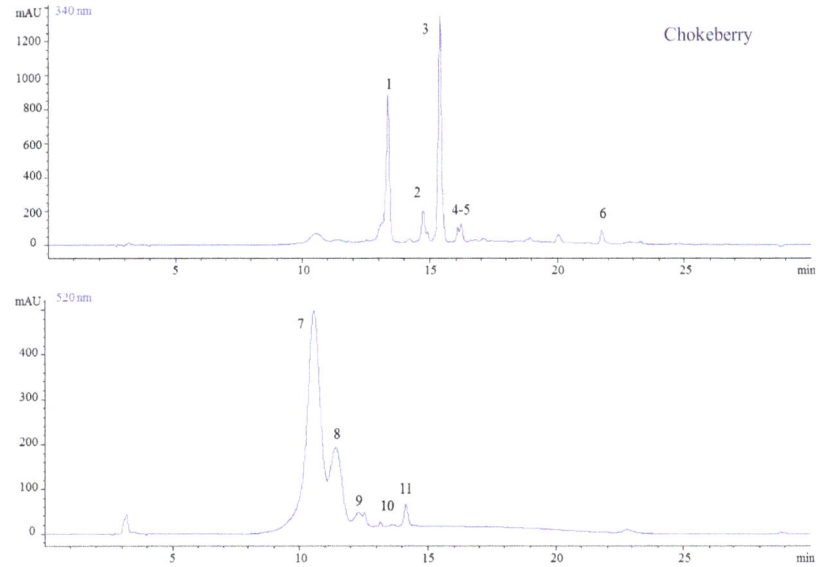

Figure 1. HPLC-DAD chromatogram of extracts from chokeberry jams (at 340 and 520 nm).

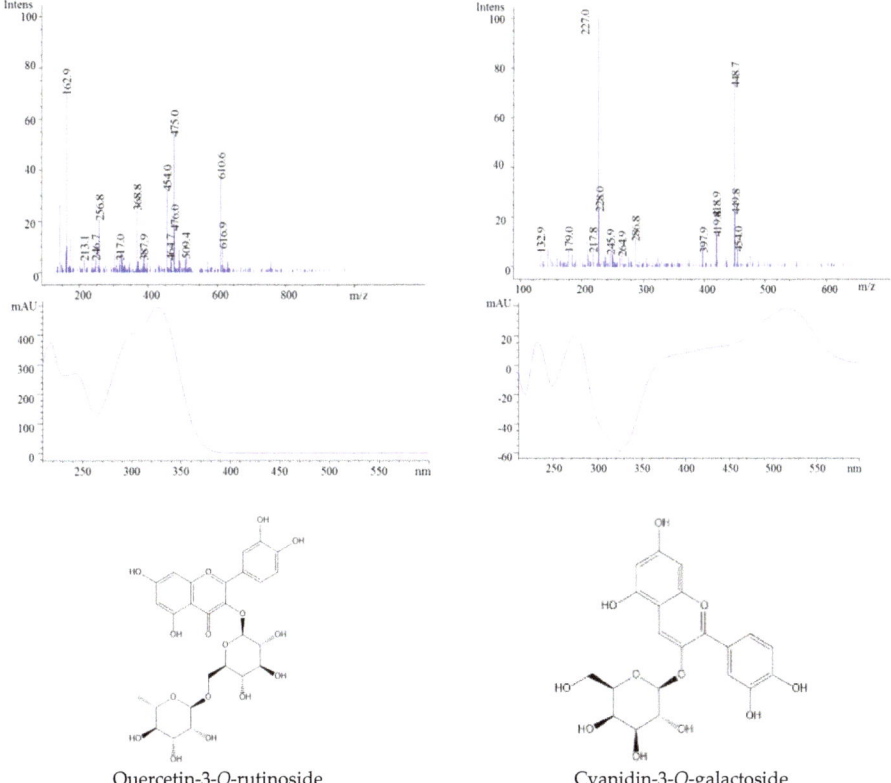

Quercetin-3-O-rutinoside   Cyanidin-3-O-galactoside

Figure 2. HPLC-MS spectra, UV/vis scanning spectra, and the chemical structures of peaks 3 and 7.

Table 1. Chromatographic, mass spectral characteristics and tentative identification of compounds compounds in berry jams by LC-PDA-ESI/MS.

Peak No.	R_t (min)	Parent Ion	Fragment Ion	MW	UV Spectra	Compound	Ref
Chokeberry							
1	13.42	181	163	180	323	Caffeic acid	
2	14.79	465	303	464	355	Quercetin-3-O-galactoside	
3	15.42	611	303	610	354	Quercetin-3-O-rutinoside (Rutin)	
4	16.11	465	303	464	355	Quercetin-3-O-glucoside	
5	16.29	-	303	302.1	364	Ellagic acid	
6	21.90	-	303	302	369	Quercetin	[22,23,25]
7	10.80	449	287	449	528	Cyanidin-3-O-galactoside	
8	11.57	419	287	419	517	Cyanidin-3-O-arabinoside	
9	12.58	419	287	454	519	Cyanidin-3-O-xyloside	
10	13.20	449	287	449	518	Cyanidin-3-O-glucoside	
11	14.31	-	287	287	528	Cyanidin	
Blackthorn							
1	13.14	181	163	180	319	Caffeic acid	
2	14.47	355	181, 163	354	325	Neochlorogenic acid	
3	15.19	611	303	610	354	Quercetin-3-O-rutinoside (rutin)	
4	21.38	303		302	369	Quercetin	[26]
5		449	287	449	528	Cyanidin-3-O-galactoside	
6	10.84	595	449, 287	595	516	Cyanidin-3-O-rutinoside	
7	11.96	609	463, 301	611	524	Peonidin-3-(6″-coumaroyl) glucoside	
Elderberry							
1	13.39	355	181, 163	354	352	Chlorogenic acid	
2	15.44	611	303	610	354	Quercetin-3-O-rutinoside	
3	16.14	465	303	464	355	Quercetin-3-O-glucoside	[27]
4	21.38	-	303	302	369	Quercetin	
5	10.94	581	449, 287	616	518	Cyanidin-3-O-sambubioside	
6	14.29	449,	287	449	518	Cyanidin-3-O-glucoside	
Blackcurrant							
1	11.16	301	139	300	252	4-Hydroxybenzoic acid-4-O-glucoside	
2	13.59	343	181, 163	343	321	Caffeic acid-4-O-glucoside	
3	13.97	595	287	594	346	Kaempferol-3-O-rutinoside	
4	14.59	627	319	626	355	Myricetin-3-O-rutinoside	
5	15.04	465	319	646	372	Myricetin-3-O-rhamnoside	
6	15.66	611	303	610	354	Quercetin-3-O-rutinoside	
7	16.37	465	303	464	355	Quercetin-3-O-glucoside	
8	16.70	357	195	194	316	Ferulic acid-4-O-glucoside	
9	17.47	449	287	448	346	Kaempferol-3-O-galactoside	
10	17.84	567	319	566	355	Myricetin-3-O-(6″-malonyl-glucoside)	[12,28,29]
11	19.25	319		300	255	Hydroxybenzoic acid-4	
12	20.25	551	303	550	358	Quercetin-3-O-(6″-malonyl-glucoside)	
13	21.99	303		302	369	Quercetin	
14	22.53	449	287	448	346	Kaempferol-3-O-glucoside	
15	22.98	287		286	365	Kaempferol	
16	10.12	465	303	465	524	Delphinidin-3-O-glucoside	
17	10.57			611	528	Delphinidin-3-O-rutinoside	
18	11.38	595	287	449	518	Cyanidin-3-O-glucoside	
19	14.38	449	287	287	514	Cyanidin	
20	15.64	303		303	520	Delphinidin	

A decrease in the content of anthocyanins was observed immediately after processing and also, during storage time as it is shown in Figure 3.

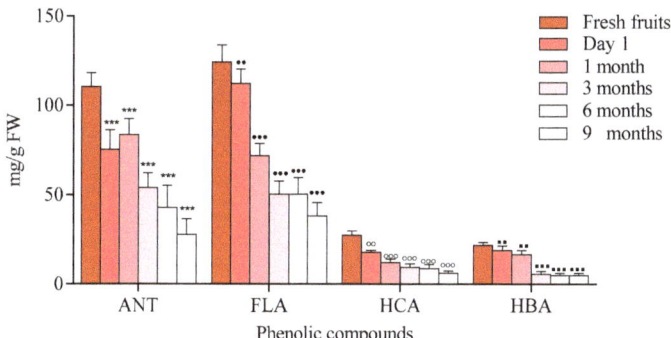

Figure 3. Phenolic compound degradation of chokeberry jams during storage, (anthocyanins (ANT), flavonols (FLA), (hydroxycinnamic acids (HCA) hydroxybenzoic acids (HBA)) Data represents the means ± SEM of at least three independent experiments (significant differences, **, ••, °°, ʺ $p < 0.01$, ***, •••, °°°, ʺʺ $p < 0.001$).

This degradation can be attributed to the hydrolytic reactions that led to the conversion of anthocyanin glycosides into chalcones, whose form can be rapidly transformed into phenolic acids and aldehydes.

Moreover, heat stable forms of polyphenol oxidase or peroxidase may play roles in the reduction of anthocyanins [30,31]. Another mechanism that may be associated with anthocyanin degradation is related to the hydrolysis of the glycoside linkages. This hydrolysis is known as the first step towards anthocyanin degradation, because high temperatures can shift the anthocyanin equilibrium towards the colorless chalcones. Chalcone degradation can occur due to the presence of oxidation reactions which can generate brown compounds or pigments that have high molecular weights. Additionally, pH values can affect the flavylium salt degradation, which is stable under highly acidic conditions. At higher pH values, salts can lose a proton and are easily transformed into an unstable pigment (quinoidal base) that is bonded to water and forms a colorless compound, commonly known as chromanol [30,32]. During processing and at the end of the storage period, anthocyanin degradation ranged from 58.90% to 74.30%. The results of the loss of anthocyanin content were lower compared with data reported previously for processed and stored black carrot jam and marmalade (87.60–95.60%). Degradation was also observed in flavonoids immediately after processing and during storage. This finding is in agreement with the previously reported data for *Rubus coreanus* Miquel berry jams [33]. The results revealed that jams prepared at pH 2.0–3.0 lost 33–35% of their anthocyanins, while the total amount of anthocyanins in jams obtained at pH 3.5–4.0 were degraded by 40–48%. In another study on blueberry jam, in contrast to other polyphenolics, the level of total flavonols was stable in response to processing, with >94% retention, compared to levels found in fresh berries [31] (Figure 3). Our study showed a degradation of HBA compound ranging from 70 to 90%. This had the highest degradation rate comparing with other existing compounds.

Chokeberries are a rich source of anthocyanins compared with other fruits. Due to this, they are usually used in the food industry as colorants or as a supplementary source of antioxidants. A recent study showed that the supplementation of strawberry jams with chokeberries and flowering quince during processing increase in the content of phenolic components in final products, especially for proanthocyanidins [34].

2.1.2. Blackthorn

These berries are becoming very popular in the food industry due to their complex and valuable phytochemical composition and also due to their easily availability in nature. The chromatographic analysis of fresh berries or jams revealed the presence of five phenolic compounds (Figure 4).

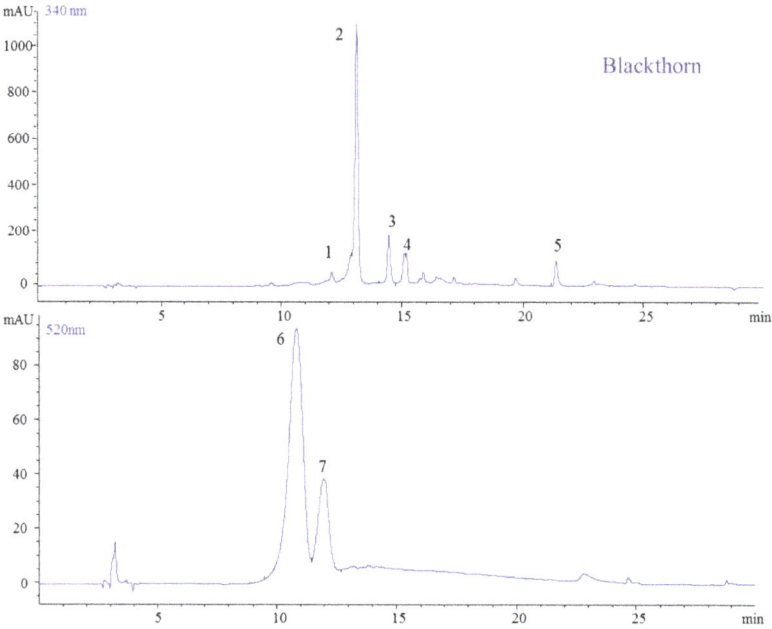

Figure 4. HPLC-DAD chromatogram of extracts from blackthorn jams (at 340 and 520 nm).

The identified compounds are summarized in Table 1. The mass spectra of peak 1 displayed a parent ion at m/z 181 and one fragment ion at m/z 163, which was identified as caffeic acid, while peak 2 had an ion at m/z 181 which was identified as neochlorogenic acid. Two more molecules were identified as quercetin (m/z 303) and quercetin-3-O-rutinoside (m/z 611). Anthocyanins were shown to be the most abundant class (fresh berries, jam), followed by flavonols and HCA. In contrast to the other berries in this study, blackthorn did not contain HBA. The identified anthocyanins were two glycosylated cyanidins and one acylated peonidin. For peak 5, in the case of cyanidins, the ESI-MS analysis indicated the presence of a molecular ion at m/z 449 corresponding to cyanidin-3-O-galactoside.

The second isolated anthocyanin showed a molecular ion at m/z 595, suggesting the presence of cyanidin-3-O-rutinoside. In this case, the ion at m/z 449 showed a loss of one molecule of rhamnoside and an ion at m/z 287, confirming the presence of aglycone cyanidin. Further, the peaks, registered with a molecular ion at m/z 603 and a fragment ion at m/z 301, were identified as peonidin 3-(6″-coumaroyl) glucoside. Peak 4 had a molecular ion at m/z 609 and two fragment ions at m/z 463 and m/z 301, which indicated the presence of peonidin 3-(6″-coumaroyl) glucoside (Figure 5). This anthocyanin identification is in agreement with Stefănuț et al., who also reported the presence of peonidin-3-O-rutinoside [26]. These differences may be attributed to the climatic conditions or harvesting time.

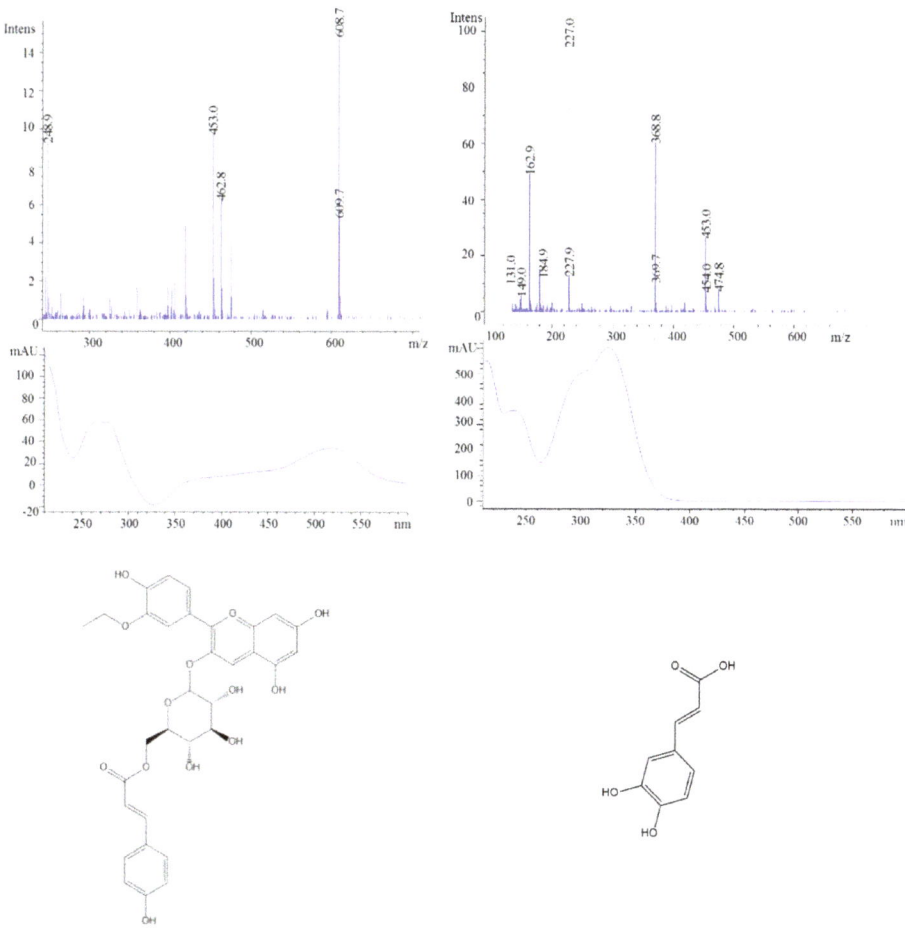

Figure 5. HPLC-MS spectra, UV/vis scanning spectra, and the chemical structures of peaks 1 and 7.

After processing, the bioactive compounds of blackthorn jam decreased (Figure 6). The amount of anthocyanins in berries decreased by 50% immediately after thermal processing compared to fresh ones and reached 82.56% after 6 months of storage. The same results were reported for black carrot (*Daucus carota*) jams and marmalades [30]. After 20 weeks of storage, the preserved anthocyanins and antioxidant capacity in samples stored at 4 °C were 53.4–81.0% and 45.2–92.0%, respectively. Time-dependent degradation of flavonols, ranging from 23 to 67%, was also observed. As in the case of HCA, the amounts of caffeic and neochlorogenic acid dramatically decreased from 41 to 81% during storage time.

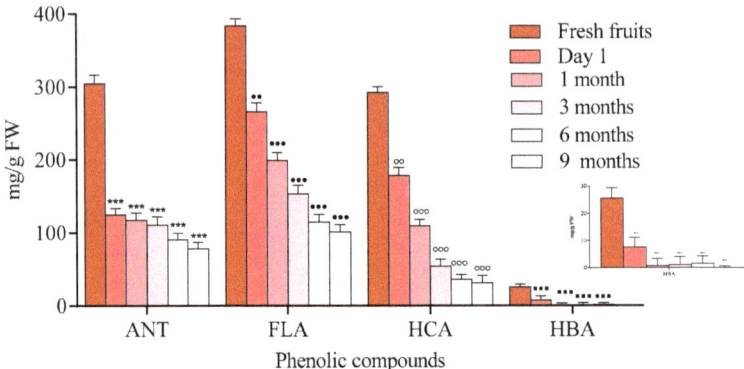

Figure 6. Phenolic compounds degradation in blackthorn jam during storage, (anthocyanins (ANT), flavonols (FLA), (hydroxycinnamic acids (HCA) hydroxybenzoic acids (HBA)). Data represents the means ± SEM of at least three independent experiments (significant differences, **, ••, ∘∘, ⁎⁎ $p < 0.01$, ***, •••, ∘∘∘, ⁎⁎⁎ $p < 0.001$).

2.1.3. Elderberry

Thus far, elderberries were not very popular for consumers due to their alkaloid content. However, this can easily be neutralized by thermal processing. Recently, an interest in elderberries has developed due to their rich polyphenolic compound content and thus, high antioxidant potential. Consequently, these berries are now becoming a very popular crop in Europe, and thus, we included them in our study. The HPLC analysis revealed that elderberry has a simple phenolic fingerprint, characterized by the presence of six compounds: two anthocyanins and four hydroxycinnamic acids (HCA) (Figure 7).

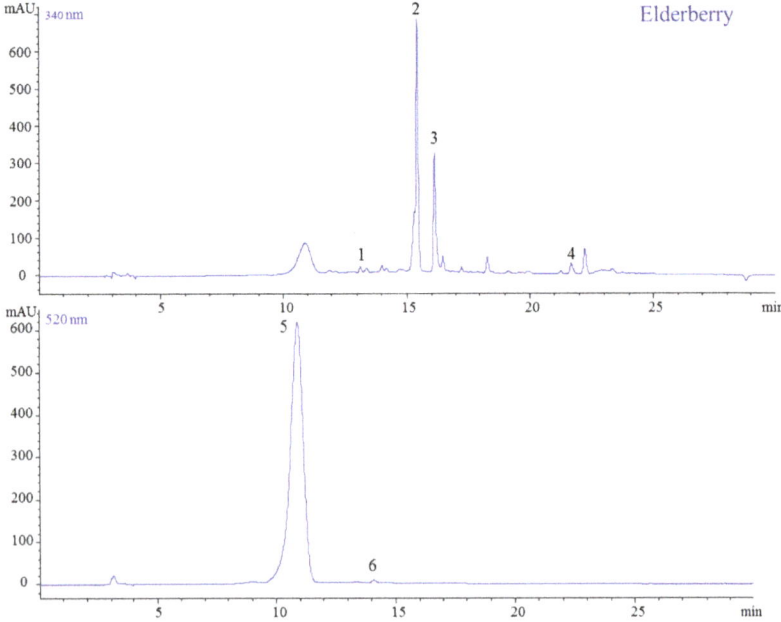

Figure 7. HPLC-DAD chromatogram of berry extracts from elderberry jams (340 and 520 nm).

The identified anthocyanins in fresh fruits and prepared jam were exclusively cyanidin-based anthocyanins, quercetin derivatives, and chlorogenic acid. Peak 1 was assigned to chlorogenic acid because it has a parent ion at m/z 355 and two fragments ions at m/z 181 and 163. The next three peaks (2, 3, 4) were found to be quercetin-3-O-rutinoside (m/z 611, 303), quercetin-3-O-glucoside (465, 303), and quercetin (303) (Figure 8). Further, the ESI-MS analysis showed the presence of molecular ions at m/z 381 corresponding to cyanidin-3-O-sambubioside, while peak 6 was identified as cyanidin-3-O-glucoside (m/z 449, 287) (Table 1, Figure 8).

Three flavonols were identified in this sample, with quercetin-3-O-rutinoside (Figure 7) being the major one, followed by quercetin-3-O-glucoside. This rank was maintained after thermal processing and storage (Figure 9).

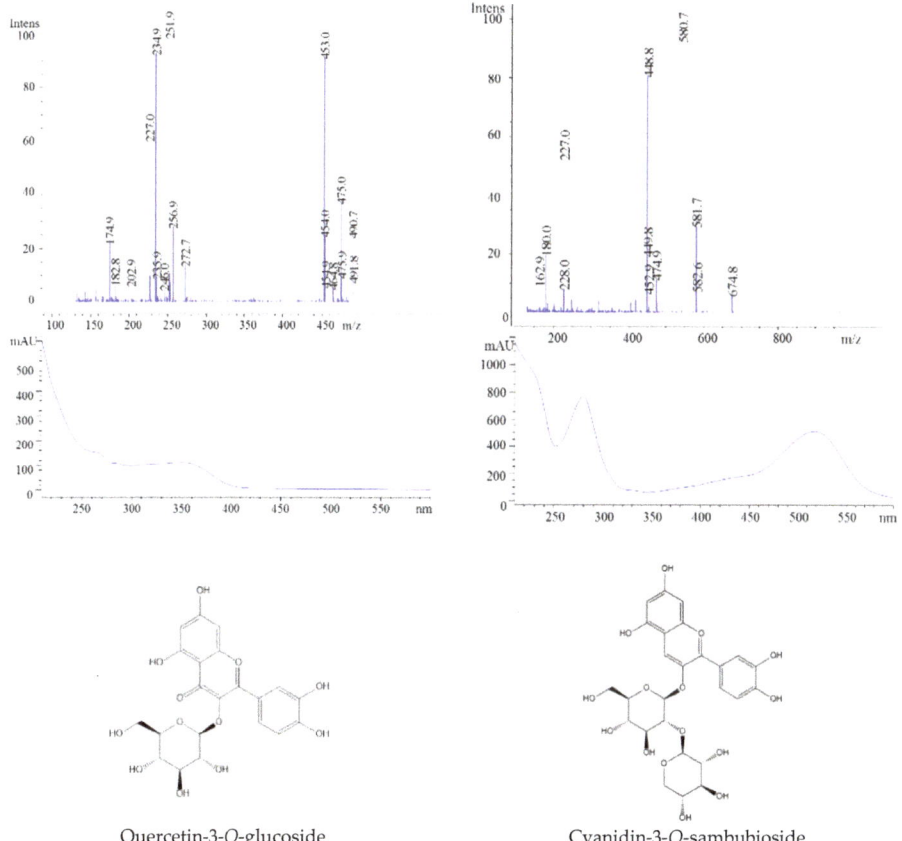

Quercetin-3-O-glucoside   Cyanidin-3-O-sambubioside

Figure 8. HPLC-MS spectra, UV/vis scanning spectra, and the chemical structures of peaks 2 and 5.

The obtained results regarding phenolic changes during processing are in agreement with the available literature [35]. The current body of literature indicates that thermal processes have a large influence on flavonoid stability, especially for rutin which has higher stability compared to its aglycon form (quercetin) [32,33]. These findings were attributed to the presence of carbanion formation because of the glycosylation of the 3-hydroxyl group in the C-ring.

Other authors also reported that glycosylated form are more stable: luteolin was found more resistant to heat than rutin or luteolin-7-glucoside when heated at 180 °C for 180 min [34]. Moreover, the highest level of polyphenolic compounds was observed in the extraction of *Orthosiphon stanmineus* leaf, with 80% methanol at 40 °C and a significant degradation of the analytes recorded at temperatures above 60 °C [16]. The results of the previously cited study also showed a significant reduction in the free radical-scavenging activity of the samples which were treated at temperatures above 60 °C. To conclude, the antioxidant capacity of the flavonoids, and therefore, their pathway to oxidative degradation is linked with their special structural features.

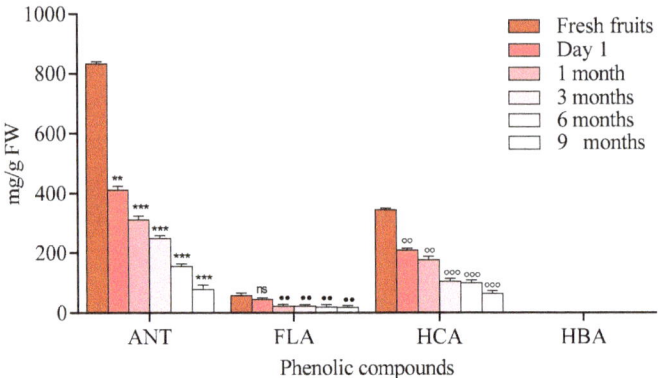

Figure 9. Phenolic compound degradation in elderberry jam during storage, (anthocyanins (ANT), flavonols (FLA), (hydroxycinnamic acids (HCA) hydroxybenzoic acids (HBA)). Data represents the means ± SEM of at least three independent experiments (significant differences, **, ••, ∘∘,″ $p < 0.01$, ***, •••, ∘∘∘,‴ $p < 0.001$).

2.1.4. The Blackcurrant

This sample had the most complex matrix of polyphenol constituents. Prior to the ESI-MS analysis, we were able to identify 20 individual compounds (Figure 10). The available literature data indicates that the polyphenolic compounds present in blackcurrant are caffeic acid, hydroxybenzoic acid, quercetin, myricetin, cyanidin, and delphinidin [28,29,36]. Table 1 presents the retention times, molecular ions, and fragmentation information for all polyphenolic compounds found in the present study. The mass spectra of peak 1 displayed a parent ion at m/z 341 and one fragment ion at m/z 139 which was identified as 4-hydroxybenzoic acid-4-O-glucoside. This sample was also characterized by the presence of 13 flavonols-mainly kaempferol-as well as quercetin or myricetin derivates. For anthocyanins, glucosides and rutinosides were the main sugar moieties of delphinidin and cyanidin identified (Table 1). Overall, the anthocyanins identified in the present study are in agreement with those detected in previous studies [12].

The first identified anthocyanin (peak 1) was delphinidin-3-O-glucoside (m/z 303), while the second isolated anthocyanin showed a parent ion at 611 and a molecular ion at m/z, suggesting the presence of delphinidin-3-O-rutinoside (Figure 11). Moreover, the ion at m/z 449 indicated the loss of one molecule of rhamnoside, and the ion at m/z 287 confirmed the presence of aglycone cyanidin (Table 1).

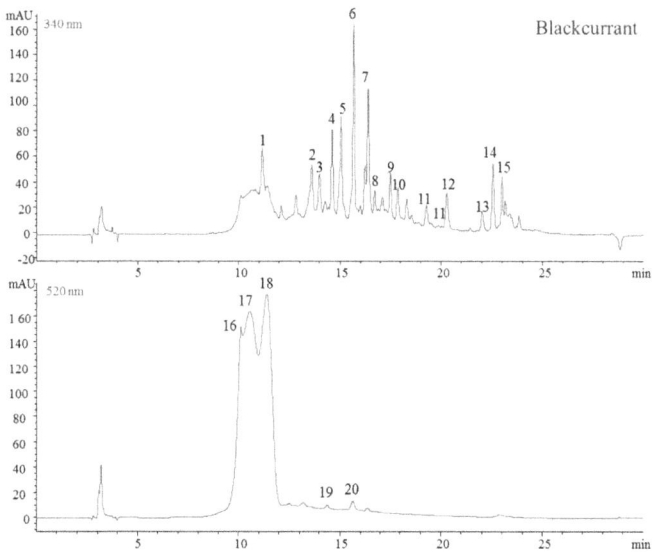

Figure 10. Chromatographic profile of berry extracts from blackcurrant jams (340 and 520 nm).

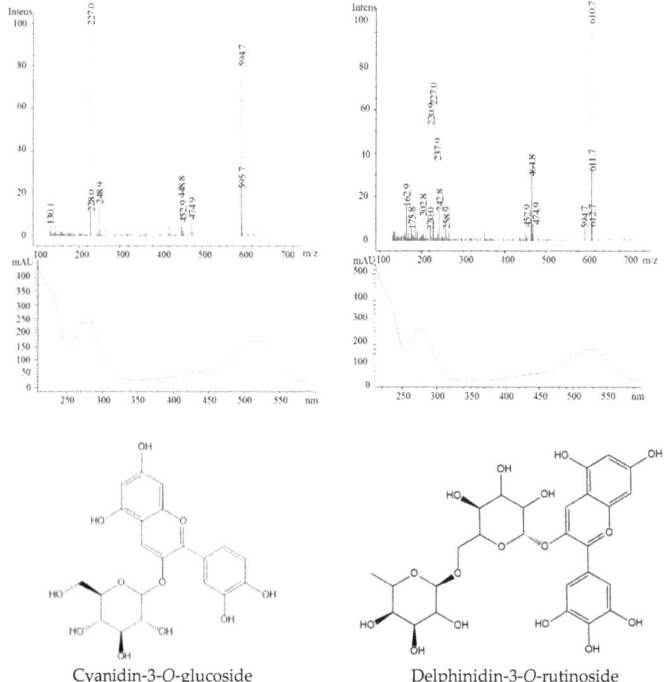

Figure 11. HPLC-MS spectra, UV/vis scanning spectra, and the chemical structures of peaks 17 and 18.

Our results indicated that heating and prolonged storage time are influencing the contents of the individual phenolic compounds, and moreover, their content decreased overall (Figure 12).

These findings are in agreement with a previous study [37] which reported that flavonoid loss may depend on the preparation method used, such as boiling, frying with oil and butter, or microwaving.

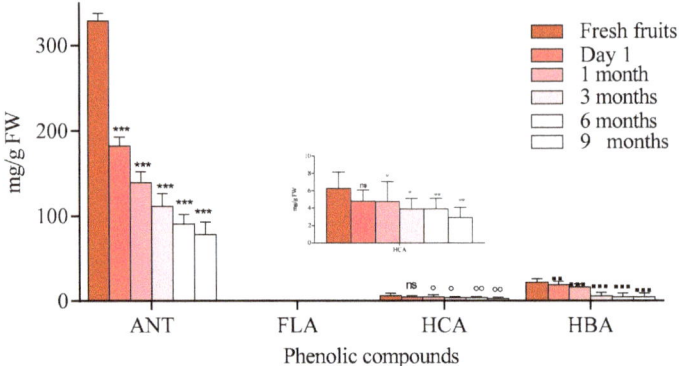

Figure 12. Phenolic compound degradation in blackcurrant jam during storage (anthocyanins (ANT), flavonols (FLA), (hydroxycinnamic acids (HCA) hydroxybenzoic acids (HBA)). Data represents the means ± SEM of at least three independent experiments (significant differences, *, •, °, · $p < 0.05$, **, ••, °°, ·· $p < 0.01$, ***, •••, °°°, ··· $p < 0.001$).

2.2. Cell Proliferation

Cell proliferation was performed by evaluating the mitochondrial succinate dehydrogenase activity of both cell lines (normal and melanoma) after applying a 24 h treatment with RPE. In the case of a normal fibroblast cell line (HFL-1), all the extracts showed a stimulation of proliferation, especially elderberry extract, while blackthorn extract exerted a less significant influence on cell proliferation. These differences could be explained by their varied phytochemical compositions. In this context we can state that elderberry extract was characterised by the presence of anthocyanins and HCA, while blackthorn, in addition to its anthocyanin and HCA contents, was shown to contain flavonols as well. Further, for the human melanoma cell line (A375), the applied treatments reduced cell proliferation after 24 h at the highest applied concentration (100 μg/mL) (Figure 13). The obtained results were well correlated with the dose concentration. Moreover, data showed that all of the applied treatments on the melanoma cell line have a cell proliferation effect ranging from 20–25%. The extract with the highest antiproliferative potential was the one obtained from blackthorn. This fact can be attributed to their phytochemical composition which is abundant in glycosylated and acylated anthocyanins (356 mg/100 g FW). In other words, there was no dose that inhibited 50% of the cultivated cells. The obtained results demonstrate that extracts rich in polyphenols have antiproliferative potential on tumour cells, while on normal cells, they have been proven to stimulate cell proliferation in a dose dependent manner.

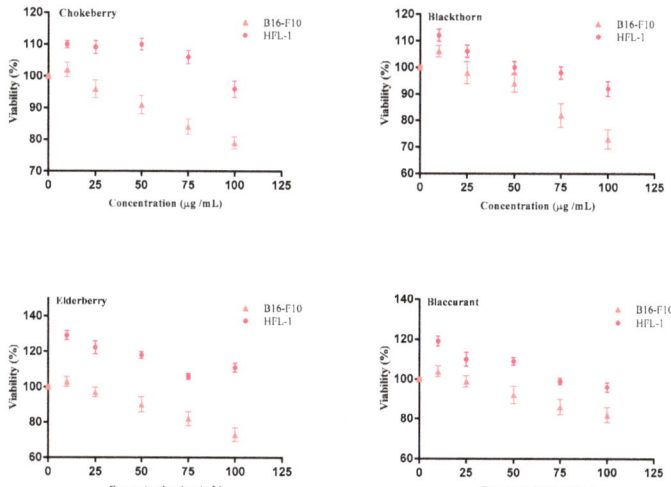

Figure 13. Effect of RPE from chokeberry, blackthorn, elderberry and blackcurrant on B16-F10 and HFL-1 cell proliferation.

This fact is in agreement with other published data [38]. However, like all natural plant metabolites, anthocyanins are unstable and highly susceptible to degradation. Their stability is highly influenced by pH, temperature, light and also the presence of complexing compounds such as other phenolic acid and flavonoids or metals ions [39]. Moreover, it is not clear how exactly anthocyanins act at cellular level, but their proprieties seem to be closely related to their antioxidant activity [40]. Bein unstable molecules, when exposed to high pH values, during the in vitro testing, anthocyanins can rapidly degrade or be breakdown in different metabolites. Very little is known about the details and the mechanisms of anthocyanin absorption and transportation when comparing with other flavonoid groups, such as flavonols. Anthocyanins exhibit complex biochemistry and much remained to be discovered about the biochemical activity of these compounds.

Currently, most investigations on anthocyanins are focusing on solving these problems, as well as anthocyanin bioavailability which seems to be very low with <1% absorption from the ingested dietary dose [41]. Moreover anthocyanins are subject to degradation in vivo, resulting in a breakdown to phenolic acids and aldehydes [42], such as protocatechuic acid (PCA) and phloroglucinol aldehyde (PGA) in the case of cyanidin. For other anthocyanins classes such as glycosylated or acylated form, the consumption and bioavailability of dietary phenolics have become a major concern in phenolic chemopreventive and cancer therapy research and these were not researched as far as we know.

3. Discussion

The obtained results revealed that during processing and storage, the bioactive compounds from all berry jams degraded over time, but they still exert antioxidant activity. Prior to the chromatographic analysis, polyphenolic compounds were identified as flavonoids (anthocyanins (ANT), flavonols (FLA)) or non-flavonoids (phenolic acids derivates of hydroxycinnamic acids (HCA) and hydroxybenzoic acids (HBA)). The polyphenolic compounds were identified by comparing the peak m/z of each molecule as well as their fragmentation and elution orders (retention time) with previously published values and available standards.

Compared to the other classes of quantified compounds, the most significant decrease was observed in HCA. This variation was expected due to the variation in the constituents and phenolic types among the different analyzed berries. These data correspond with similar conclusions of previous experiments reported regarding polyphenols antioxidant activity and their thermal degradation [43].

Moreover any processing of berries (especially thermal) and also storage were proved to be responsible for the significant losses of polyphenols. In a recent study, processing methods had insignificant effects on blueberry ellagitannins, but juice processing of berries resulted in total ellagitannin losses of about 70–82% [44]. Same author reported that storage at 25 degrees C of all processed products resulted in dramatic losses in monomeric anthocyanins with as much as 75% losses of anthocyanins throughout storage [45]. Another study, reported that thermal processes blackberries, showed a decreased content of anthocyanins (cyanidin-3-glucoside (by 52%) and cyanidin-3-malonyl glucoside (64%) respectively). They also reported that anthocyanins continue to decline during storage, especially when temperatures were high [46]. The obtained values for each type of berry of processed product are not easy to compare with literature available data due to the source of the berries or fruit. Their initial amount of polyphenols may vary with cultivation type, variety or climatic condition.

For the in vitro test we have obtained promising results which can be compared with available published data. Many studies have proved that anthocyanins present beneficial effects for human health [47]. Because of their physiological activities, the consumption of anthocyanins may play a significant role in preventing lifestyle-related diseases such as cancer, diabetes, cardiovascular and neurological disease. However, the exact roles of the anthocyanins in human health maintenance versus other phytochemicals in a complex mixture from a fruit extract or whole food have not been completely sorted out. In vitro studies have shown various beneficial effects of anthocyanins regarding human health, but without doubt, in vivo, epidemiological and clinical trials would be more accurate. However, to the best of our knowledge, no report exists on the effect of processing on the phenolic compounds content of homemade jams from chokeberry, elderberry, blackcurrant or blackthorn.

4. Materials and Methods

All solvents, reagents, and standards used to perform the experiments were of analytical grade and purchased from Sigma-Aldrich (Darmstadt, Germany) The anthocyanin standards cyanidin-3-*O*-glucoside chloride, pelargonidin-3-*O*-glucoside chloride, cyanidin-3-*O*-galactoside (purity 90%), cyanidin-3-*O*-arabinoside (purity 97%), cyanidin-3-*O*-glucoside (purity 95%), and cyanidin (purity 95%) were purchased from Polyphenols AS (Sandnes, Norway). Chlorogenic acid, caffeic acid, quercetin-3-*O*-rutinoside, quercetin-3-*O*-glucoside, ellagic acid, and myricetin were also purchased from Sigma-Aldrich (Darmstadt, Germany).

4.1. Sampling Procedure

Berry fruits (chokeberry, elderberry, blackcurrant, and blackthorn) were purchased from local farmers near Cluj-Napoca, Romania. Immediately after harvesting, the berries were frozen at −18 °C for future analyses. Basically, a common and simple jam-making procedure was followed in this study. Jams were prepared from berries using 250 g of sugar and 500 g of chopped berries, this being the most common ratio found in homemade jam products. The obtained mixture was heated in a gas stove (85 °C) for 15 min each day over 3 consecutive days. After boiling on the 3rd day, the jams were allowed to cool down to room temperature before being placed in glass jars (45 g). The obtained jams were analyzed immediately after preparation, and the remaining jams were divided into four batches and stored in the dark at 4 °C. Samples were analyzed after 1, 3, 6, and 9 months of storage.

4.2. Extraction of Anthocyanin and Non-Anthocyanin Phenolics from Fresh Berries and Berry Jam

For the extraction of polyphenols, 5 g of fresh berries of each type were ground using an ultraturrax (Miccra D-9 KT Digitronic, Heitersheim, Germany). Additionally, the same amount of berry jams was homogenized and weighed, followed by the addition of 10 mL of methanol containing hydrochloric acid (0.3% v/v). The obtained mixtures were sonicated for 20 min in the dark and then centrifuged at 5000 rpm for 5 min. The supernatant was collected, and the extraction process was repeated until the samples were colorless. The extracts obtained for each sample were concentrated at 35 °C under reduced pressure (Rotavapor R-124, Buchi, Flawil, Switzerland) and then filtered through a

0.45 µm Millipore filter. All the sample preparation steps were carried out in subdued light and under controlled conditions.

4.3. RP-HPLC-PDA Identification and Quantification of Phenolic Compounds

HPLC analysis was performed on a Shimadzu (Kyoto, Japan) system equipped with a binary pump delivery system (model LC-20 AT Prominence), a degasser (model DGU-20 A3 Prominence), a UV–VIS diode array detector (model SPD-M20), and a Luna C-18 column (film thickness, 5 µm; 25 cm, 4.6 mm) (Phenomenex, Torrance, CA, USA). The mobile phases were formic acid (4.5%) in double-distilled water (solvent A) and acetonitrile (solvent B). The gradient elution system was as follows: 10% B, 0–9 min; 12% B, 9–17 min; 25% B, 17–30 min; 90% B, 30–50 min; and 10% B, 50–55 min. The flow rate was 0.8 mL/min, and all analyses were performed at 35°C. Identification and peak assignments were conducted based on their retention times UV-VIS spectra, standards and available literature. The chromatograms were monitored at 340 and 520 nm. Anthocyanin quantification was conducted using a cyanidin-3-O-galactoside standard curve while for flavanol and phenolic acid was assessed using a rutin or chlorogenic acid standard curve.

4.4. HPLC-PDA/-ESI-MS Identification and Quantification of Phenolic Compounds

To confirm the identified compounds, an ESI-MS analysis was also conducted. The ESI-MS analysis was performed using an Agilent 1200 system equipped with a binary pump delivery system (LC-20 AT, Prominence), a degasser (DGU-20 A3, Prominence), a diode array SPD-M20 A UV–VIS detector (DAD), and an Eclipse XDB C18 column (4 µm, 4.6 × 150 mm) was used. The mobile phases used the following solvents: (A) bidistilled water and 0.1% acetic acid/acetonitrile (99/1 v/v), and (B) acetonitrile and acetic acid 0.1%. The gradient elution system conditions were as follows: 0–2 min, isocratic with 5% (v/v) eluent B; 2–18 min, linear gradient from 5% to 40% (v/v) eluent B; 18–20 min, linear gradient from 40% to 90% (v/v) eluent B; 20–24 min, isocratic on 90% (v/v) eluent B; 24–25 min, linear gradient from 90% to 5% (v/v) eluent B; 25–30 min, isocratic on 5% (v/v) eluent B. The flow rate was 0.5 mL/min, and the column temperature was maintained at 25° C. The chromatograms were monitored at 280 and 340 nm, respectively. The identification of compounds was conducted based on their retention times, UV-VIS spectra, standards (chlorogenic acid, caffeic acid, quercetin-rutinoside, quercetin-glucoside, ellagic acid, and myricetin, all purchased from Sigma-Aldrich, and published data. The mass spectrometric data were obtained using a single quadrupole 6110 mass spectrometer (Agilent Technologies, Chelmsford, MA, USA) equipped with an ESI probe with scanning range between 280 to 1000 m/z. The measurements were performed in the positive mode, with an ion spray voltage of 3000 V and a capillary temperature of 350 °C.

4.5. Cell Culture

The metastatic B16-F10 murine melanoma cell line was purchased from ATCC (Rockville, MD, USA) and grown under standard conditions. More specifically the cells were cultivated in DMEM (Dulbecco's Modified Eagle Medium) medium containing 4.5 g/L glucose, 10% FBS supplemented with 2 mM glutamine, 1% penicillin, and streptomycin. The non-tumor model (HFL-1 human fetal lung fibroblast cell line, ATCC) was cultivated in a F-12K (Kaighn's Modification of Ham's F-12 Medium) medium containing 10% FBS and 1% penicillin/streptomycin. Both cell lines were maintained under standard conditions at 37 °C, 5% CO_2 and 95% relative humidity.

4.6. Analysis of Cell Proliferation

For proliferation analysis, both cell lines were plated at a density of 8×10^3 cells/well in a 96-well microplate and cultured in complete medium for 24 h. The medium was then replaced with a complete medium containing, or not containing rich polyphenolic extracts (RPE) at various concentrations (0–100 µg/mL) for 24 h at 37 °C with 5% CO_2. The RPE stock solution was prepared with a complete medium containing 0.3% DMSO. The treatment was applied for 24 h at 37 °C with 5% CO_2. To assess the cell viability after treatment with RPE we used a standard procedure. Briefly, the cell culture medium was removed and freshly prepared MTT reagent (0.5 mg/mL) was added to each well. After 2 h of incubation at 37 °C, the MTT solution was carefully removed, and DMSO was added in order to dissolve the formazan crystals that had formed in the mitochondria. The solubilized formazan formed in the viable cells was measured at 550 and 630 nm (for the sample and background, respectively) using the microplate reader, HT BioTek Synergy (BioTek Instruments, Winooski, VT, USA). The results are expressed as the survival percentage with respect to an untreated control. The control cells were assessed to be 100% viable.

4.7. Statistical Analysis

Data are expressed as the mean ± standard error of mean (SEM) of three analyses of each sample. Analysis of variance (ANOVA) and Dunnett's multiple comparisons test were used to determine significant differences between values ($p < 0.05$).

Funding: This paper was published under the frame of two national grants financed by Romanian National Authority for Scientific Research (UEFISCDI) project number PN-III-P2-2.1-PED-2016-1002, 186PED, 01/09/2017.

Acknowledgments: The author is grateful to Florica Ranga for running the LS-MS samples.

Conflicts of Interest: The authors declare no conflict of interest.

Abbreviations

3-(4,5-Dimethylthiazol-2-yl)-2,5-Diphenyltetrazolium Bromide	MTT
anthocyanins	ANT
Flavonols	FLA
Foetal bovin serum	FBS
Hydroxybenzoic acids	HBA
Hydroxycinnamic acids	HCA
Metastatic murine melanoma cell line	B16-F10
Normal fibroblast cell line	HFL-1
Rich polyphenolic extracts	RPE

References

1. Blando, F.; Calabriso, N.; Berland, H.; Maiorano, G.; Gerardi, C.; Carluccio, M.; Andersen, Ø. Radical scavenging and anti-inflammatory activities of representative anthocyanin groupings from pigment-rich fruits and vegetables. *Int. J. Mol. Sci.* **2018**, *19*, 169. [CrossRef] [PubMed]
2. Jurikova, T.; Mlcek, J.; Skrovankova, S.; Sumczynski, D.; Sochor, J.; Hlavacova, I.; Snopek, L.; Orsavova, J. Fruits of black chokeberry aronia melanocarpa in the prevention of chronic diseases. *Molecules* **2017**, *22*, 944. [CrossRef] [PubMed]
3. Lin, D.; Xiao, M.; Zhao, J.; Li, Z.; Xing, B.; Li, X.; Kong, M.; Li, L.; Zhang, Q.; Liu, Y.; et al. An overview of plant phenolic compounds and their importance in human nutrition and management of type 2 diabetes. *Molecules* **2016**, *21*, 1374. [CrossRef] [PubMed]
4. Quintin, D.; Garcia-Gomez, P.; Ayuso, M.; Sanmartin, A.M. Active biocompounds to improve food nutritional value. *Trends Food Sci. Technol.* **2018**. [CrossRef]
5. Berger, R.G. Biotechnology of flavours—The next generation. *Biotechnol. Lett.* **2009**, *31*, 1651–1659. [CrossRef] [PubMed]
6. Brewer, M.S. Natural antioxidants: Sources, compounds, mechanisms of action, and potential applications. *Compr. Rev. Food Sci. Food Saf.* **2011**, *10*, 221–247. [CrossRef]
7. Chhikara, N.; Kushwaha, K.; Sharma, P.; Gat, Y.; Panghal, A. Bioactive compounds of beetroot and utilization in food processing industry: A critical review. *Food Chem.* **2018**, *272*, 192–200. [CrossRef]
8. Palmieri, M.G.S.; Cruz, L.T.; Bertges, F.S.; Húngaro, H.M.; Batista, L.R.; da Silva, S.S.; Fonseca, M.J.V.; Rodarte, M.P.; Vilela, F.M.P.; Amaral, M.D.P.H.D. Enhancement of antioxidant properties from green coffee as promising ingredient for food and cosmetic industries. *Biocatal. Agric. Biotechnol.* **2018**, *16*, 43–48. [CrossRef]

9. Nirmala, C.; Bisht, M.S.; Bajwa, H.K.; Santosh, O. Bamboo: A rich source of natural antioxidants and its applications in the food and pharmaceutical industry. *Trends Food Sci. Technol.* **2018**, *77*, 91–99. [CrossRef]
10. Młynarczyk, K.; Walkowiak-Tomczak, D.; Łysiak, G.P. Bioactive properties of *Sambucus nigra* L. As a functional ingredient for food and pharmaceutical industry. *J. Funct. Foods* **2018**, *40*, 377–390. [CrossRef]
11. Ganesan, K.; Xu, B. A critical review on polyphenols and health benefits of black soybeans. *Nutrients* **2017**, *9*, 455. [CrossRef] [PubMed]
12. Diaconeasa, Z.; Leopold, L.; Rugina, D.; Ayvaz, H.; Socaciu, C. Antiproliferative and antioxidant properties of anthocyanin rich extracts from blueberry and blackcurrant juice. *Int. J. Mol. Sci.* **2015**, *16*, 2352–2365. [CrossRef] [PubMed]
13. Decareau, R.; Livingston, G.E.; Fellers, C.R. Color changes in strawberry jellies. *Food Res.* **1956**, *10*, 125–128.
14. Markakis, P. (Ed.) Stability of anthocyanins in foods. In *Anthocyanins as Food Colors*; Academic Press: New York, NY, USA, 1982; pp. 163–181.
15. Pilando, L.S.; Wrolstad, R.E.; Heatherbell, D.A. Influence of fruit composition, maturity and mold contamination on the color and appearance of strawberry wine. *J. Food Sci.* **1985**, *50*, 1121–1125. [CrossRef]
16. García-Viguera, C.; Zafrilla, P.; Artés, F.; Romero, F.; Abellán, P.; Tomás-Barberán, F.A. Colour and anthocyanin stability of red raspberry jam. *J. Sci. Food Agric.* **1998**, *78*, 565–573. [CrossRef]
17. García-Viguera, C.; Zafrilla, P.; Romero, F.; Abellán, P.; Artés, F.; Tomás-Barberán, F.A. Color stability of strawberry jam as affected by cultivar and storage temperature. *J. Food Sci.* **1999**, *64*, 243–247. [CrossRef]
18. Garzón, G.A.; Wrolstad, R.E. Comparison of the stability of pelargonidin-based anthocyanins in strawberry juice and concentrate. *J. Food Sci.* **2002**, *67*, 1288–1299. [CrossRef]
19. Patras, A.; Brunton, N.P.; Tiwari, B.K.; Butler, F. Stability and degradation kinetics of bioactive compounds and colour in strawberry jam during storage. *Food Bioprocess Technol.* **2011**, *4*, 1245–1252. [CrossRef]
20. Amaro, L.F.; Soares, M.T.; Pinho, C.; Almeida, I.F.; Ferreira, I.M.; Pinho, O. Influence of cultivar and storage conditions in anthocyanin content and radical-scavenging activity of strawberry jams. *World Acad. Sci. Eng. Technol. Int. J. Nutr. Food Eng.* **2012**, *6*, 112–116.
21. Mikulic-Petkovsek, M.; Slatnar, A.; Stampar, F.; Veberic, R. HPLC-MSn identification and quantification of flavonol glycosides in 28 wild and cultivated berry species. *Food Chem.* **2012**, *135*, 2138–2146. [CrossRef] [PubMed]
22. Bursac Kovacevic, D.; Gajdos Kljusuric, J.; Putnik, P.; Vukusic, T.; Herceg, Z.; Dragovic-Uzelac, V. Stability of polyphenols in chokeberry juice treated with gas phase plasma. *Food Chem.* **2016**, *212*, 323–331. [CrossRef] [PubMed]
23. Taheri, R.; Connolly, B.A.; Brand, M.H.; Bolling, B.W. Underutilized chokeberry (*Aronia melanocarpa, Aronia arbutifolia, Aronia prunifolia*) accessions are rich sources of anthocyanins, flavonoids, hydroxycinnamic acids, and proanthocyanidins. *J. Agric. Food Chem.* **2013**, *61*, 8581–8588. [CrossRef] [PubMed]
24. Cebulak, T.; Oszmianski, J.; Kapusta, I.; Lachowicz, S. Effect of UV-C radiation, ultra-sonication electromagnetic field and microwaves on changes in polyphenolic compounds in chokeberry (*Aronia melanocarpa*). *Molecules* **2017**, *22*, 1161. [CrossRef] [PubMed]
25. Ştefănuţ, M.N.; Căta, A.; Pop, R.; Moşoarcă, C.; Zamfir, A.D. Anthocyanins hplc-dad and ms characterization, total phenolics, and antioxidant activity of some berries extracts. *Anal. Lett.* **2011**, *44*, 2843–2855. [CrossRef]
26. Veberic, R.; Jakopic, J.; Stampar, F.; Schmitzer, V. European elderberry (*Sambucus nigra* L.) rich in sugars, organic acids, anthocyanins and selected polyphenols. *Food Chem.* **2009**, *114*, 511–515. [CrossRef]
27. Rubinskiene, M.; Jasutiene, I.; Venskutonis, P.R.; Viskelis, P. HPLC determination of the composition and stability of blackcurrant anthocyanins. *J. Chromatogr. Sci.* **2005**, *43*, 478–482. [CrossRef] [PubMed]
28. Mattila, P.H.; Hellström, J.; Karhu, S.; Pihlava, J.-M.; Veteläinen, M. High variability in flavonoid contents and composition between different north-european currant (*Ribes* spp.) varieties. *Food Chem.* **2016**, *204*, 14–20. [CrossRef] [PubMed]
29. Kamiloglu, S.; Pasli, A.A.; Ozcelik, B.; Van Camp, J.; Capanoglu, E. Colour retention, anthocyanin stability and antioxidant capacity in black carrot (*Daucus carota*) jams and marmalades: Effect of processing, storage conditions and in vitro gastrointestinal digestion. *J. Funct. Foods* **2015**, *13*, 1–10. [CrossRef]
30. Howard, L.R.; Castrodale, C.; Brownmiller, C.; Mauromoustakos, A. Jam processing and storage effects on blueberry polyphenolics and antioxidant capacity. *J. Agric. Food Chem.* **2010**, *58*, 4022–4029. [CrossRef] [PubMed]

31. Rababah, T.M.; Al-Mahasneh, M.A.; Kilani, I.; Yang, W.; Alhamad, M.N.; Ereifej, K.; Al-U'datt, M. Effect of jam processing and storage on total phenolics, antioxidant activity, and anthocyanins of different fruits. *J. Sci. Food Agric.* **2011**, *91*, 1096–1102. [CrossRef] [PubMed]
32. Lee, D.J.; Lee, H.; Lee, S.-H.; Lee, C.Y.; Kim, D.-O. Effects of jam processing on anthocyanins and antioxidant capacities of rubus coreanus miquel berry. *Food Sci. Biotechnol.* **2013**, *22*, 1607–1612. [CrossRef]
33. Wojdyło, A.; Oszmiański, J.; Bober, I. The effect of addition of chokeberry, flowering quince fruits and rhubarb juice to strawberry jams on their polyphenol content, antioxidant activity and colour. *Eur. Food Res. Technol.* **2008**, *227*, 1043–1051. [CrossRef]
34. Buchner, N.; Krumbein, A.; Rohn, S.; Kroh, L.W. Effect of thermal processing on the flavonols rutin and quercetin. *Rapid Commun. Mass Spectrom. RCM* **2006**, *20*, 3229–3235. [CrossRef] [PubMed]
35. Mattila, P.H.; Hellstrom, J.; McDougall, G.; Dobson, G.; Pihlava, J.M.; Tiirikka, T.; Stewart, D.; Karjalainen, R. Polyphenol and vitamin C contents in European commercial blackcurrant juice products. *Food Chem.* **2011**, *127*, 1216–1223. [CrossRef] [PubMed]
36. Ioku, K.; Aoyama, Y.; Tokuno, A.; Terao, J.; Nakatani, N.; Takei, Y. Various cooking methods and the flavonoid content in onion. *J. Nutr. Sci. Vitaminol.* **2001**, *47*, 78–83. [CrossRef] [PubMed]
37. Wang, E.; Liu, Y.; Xu, C.; Liu, J. Antiproliferative and proapoptotic activities of anthocyanin and anthocyanidin extracts from blueberry fruits on B16-F10 melanoma cells. *Food Nutr. Res.* **2017**, *61*, 1325308. [CrossRef] [PubMed]
38. Trouillas, P.; Sancho-García, J.C.; De Freitas, V.; Gierschner, J.; Otyepka, M.; Dangles, O. Stabilizing and modulating color by copigmentation: Insights from theory and experiment. *Chem. Rev.* **2016**, *116*, 4937–4982. [CrossRef] [PubMed]
39. He, J.; Giusti, M.M. Anthocyanins: Natural colorants with health-promoting properties. *Annu. Rev. Food Sci. Technol.* **2010**, *1*, 163–187. [CrossRef] [PubMed]
40. Bresciani, L.; Martini, D.; Mena, P.; Tassotti, M.; Calani, L.; Brigati, G.; Brighenti, F.; Holasek, S.; Malliga, D.-E.; Lamprecht, M.; et al. Absorption profile of (poly)phenolic compounds after consumption of three food supplements containing 36 different fruits, vegetables, and berries. *Nutrients* **2017**, *9*, 194. [CrossRef] [PubMed]
41. Vitaglione, P.; Donnarumma, G.; Napolitano, A.; Galvano, F.; Gallo, A.; Scalfi, L.; Fogliano, V. Protocatechuic acid is the major human metabolite of cyanidin-glucosides. *J. Nutr.* **2007**, *137*, 2043–2048. [CrossRef] [PubMed]
42. Volf, I.; Ignat, I.; Neamtu, M.; Popa, V.I. Thermal stability, antioxidant activity, and photo-oxidation of natural polyphenols. *Chem. Pap.* **2014**, *68*, 121–129. [CrossRef]
43. Hager, T.J.; Howard, L.R.; Prior, R.L. Processing and storage effects on the ellagitannin composition of processed blackberry products. *J. Agric. Food Chem.* **2010**, *58*, 11749–11754. [CrossRef] [PubMed]
44. Hager, T.J.; Howard, L.R.; Prior, R.L. Processing and storage effects on monomeric anthocyanins, percent polymeric color, and antioxidant capacity of processed blackberry products. *J. Agric. Food Chem.* **2008**, *56*, 689–695. [CrossRef] [PubMed]
45. Gancel, A.-L.; Feneuil, A.; Acosta, O.; Pérez, A.M.; Vaillant, F. Impact of industrial processing and storage on major polyphenols and the antioxidant capacity of tropical highland blackberry (*Rubus adenotrichus*). *Food Res. Int.* **2011**, *44*, 2243–2251. [CrossRef]
46. Diaconeasa, Z.; Ayvaz, H.; Rugina, D.; Leopold, L.; Stanila, A.; Socaciu, C.; Tabaran, F.; Luput, L.; Mada, D.C.; Pintea, A.; et al. Melanoma inhibition by anthocyanins is associated with the reduction of oxidative stress biomarkers and changes in mitochondrial membrane potential. *Plant Foods Hum. Nutr.* **2017**, *72*, 404–410. [CrossRef] [PubMed]
47. Ma, L.; Sun, Z.; Zeng, Y.; Luo, M.; Yang, J. Molecular mechanism and health role of functional ingredients in blueberry for chronic disease in human beings. *Int. J. Mol. Sci.* **2018**, *19*, 2785. [CrossRef] [PubMed]

Sample Availability: Samples of the compounds are not available from the authors.

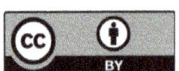

© 2018 by the author. Licensee MDPI, Basel, Switzerland. This article is an open access article distributed under the terms and conditions of the Creative Commons Attribution (CC BY) license (http://creativecommons.org/licenses/by/4.0/).

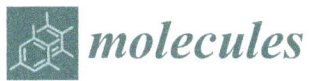

Communication

From Plant Compounds to Botanicals and Back: A Current Snapshot

Alessandra Durazzo *, Laura D'Addezio, Emanuela Camilli, Raffaela Piccinelli, Aida Turrini *, Luisa Marletta, Stefania Marconi, Massimo Lucarini, Silvia Lisciani, Paolo Gabrielli, Loretta Gambelli, Altero Aguzzi and Stefania Sette

CREA-Research Centre for Food and Nutrition, 00178 Rome, Italy; laura.daddezio@crea.gov.it (L.D.); emanuela.camilli@crea.gov.it (E.C.); raffaela.piccinelli@crea.gov.it (R.P.); luisa.marletta@crea.gov.it (L.M.); stefania.marconi@crea.gov.it (S.M.); massimo.lucarini@crea.gov.it (M.L.); silvia.lisciani@crea.gov.it (S.L.); paolo.gabrielli@crea.gov.it (P.G.); loretta.gambelli@crea.gov.it (L.G.); altero.aguzzi@crea.gov.it (A.A.); stefania.sette@crea.gov.it (S.S.)
* Correspondence: alessandra.durazzo@crea.gov.it (A.D.); aida.turrini@crea.gov.it (A.T.); Tel.: +39-065-149-4430 (A.D.); +39-065-149-4440 (A.T.)

Academic Editor: Derek J. McPhee
Received: 4 July 2018; Accepted: 21 July 2018; Published: 24 July 2018

Abstract: This work aims at giving an updated picture of the strict interaction between main plant biologically active compounds and botanicals. The main features of the emerging class of dietary supplements, the botanicals, are highlighted. Focus is also on the definition of actual possibilities of study approach and research strategies. Examples of innovative directions are given: assessment of interaction of bioactive compounds, chemometrics and the new goal of biorefineries. Current models of existing databases, such as plant metabolic pathways, food composition, bioactive compounds, dietary supplements, and dietary markers, are described as usable tools for health research. The need for categorization of botanicals as well as for the implementation of specific and dedicated databases emerged, based on both analytical data and collected data taken from literature throughout a harmonized and standardized approach for the evaluation of an adequate dietary intake.

Keywords: dietary supplements; botanicals; bioactive compounds; antioxidants; study approach; integrated food research; dedicated databases; dietary assessment

---

1. The Emerging Class of Dietary Supplements: A Mini Overview of Botanicals Features

The field of food supplements appears varied and growing: a wider spectrum of new products appears on the market every year. This reflects a new reorganization of the market for dietary supplements, resulting from new strategies, technologies and also the changes in the regulation applied to nutrition and to health claims. The growth of this sector is encouraged by greater consumer interest in improving physical and mental wellbeing and health status, often to compensate for an incorrect lifestyle [1–3]; as reported by Ekor, [4], over four billion people of the world's population use herbal supplements as products of medical care; there is a great and widespread growth in the consumption of herbal remedies [5], related generally to their easy availability, but also to the easy and false perception or idea, that many people feel that what is "natural" is supposed to be healthful and safety, never toxic or side effects.

With the term botanicals is here indicated herbal remedies, herbal drugs, herbal medicinal products, herbal medicines, botanical drugs as synonyms; numerous are the definitions of the term botanicals in relation to the different fields (i.e., pharmacy, botany, medicine, nutrition) [6–8]. Herbal medicinal products are referred to "any medicinal product, exclusively containing as active ingredients one or more herbal substances or one or more herbal preparations, or one or more such herbal substances in combination with one or more such herbal preparations" as introduced in 2004 by Directive 2004/24/EC of the European Parliament and of the Council of 31 March 2004 [9].

Here the definition by the World Health Organization (WHO) is also reported as follows "Herbal medicines include herbs, herbal materials, herbal preparations and finished herbal products, that contain as active ingredients parts of plants, or other plant materials, or combinations" [10].

Botanicals are made of single herbs or by mixing different herbs, from raw material of whole plants or parts of them, and include flowering herbs, leaves, leaf exudate, fruits, berries, roots, rhizomes, fungi, microorganisms, algae.

Starting from these materials, numerous and different techniques and procedures i.e., extraction, distillation, purification, fractionation, concentration, fermentation, etc. are used to obtain botanical substances (single active compounds or more compounds of a chemical class) and preparations/formulation (i.e., extracts, tinctures, powders). Botanicals are prepared through a complex, specific and detailed procedure of preparation process, and on this matter reference and regulation books are available [6,11–13].

In this regard, as described by Alamgir, [14], in a recent 2017 work, it is important to distinguish between pharmacopoeia reference books for the preparation of quality medicines, and herbal and therapeutic compendium, an accurate description of botanicals, as Materia Medica [14].

Moreover, the WHO has developed a portal [15], that contains 5845 medicines and health product-related publications taken from WHO, other United Nations (UN) partners, global Non-Governmental Organizations (NGOs), development agencies and their partners, countries and academics, and is updated monthly [16]. It is important to mention the guidance document formulated by the European Food Safety Authority (EFSA) with a science-based approach, on how to assess the safety of botanicals and of botanical preparations/formulations to be used in the food sector; in particular, a list of the main categories of botanicals and safe botanical preparations/formulations was established [6,7].

The recent study of Breemen et al. [17] summarized and well described the main steps for the development of botanical dietary supplements, underlying how these steps should be similar to those of pharmaceuticals: definition of action mechanism of main bioactive compounds, chemical standardization related to the main compounds and biological standardization linked to pharmacological activity, bioavailability studies, toxicity evaluation, preclinical evaluation, clinical studies of safety and efficacy.

2. Study Approach about Botanicals and Their Main Plant Compounds: Up-to-Date, Current and Innovative Directions

In this paragraph examples of actual possibilities and innovative directions of research strategy are given: assessment of interaction of bioactive compounds; chemometrics; new goal of biorefinery.

2.1. Main Plant Compounds and Their Interactions Assessment

Plants are the source of a magnificent spectrum of compounds and, in this order, are defined as one of the most efficient chemical systems known [18]: 200,000–1,000,000 different metabolites are estimated to be synthetized in the plant kingdom [18].

The diversity of plant compounds derived from the infinite combinations of fundamental functional groups such as hydroxyls, alcohols, aldehydes, alkyls, benzyl rings, steroids that originate compounds with peculiar chemical and physical characteristics (i.e., solubility, melting point, and reactivity) [19].

The combined and concerted action of phytochemicals, (i.e., polyphenols, carotenoids, glucosinolates, lignans, etc.) gives the potential beneficial properties of each plant matrix [20,21]; these concerted interactions are responsible for a large spectra of physiological and biological functions (i.e., anti-inflammatory, antioxidant, anti-allergic, antimicrobial, anti-atherogenic, etc.) [22]. Many original researches and reviews are present in literature on the relationship compound-activity [23,24] as well as chemical class and related bioactivity, i.e., alkaloids [25,26], saponins [27], terpenoids [28], polyphenols [29,30], etc.

As defined by Biesalski et al. [31], "bioactive compounds" are compounds that occur in nature, part of the food chain, that has the ability to interact with one or more compounds of the living tissue, by showing an effect on human health.

The identification, isolation and quantification of bioactive compounds as well as the assessment of their interactions, in the specific case the definition of herb-drug ones, could be considered as the main steps in the study of the potential beneficial plants' properties.

In this regard, it is important to underline how the quantification of bioactive compounds present in the plant extracts is required as starting point. This output involves the applications of a large spectra of techniques as described by several authors [32–35]. As instance, Sasidharan et al. 2010 [32] summarized the main analytical techniques for the ingredient characterization in herbal preparations, by highlighting the relevance of extraction procedures. Ingle et al. [34] categorized in a detailed manner the main techniques of extraction and analysis for botanicals. Ganzera et al. [33] focused on recent perspectives and application in botanicals of HPLC/MS. Pandey and Tripathi, [35] defined and exploited the standardization in drug analysis.

The concerted actions of compounds bioactivity and the related activities of food extracts, were clearly studied and discussed by Durazzo, [20]; the author underlined how two complementary approaches can be applied: either the evaluation of bioactivities of pure compounds and/or their mixtures or the isolation of different biologically active compound-rich extracts and how these fractions contribute to the total activity of food extract.

2.2. Integrated Research, Emerging Technologies and Chemometrics

Among recent approaches with rapid and green procedures, direct analysis such as fluorescence, near infrared (NIR), mid infrared (MIR), nuclear magnetic resonance (NMR) spectroscopies, infrared spectroscopy, multi-elemental analysis, isotopic ratio mass spectrometry, etc. produce large datasets representing the input for multivariate data analysis methods. Therefore, studies on the evaluation of bioactive components are generally integrated into a multidisciplinary system of detection and analysis, generating data matrices for the application of statistical methods like in the chemometrics science.

Moving from bioactive components to botanicals, chemometrics opened a new scenario for herbal drugs [36]; the chemometric approach represents a valid tool in the following actions: authentication of individual herbs, monitoring of the quality of herbs and herb medicines, identification of chemical constituents, detection of adulteration or contamination of herbs, production of standardized formulations.

In the past, two were the main approaches for quality control of herbal medicines, the 'component-based' and 'pattern-based' ones [37,38]. The first approach was focused on the study of specific compounds with defined properties (i.e., marker approach and multi-compound approach), whereas the latter one studied all detectable compounds (i.e., the pattern approach and the multi-pattern approach).

Considering the complexity of herbal ingredients used for testing, the markers do not allow an adequate evaluation of the quality assurance of the herbal materials in all cases; generally, one or two markers are necessary for quality control and authenticity of herbal medicines. The lack of a unique marker did not allow a total overview of an herbal product representing a real problem when qualitatively differentiating them.

An emerging intervention strategy is given by the fingerprint analysis and chemometric technique that make feasible the comparison of compositions in nutrients and bioactive compounds in numerous and different samples, i.e., using all the components detected through their whole chromatograms acquired from spectroscopy, liquid chromatography, gas chromatography, mass spectrometry, and so on. Indeed, this new approach allows the workflow for chemistry, manufacturing, the quality assessment and controls of botanical drugs. In this regard, the recent work of Harnly et al. [39] provided an overview on how to detect the transition of chemical composition from botanical ingredients to resulting products by using chemometrics, differentiating them quickly.

In this context, the identification and formulation of innovative types of quality markers is required and, in this direction, multi-compound, multi-target and multi-pathway studies are being carried out.

In a recent work, Yang et al. [40] proposed the use of bioactive chemical markers, a cluster of chemo-markers showing similar pharmacological activities and comparable to the whole botanical drug: bioactive chemical markers based strategy was formulated and applied to *Xuesaitong Injection*.

As another example in this direction, Zhang et al. [41] gave a general prototype combining the chromatographic fingerprint of bioactive compounds and bioactivity assay to elucidate the relationship spectrum–effect, in a traditional Chinese plant, *Acalypha australis* Linn.

Also Abubakar et al. [42] in an effective research have proposed and discussed DNA barcoding in combination with chromatography fingerprints for the authentication of botanical ingredients in herbal medicines.

The current review of Sánchez-Vidaña et al. [43] emphasized how novel advanced technologies in the field of traditional Chinese medicine research are required for the implementation of separation methods, standardization techniques, quality control, the understanding of the action mechanism of single compounds, clinical validation assays; in this order, the application of omic technologies represents a promising approach in phytotherapy [38,39,43,44].

2.3. Food Waste as Source of Bioactive Compounds: A New Goal of Circular Bioeconomy and Biorefinery

Another innovative direction concerning the botanicals research is given by the diffusion of use of food waste as a sustainable alternative source of biologically active compounds. The "Universal Recovery Strategy" for the commercial recapture of valuable compounds from food wastes is a new goal of the circular bioeconomy and the biorefinery concept [45–49]. The bioactive compounds are nowadays recycled inside food chain from field to fork [50,51]: they are extracted, recovered and reutilized from food byproducts to formulate functional foods and nutraceuticals [52]. The agro-industrial field gives a great opportunity when considering the large quantities of waste and by-products generated every year in the processing of fruit and vegetables. In particular, by-products of plant food processing represent a promising source of biologically active compounds, which may be used for their favorable technological or biological properties; moreover, the use of new technologies is utilized to reinforce and increase the "Green Economy" in agriculture and agro-industry [53,54].

It is worth mentioning the work of Pfaltzgraff et al. [55] that described and schematized well the components (i.e., pectin, sugars, starch, collagen, amino acids, polyphenols) present in food supply chain residues (i.e., tomato pomace, wheat straw, rice husks, spent Brewer's grain) and their uses in common consumer applications. Another interesting review is the work of Baiano et al. [56], that gave detailed and updated description of the type and amounts of food wastes and their legislation as well as conventional and innovative techniques for the extraction of bioactive compounds; also the future trends in nutraceutical, cosmetic, pharmaceutical sectors were discovered [56].

3. From Metabolic Pathways to Bioactive Compound Databases: Tools towards Health

Current models of specialized databases represent effective tools to study the relationship between plant natural compounds and botanicals. In this paragraph, an updated description and a shot of the current state are given and discussed: plant metabolic pathways databases; food composition databases; bioactive compound databases; dietary supplements databases; dietary markers databases. Several and different tools are being developed for secondary metabolic pathways, biological activities, chemical structures, ethnobotanical uses, content in foods, and pharmacology; they represent open source and queryable that can serve as updated sources of information [57].

As starting point, recent examples of plant metabolic pathway tools are given by KEGG Bioinformatics Resource [58]—a tool for interconnection between Plant Genomics and Metabolomics data—and by Plant Reactome [59]—a database that gives bioinformatics tools for visualization, analysis and interpretation of plant metabolic pathways—all aiming to support modelling, systems biology, genome annotation and analysis, basic research and education.

Moving into the nutrition scenario, food composition databases represent the main tools for numerous interventions: elaboration of food consumption data, allowing to convert them into nutrient intake; evaluation of the nutritional and health status of a population; carrying out of epidemiological studies; formulation of diets at the individual and/or population level; epidemiological and clinical research; nutritional education; support industrial and handicraft companies for the labeling [60–62]. The European Food Information Resource (EuroFIR) Network of Excellence and Nexus projects (2005–2013) put the basis of harmonization of Food Composition Databases through standardized protocols and food description system i.e., LanguaL™ [63]. The EuroFIR-AISBL, an international non-profit Association, provides a widespread resource at European level for compilers and users of food composition data throughout a large set of online tools, i.e., FoodEXplorer, Food Basket, eBAsis, PlantaLibra [64]. FoodEXplorer online tool is a virtual platform that combines 30 national standardized and specialized food composition databases (Europe, the United States, Canada Australia, Japan), including more than 40,000 foods [60]. The International Network of Food Data Systems (INFOODS) by FAO, contributes to improve the accessibility, reliability and management of food composition data at worldwide level [65].

For bioactive compounds, the major public, core comprehensive databases are: the United States Department of Agriculture (USDA) databases [66]; the Phenol-Explorer database [67,68]; Bioactive Substances in Food Information Systems (eBASIS) [69–71]; ePlantLIBRA database [72].

The USDA database was developed in 2004 and it is based on a compilation of data from literature and expanded in recent years to include flavonoids, proanthocyanidins and isoflavones [73–75].

Phenol-Explorer represents the first comprehensive open access database on content of polyphenols in foods; several updates on pharmacokinetic and metabolites, effect of food processing and cooking were carried out [76,77]. Five steps—literature search, data compilation, data evaluation, data aggregation, data exportation to the MySQL database (used by the web interface)—were carried out during the procedure of development of the Phenol-Explorer database. Composition data were taken from the peer-reviewed scientific publications and evaluated, then they were aggregated to obtain mean values.

The eBASIS, the first EU harmonized database, combines composition data and biological effects on over 300 major European plant foods of 24 compound classes, e.g., glucosinolates, phytosterols, polyphenols, isoflavones, glycoalkaloids, xanthine alkaloids [70,71]. EuroFIR eBASIS resource represents a collection of data from peer-reviewed literature evaluated critically by experts and inserted as raw data.

Nowadays, there is the need to include extractable and non-extractable phytochemicals in bioactive compounds databases [78] for a better dietary intake assessment: extractable compounds are those that are present in free forms and are solubilized by aqueous–organic solvents, whereas non-extractable compounds are bound forms, remaining in the residue of aqueous-organic extract. In this direction, development and expansion of eBasis structure was addressed [79].

Concerning the specialties of food supplements, ePlantLIBRA database [80], developed within the PlantLIBRA (PLANT food supplements: Levels of Intake, Benefit and Risk Assessment) project, represents a comprehensive and searchable database, with up-to-date information on bioactive compounds specific for plant food supplements, reporting health benefits, adverse effects, contaminants and residues. In order to search, extract, and export the data, ePlantLIBRA database was structured as user-friendly, efficient and flexible interface, by including also links to the original references [72]. As reported by Plumb et al. [80] in ePlantLIBRA, data from over 570 publications have been evaluated for quality, by covering seventy plant food supplements or their botanical ingredients.

Considering the importance of dietary supplements in the evaluation of dietary intake, as revealed during the National Health and Nutrition Examination Survey, NHANES, a dietary supplement label database [81,82] was developed and launched in 2013 by the Academy of Nutrition and Dietetics in the United States: now it contains supplement label information (brand name, ingredients, amount per serving, and manufacturer contact information) of about 50,000 dietary supplements present in the U.S. marketplace and consumed [11,83]. Browsing options were developed and organized to search by product, ingredient or contact of manufacturer, by representing a useful tool for consumers, professionals, researchers [83,84].

In this context, recently, at European level, within the PD Manager Project [85], information on the composition of dietary supplements taken from labels, and according to the Italian market were collected and updated for the development of a Dietary Supplement Label Database [86]: 212 items were inserted, by trying to give a uniform and representative picture of the main classes of dietary supplements consumed in Italy, and 82 descriptors were included, in addition to nutritional information: Brand name, Food group, Distributor, Producer, Packaging sizes, Unit weights, Data source, Additional remarks [86]. It is important to underline that for each item a code was assigned following the food classification system FoodEx2 developed by EFSA [87], to allow the standardization and harmonization of data among different countries; feedbacks and proposal for FoodEx2 revision 2 implementation, with focus on dietary supplements, [88] as well as a constant update and implementation of Dietary Supplement Label Database are ongoing [89].

At the same time the understanding of activities and benefits of bioactive compounds in humans is essential; however, the evidence derived from human intervention gave limited and conflicting results, partly due to differences in absorption, distribution, metabolism and excretion between individuals [90]. The recent work by Dragsted et al. [91] underlined the importance of databases for dietary biomarkers for the main food groups and new data on non-nutrients compounds and their metabolites. The Human Metabolome Database or HMDB 4.0 [92] is a web metabolomic database on human metabolites [93]. PhytoHub is a freely electronic database containing detailed information about all phytochemicals commonly ingested with diet and their metabolites [94,95].

4. Conclusions

During the last decade botanicals, the newest class of dietary supplements, have emerged and their use is spreading among consumers, although they should not replace a correct lifestyle and/or a healthy diet. The scientific community is addressing towards the development and assessment of methodologies to isolate and standardize fractions with specified bioactivities from medicinal plants. Emerging technologies combined with chemometrics are being applied to medicinal plants in an innovative and integrated research approach, also in the directions of circular economy and biorefineries.

In addition, studies on the description and exploitation of bioactive compounds in medicinal plants as well as on physiological mechanism and bioaccessibility of compounds are being carried out.

The overall goal is the categorization and classification of botanicals as well as the development and implementation of dedicated databases, based on specific analytical and collected data, and achieved throughout a harmonized and standardized approach in order to evaluate a correct dietary intake.

It is important to underline how nowadays the "botanicals" class is expanding from herbs and medicinal plants to also include some foods, i.e., artichoke, garlic, etc. This suggests enhancing the value of foods by also investigating their functional/nutraceutical characteristics, in order to integrate intrinsic nutritional properties.

Author Contributions: A.D., L.M., A.T., S.S., L.D., E.C., R.P. have conceived and designed the work. All authors have made a substantial contribution to the revision of work, and approved it for publication.

Funding: The present work has been performed within the sub-contract agreement 'ITALIAN AND GREEK FOOD, RECIPES AND DIETARY SUPPLEMENTS COMPOSITION DATABASES AND DAILY REFERENCE VALUES FOR ITALY AND GREECE' (PD_manager) awarded by EuroFIR.

Acknowledgments: The authors thank Romana Roccaldo for the linguistic revision and the editing of this paper.

Conflicts of Interest: The authors declare that the research was conducted in the absence of any commercial or financial relationships that could be construed as a potential conflict of interest.

References

1. Tallini, A. Health is state of physical, mental, and social wellbeing. *Br. Med. J.* **2011**, *343*, d5358. [CrossRef] [PubMed]
2. Giammarioli, S. Indagini sui consumi degli integratori alimentari in Italia. In Proceedings of the SANIT—XI Edizione, Integratori Alimentari: Attualità e Prospettive Future, Roma, Italy, 14–17 December 2014.
3. Bircher, J.; Hahn, E.G. Understanding the nature of health: New perspectives for medicine and public health. Improved wellbeing at lower costs. *F1000 Res.* **2016**, *5*, 167. [CrossRef] [PubMed]
4. Ekor, M. The growing use of herbal medicines: Issues relating to adverse reactions and challenges in monitoring safety. *Front. Pharmacol.* **2013**, *4*, 177. [CrossRef] [PubMed]
5. Shaw, D.; Graeme, L.; Pierre, D.; Elizabeth, W.; Kelvin, C. Pharmacovigilance of herbal medicine. *J. Ethnopharmacol.* **2012**, *140*, 513–518. [CrossRef] [PubMed]
6. EFSA Scientific Committee. Guidance on safety assessment of botanicals and botanical preparations intended for use as ingredients in food supplements, on request of EFSA. *EFSA J.* **2009**, *7*, 1249.
7. European Food safety Authority. Compendium of botanicals reported to contain naturally occuring substances of possible concern for human health when used in food and food supplements. *EFSA J.* **2012**, *10*, 2663.
8. U.S. Department of Health and Human Services Food and Drug Administration Center for Drug Evaluation and Research (CDER). Botanical Drug Development Guidance for Industry. December 2016 Pharmaceutical Quality/CMC Revision 1. Available online: https://www.fda.gov/Drugs/GuidanceComplianceRegulatoryInformation/Guidances/default.htm (accessed on 24 May 2018).
9. European Commission. Herbal Medicinal Products. Available online: https://ec.europa.eu/health/human-use/herbal-medicines_en (accessed on 24 May 2018).
10. World Health Organization, Programme on Traditional Medicine. *General Guidelines for Methodologies on Research and Evaluation of Traditional Medicines*; World Health Organization: Geneva, Switzerland, 2000; 71p.
11. Brown, A.C. An overview of herb and dietary supplement efficacy, safety and government regulations in the United States with suggested improvements. Part 1 of 5 series. *Food Chem. Toxicol.* **2017**, *107*, 449–471. [CrossRef] [PubMed]
12. Ma, C.; Oketch-Rabah, H.; Kim, N.-C.; Monagas, M.; Bzhelyansky, A.; Sarma, N.; Giancaspro, G. Quality specifications for articles of botanical origin from the United States Pharmacopeia. *Phytomedicine* **2018**, *45*, 105–119. [CrossRef] [PubMed]
13. Qu, L.; Zou, W.; Wang, T.; Wang, M. European regulation model for herbal medicine: The assessment of the EU monograph and the safety and efficacy evaluation in marketing authorization or registration in Member States. *Phytomedicine* **2018**, *42*, 219–225. [CrossRef] [PubMed]
14. Alamgir, A.N.M. Pharmacopoeia and herbal monograph, the aim and use of WHO's herbal monograph, WHO's guide lines for herbal monograph, pharmacognostical research and monographs of organized, unorganized drugs and drugs from animal sources. In *Therapeutic Use of Medicinal Plants and Their Extracts*; Rainsford, K.D., Ed.; Springer International Publishing: Cham, Switzerland, 2017; pp. 295–353, ISBN 978-3-319-63861-4.
15. World Health Organization. Essential Medicines and Health Products Information Portal. Available online: http://apps.who.int/medicinedocs/en/ (accessed on 05 June 2018).
16. Shankar, P.R. Essential medicines and health products information portal. *J. Pharmacol. Pharmacother.* **2014**, *5*, 74–75. [CrossRef] [PubMed]
17. Van Breemen, R.B. Development of safe and effective botanical dietary supplements. *J. Med. Chem.* **2015**, *58*, 8360–8372. [CrossRef] [PubMed]
18. Saito, K.; Matsuda, F. Metabolomics for functional genomics, systems biology, and biotechnology. *Annu. Rev. Plant Biol.* **2010**, *61*, 463–489. [CrossRef] [PubMed]
19. Roessner, U.; Beckles, D.M. Metabolite measurements. In *Plant Metabolic Networks*; Schwender, J., Ed.; Springer Verlag: New York, NY, USA, 2009; pp. 39–69. ISBN 978-0-387-78745-9.

20. Durazzo, A. Study approach of antioxidant properties in foods: Update and considerations. *Foods* **2017**, *6*, 17. [CrossRef] [PubMed]
21. Liu, F.; Ma, C.; Gao, Y.; McClements, D.J. Food-grade covalent complexes and their application as nutraceutical delivery systems: A review. *Compr. Rev. Food Sci. Food Saf.* **2017**, *16*, 76–95. [CrossRef]
22. Scalbert, A.; Manach, C.; Morand, C.; Rémésy, C.; Jiménez, L. Dietary polyphenols and the prevention of diseases. *Crit. Rev. Food Sci. Nutr.* **2005**, *45*, 287–306. [CrossRef] [PubMed]
23. Sun, J. D-limonene: Safety and clinical applications. *Altern. Med. Rev.* **2007**, *12*, 259–264. [PubMed]
24. Sureda, A.; Sanches Silva, A.; Sánchez-Machado, D.I.; López-Cervantes, J.; Daglia, M.; Nabavi, S.F.; Nabavi, S.M. Hypotensive effects of genistein: From chemistry to medicine. *Chem. Biol. Interact.* **2017**, *268*, 37–46. [CrossRef] [PubMed]
25. Yadav, M.; Chatterji, S.; Gupta, S.K.; Watal, G. Preliminary phytochemical screening of six medicinal plants used in traditional medicine. *Int. J. Pharm. Pharmaceut. Sci.* **2014**, *6*, 539–542.
26. Kuete, V. Health effects of alkaloids from African medicinal plants. In *Toxicological Survey of African Medicinal Plants*; Kuete, V., Ed.; Elsevier: New York, NY, USA, 2014; pp. 611–633, ISBN 9780128000182.
27. Song, X.; Hu, S. Adjuvant activities of saponins from traditional Chinese medicinal herbs. *Vaccine* **2009**, *27*, 4883–4890. [CrossRef] [PubMed]
28. Zhou, M.; Zhang, R.H.; Wang, M.; Xu, G.B.; Liao, S.G. Prodrugs of triterpenoids and their derivatives. *Eur J. Med. Chem.* **2017**, *131*, 222–236. [CrossRef] [PubMed]
29. Du, G.; Sun, L.; Zhao, R.; Du, L.; Song, J.; Zhang, L.; He, G.; Zhang, Y.; Zhang, J. Polyphenols: Potential source of drugs for the treatment of ischaemic heart disease. *Pharmacol. Ther.* **2016**, *162*, 23–34. [CrossRef] [PubMed]
30. Kim, Y.; Keogh, J.B.; Clifton, P.M. Polyphenols and glycemic control. *Nutrients* **2016**, *8*, 17. [CrossRef] [PubMed]
31. Biesalski, H.K.; Dragsted, L.O.; Elmadfa, I.; Grossklaus, R.; Müller, M.; Schrenk, D.; Walter, P.; Weber, P. Bioactive compounds: Definition and assessment of activity. *Nutrition* **2009**, *25*, 1202–1205. [CrossRef] [PubMed]
32. Sasidharan, S.; Chen, Y.; Saravanan, D.; Sundram, K.M.; Yoga Latha, L. Extraction, isolation and characterization of bioactive compounds from plants' extracts. *Afr. J. Tradit. Complement. Altern. Med.* **2011**, *8*, 1–10. [CrossRef] [PubMed]
33. Ganzera, M.; Sturm, S. Recent advances on HPLC/MS in medicinal plant analysis-An update covering 2011–2016. *J. Pharm. Biomed. Anal.* **2017**, *147*, 211–233. [CrossRef] [PubMed]
34. Ingle, K.P.; Deshmukh, A.G.; Padole, D.A.; Dudhare, M.S.; Moharil, M.P.; Khelurkar, VC. Phytochemicals: Extraction methods, identification and detection of bioactive compounds from plant extracts. *J. Pharmacogn. Phytochem.* **2017**, *6*, 32–36.
35. Pandey, A.; Tripathi, S. Concept of standardization, extraction and pre phytochemical screening strategies for herbal drug. *J. Pharmacogn. Phytochem.* **2014**, *2*, 115–119.
36. Bansal, A.; Chhabra, V.; Rawal, R.K.; Sharma, S. Chemometrics: A new scenario in herbal drug standardization. *J. Pharm. Anal.* **2014**, *4*, 223–233. [CrossRef] [PubMed]
37. Mok, D.K.W.; Chau, F.T. Chemical information of Chinese medicines: A challenge to chemist. *Chemom. Intell. Lab. Syst.* **2006**, *82*, 210–217. [CrossRef]
38. Zeng, Z.; Chau, F.T.; Chan, H.Y.; Cheung, C.Y.; Lau, T.Y.; Wei, S.; Mok, D.K.; Chan, C.O.; Liang, Y. Recent advances in the compound-oriented and pattern-oriented approaches to the quality control of herbal medicines. *Chin. Med.* **2008**, *3*, 9. [CrossRef] [PubMed]
39. Harnly, J.; Lu, Y.; Sun, J.; Chen, C. Botanical supplements: Detecting the transition from ingredient to product. *J. Food Compos. Anal.* **2017**, *64*, 85–92. [CrossRef]
40. Yang, Z.; Shao, Q.; Ge, Z.; Ai, N.; Zhao, X.; Fan, X. A bioactive chemical markers based strategy for quality assessment of botanical drugs: Xuesaitong injection as a case study. *Sci. Rep.* **2017**, *7*, 2410. [CrossRef] [PubMed]
41. Zhang, X.; Zhang, L.-F.; Cai, C.-Y.; Xue, F.-Q.; Xiao, S. An approach for searching bioactive compounds from traditional Chinese plant food and herb medicines by investigating spectrum–effect relationships. *Curr. Pharm. Anal.* **2017**, *13*, 417–426. [CrossRef]

42. Abubakar, B.M.; Salleh, F.M.; Omar, M.S.S.; Wagiran, A. Review: DNA barcoding and chromatography fingerprints for the authentication of botanicals in herbal medicinal products. *Evid. Based Complement. Alternat. Med.* **2017**, *2017*, 1352948. [CrossRef]
43. Sánchez-Vidaña, D.I.; Rajwani, R.; Wong, M.S. The use of omic technologies applied to traditional chinese medicine research. *Evid. Based Complement. Alternat. Med.* **2017**, *2017*, 6359730. [CrossRef] [PubMed]
44. Mumtaz, M.W.; Hamid, A.A.; Akhtar, M.T.; Anwar, F.; Rashid, U.; Al-Zuaidy, M.H. An overview of recent developments in metabolomics and proteomics—Phytotherapic research perspectives. *Front. Life Sci.* **2017**, *10*, 1–37. [CrossRef]
45. Galanakis, C.M. Recovery of high added-value components from food wastes: Conventional, emerging technologies and commercialized applications. *Trends Food Sci. Technol.* **2012**, *6*, 68–87. [CrossRef]
46. Galanakis, C.M.; Cvejic, J.; Verardo, V.; Segura Carretero, A. Food use for social innovation by optimizing food waste recovery strategies. In *Innovation Strategies in the Food Industry. Tools for Implementation*; Galanakis, C.M., Ed.; Academic Press: London, UK, 2016; pp. 211–236.
47. Lin, C.S.K.; Koutinas, A.A.; Stamatelatou, K.; Mubofu, E.B.; Matharu, A.S.; Kopsahelis, N.; Pfaltzgraff, L.A.; Clark, J.H.; Papanikolaou, S.; Kwan, T.H.; et al. Current and future trends in food waste valorization for the production of chemicals, materials and fuels: A global perspective. *Biofuels Bioprod. Bioref.* **2014**, *8*, 686–715. [CrossRef]
48. Stahel, W.R. The circular economy. *Nature* **2016**, *531*, 435–438. [CrossRef] [PubMed]
49. Kumar, H.; Yadav, A.N.; Kumar, V.; Vyas, P.; Dhaliwal, H.S. Food waste: A potential bioresource for extraction of nutraceuticals and bioactive compounds. *Bioresour. Bioprocess* **2017**, *4*, 18. [CrossRef]
50. Banach, M.; Mikhailidis, D.P.; Serban, M.C.; Sahebkar, A. Editorial: Natural products as the integral part of the therapy? *Curr. Pharm. Des.* **2017**, *23*, 2411–2413. [CrossRef] [PubMed]
51. Thompson, P.B. *From Field to Fork, Food Ethics for Everyone*; Oxford University Press: New York, NY, USA, 2015; 346p, ISBN 9780199391684.
52. Varzakas, T.; Zakynthinos, G.; Verpoort, F. Plant food residues as a source of nutraceuticals and functional foods. *Foods* **2016**, *5*, 88. [CrossRef] [PubMed]
53. Romani, A.; Ciani Scarnicci, M.; Scardigli, A.; Paiano, A. Circular Economy as a New Model for the Exploitation of the Agroindustrial Biomass. In Proceedings of the 20th IGWT Symposium, Commodity Science in a Changing World, Varna, Bulgaria, 12–16 September 2016.
54. Romani, A.; Pinelli, P.; Ieri, F.; Bernini, R. Sustainability, Innovation and Green Chemistry in the Production and Valorization of Phenolic Extracts from *Olea europaea* L. *Sustainability* **2016**, *8*, 1002. [CrossRef]
55. Pfaltzgraff, L.A.; De bruyn, M.; Cooper, E.C.; Budarin, V.; Clark, J.H. Food waste biomass: A resource for high-value Chemicals. *Green Chem.* **2013**, *15*, 307–314. [CrossRef]
56. Baiano, A. Recovery of biomolecules from food wastes—A review. *Molecules* **2014**, *19*, 14821–14842. [CrossRef] [PubMed]
57. Cheng, D.M.K. Phytochemistry. In *Ethnobotany: A Phytochemical Perspective*; Schmidt, B.M., Cheng, D.M.K., Eds.; John Wiley & Sons Ltd.: Chichester, UK, 2017; pp. 111–140.
58. Kanehisa, M. KEGG bioinformatics resource for plant genomics and metabolomics. *Methods Mol. Biol.* **2016**, *1374*, 55–70. [CrossRef] [PubMed]
59. Naithani, S.; Preece, J.; D'Eustachio, P.; Gupta, P.; Amarasinghe, V.; Dharmawardhana, P.D.; Wu, G.; Fabregat, A.; Elser, J.L.; Weiser, J.; et al. Plant Reactome: A resource for plant pathways and comparative analysis. *Nucleic Acids Res.* **2017**, *45*, 1029–1039. [CrossRef] [PubMed]
60. Finglas, P.; Berry, R.; Astley, S. Assessing and improving the quality of food composition databases for nutrition and health applications in Europe: The contribution of EuroFIR. *Adv. Nutr.* **2014**, *5*, 608S–614S. [CrossRef] [PubMed]
61. Finglas, P.; Roe, M.; Pinchen, H.; Astley, S. The contribution of food composition resources to nutrition science methodology. *Nutr. Bull.* **2017**, *42*, 198–206. [CrossRef]
62. Gurinović, M.; Zeković, M.; Milešević, J.; Nikolić, M.; Glibetić, M. Nutritional Assessment. *Ref. Module Food Sci.* **2017**, 1–14. [CrossRef]
63. LanguaL™—The International Framework for Food Description. Available online: http://www.langual.org/ (accessed on 7 June 2018).
64. EuroFIR AISBL. EuroFIR—European Food Information Resource. Available online: http://www.eurofir.org/ (accessed on 7 June 2018).

65. FAO. International Network of Food Data Systems (INFOODS). 2017. Available online: www.fao.org/infoods/infoods/en/ (accessed on 10 November 2017).
66. USDA Food Composition Databases. Available online: https://ndb.nal.usda.gov/ndb/ (accessed on 7 June 2018).
67. Phenol-Explorer—Database on Polyphenol Content in Foods. Available online: http://phenol-explorer.eu/ (accessed on 8 June 2018).
68. Neveu, V.; Perez-Jiménez, J.; Vos, F.; Crespy, V.; du Chaffaut, L.; Mennen, L.; Knox, C.; Eisner, R.; Cruz, J.; Wishart, D.; et al. Phenol-Explorer: An online comprehensive database on polyphenol contents in foods. *J. Biol. Databases Curation* **2010**, *2010*, bap024. [CrossRef] [PubMed]
69. eBASIS—Bioactive Substances in Food Information System. Available online: http://ebasis.eurofir.org/Default.asp (accessed on 8 June 2018).
70. Kiely, M.; Black, L.J.; Plumb, J.; Kroon, P.A.; Hollman, P.C.; Larsen, J.C.; Speijers, G.J.; Kapsokefalou, M.; Sheehan, D.; Gry, J.; et al. EuroFIR eBASIS: Application for health claims submissions and evaluations. *Eur. J. Clin. Nutr.* **2010**, *64*, S101–S107. [CrossRef] [PubMed]
71. Plumb, J.; Pigat, S.; Bompola, F.; Cushen, M.; Pinchen, H.; Nørby, E.; Astley, S.; Lyons, J.; Kiely, M.; Finglas, P. eBASIS (Bioactive Substances in Food Information Systems) and bioactive intakes: Major updates of the bioactive compound composition and beneficial bio effects database and the development of a probabilistic model to assess intakes in Europe. *Nutrients* **2017**, *9*, 320. [CrossRef] [PubMed]
72. Bucchini, L.; Rodarte, A.; Restani, P. The PlantLIBRA project: How we intend to innovate the science of botanicals. *Food Funct.* **2011**, *2*, 769–773. [CrossRef] [PubMed]
73. Bhagwat, S.; Haytowitz, D.B.; Holden, J.M. *USDA Database for the Isoflavone Content of Selected Foods, Release 2.0*; U.S. Department of Agriculture, Agricultural Research Service, Nutrient Data Laboratory: Beltsville, MD, USA, 2008. Available online: https://data.nal.usda.gov/dataset/usda-database-isoflavone-content-selected-foods-release-20_108 (accessed on 10 November 2017).
74. Bhagwat, S.; Haytowitz, D.B.; Holden, J.M. *USDA Database for the Flavonoid Content of Selected Foods. Release 3.1*; U.S. Department of Agriculture, Agricultural Research Service, Nutrient Data Laboratory: Beltsville, MD, USA, 2014. Available online: https://data.nal.usda.gov/dataset/usda-database-flavonoid-content-selected-foods-release-31-may-2014_109 (accessed on 10 November 2017).
75. Bhagwat, S.; Haytowitz, D. *USDA Database for the Proanthocyanidin Content of Selected Foods, Release 2*; U.S. Department of Agriculture, Agricultural Service, Nutrient Data Laboratory: Beltsville, MD, USA, 2015. Available online: https://data.nal.usda.gov/dataset/usda-database-proanthocyanidin-content-selected-foods-release-2-2015/resource/df39fc45-5fb2 (accessed on 10 November 2017).
76. Rothwell, J.A.; Urpi-Sarda, M.; Boto-Ordonez, M.; Knox, C.; Llorach, R.; Eisner, R.; Cruz, J.; Neveu, V.; Wishart, D.; Manach, C.; et al. Phenol-Explorer 2.0: A major update of the Phenol-Explorer database integrating data on polyphenol metabolism and pharmacokinetics in humans and experimental animals. *J. Biol. Databases Curation* **2012**, *2012*, bas031. [CrossRef] [PubMed]
77. Rothwell, J.A.; Perez-Jimenez, J.; Neveu, V.; Medina-Remon, A.; M'Hiri, N.; Garcia-Lobato, P.; Manach, C.; Knox, C.; Eisner, R.; Wishart, D.S.; et al. Phenol-Explorer 3.0: A major update of the Phenol-Explorer database to incorporate data on the effects of food processing on polyphenol content. *J. Biol. Databases Curation* **2013**, *2013*, bat070. [CrossRef] [PubMed]
78. Durazzo, A. Extractable and non-extractable polyphenols: An overview. In *Non-Extractable Polyphenols and Carotenoids: Importance in Human Nutrition and Health. Food Chemistry, Function and Analysis Series n. 5*; Saura-Calixto, F., Pérez-Jiménez, J., Eds.; Royal Society of Chemistry: London, UK, 2018; ISBN 2398-0656.
79. Durazzo, A.; Plumb, J.; Lucarini, M.; Fernandez-Lopez, G.; Camilli, E.; Turrini, A.; Finglas, P.; Marletta, L. *Extractable and Non-Extractable Antioxidants at the Interface of eBASIS Structure: Database Development and Expansion*; EuroFIR Food Forum: Brussels, Belgium, 2018.
80. Plumb, J.; Lyons, J.; Nørby, K.; Thomas, M.; Nørby, E.; Poms, R.; Bucchini, L.; Restani, P.; Kiely, M.; Finglas, P.; et al. PlantLIBRA Consortia. ePlantLIBRA: A composition and biological activity database for bioactive compounds in plant food supplements. *Food Chem.* **2016**, *193*, 121–127. [CrossRef] [PubMed]
81. National Institutes of Health. DSLD—Dietary Supplement Label Database. Available online: https://ods.od.nih.gov/Research/Dietary_Supplement_Label_Database.aspx (accessed on 8 June 2018).
82. DSLD—Dietary Supplement Label Database. Available online: https://dsld.nlm.nih.gov/dsld/ (accessed on 8 June 2018).

83. Dwyer, J.T.; Saldanha, L.G.; Bailen, R.A.; Bailey, R.L.; Costello, R.B.; Betz, J.M.; Chang, F.F.; Goshorn, J.; Andrews, K.W.; Pehrsson, P.R.; et al. A free new dietary supplement label database for registered dietitian nutritionists. *J. Acad. Nutr. Diet.* **2014**, *114*, 1512–1517. [CrossRef] [PubMed]
84. Potischman, N.; Salazar, S.; Susser, J.; Saldanha, L.S.J.; Dwyer, J.; Kuzak, A.; Betz, J.; Bailen, R. Testing usability of the Dietary Supplement Label Database (DSLD): A resource for consumers, professionals, and researchers. *J. Nutr. Educ. Behav.* **2017**, *49*, S99. [CrossRef]
85. PD_Manager Project. Available online: www.parkinson-manager.eu (accessed on 8 June 2018).
86. Durazzo, A.; Camilli, E.; Sette, S.; D'Addezio, L.; Marletta, L.; Turrini, A. *Dietary Supplement Label Database Development: Approach Description and Preliminary Results*; EuroFIR Food Forum: Bruxelles, Belgium, 2016.
87. European Food Safety Authority. Classification and description system FoodEx2 (revision 2). *EFSA J.* **2015**, *EN-804*, 1–90.
88. Durazzo, A.; D'Addezio, L.; Camilli, E.; Piccinelli, R.; Marletta, L.; Turrini, A.; Sette, S. Feedbacks and Proposal for FoodEx2 revision 2 implementation: Focus on Dietary supplements. In Proceedings of the EuroFIR Food Forum, Brussels, Belgium, 10–12 April 2018.
89. Durazzo, A.; Camilli, E.; D'Addezio, L.; Piccinelli, R.; Lisciani, S.; Marletta, L.; Turrini, A.; Sette, S. Una finestra sugli integratori alimentari in Italia: Sviluppo di un database dedicato. In Proceedings of the XXVIII Congresso Nazionale di Scienze Merceologiche, Firenze, Italy, 21–23 February 2018; pp. 408–411.
90. Manach, C.; Milenkovic, D.; van de Wiele, T.; Rodriguez-Mateos, A.; de Roos, B.; Garcia-Conesa, M.T.; Landberg, R.; Gibney, E.R.; Heinonen, M.; Tomás-Barberán, F.; et al. Addressing the inter-individual variation in response to consumption of plant food bioactives: Towards a better understanding of their role in healthy aging and cardiometabolic risk reduction. *Mol. Nutr. Food Res.* **2017**, *61*, 1–16. [CrossRef] [PubMed]
91. Dragsted, L.O.; Gao, Q.; Praticò, G.; Manach, C.; Wishart, D.S.; Scalbert, A.; Feskens, E.J.M. Dietary and health biomarkers—Time for an update. *Genes Nutr.* **2017**, *12*, 24. [CrossRef] [PubMed]
92. HMDB—Human Metabolome Database. Available online: www.hmdb.ca (accessed on 8 June 2018).
93. Wishart, D.S.; Feunang, Y.D.; Marcu, A.; Guo, A.C.; Liang, K.; Vázquez-Fresno, R.; Sajed, T.; Johnson, D.; Li, C.; Karu, N.; et al. HMDB 4.0: The human metabolome database for 2018. *Nucleic Acids Res.* **2017**, *46*, D608–D617. [CrossRef] [PubMed]
94. PhytoHub Database. Available online: www.phytohub.eu (accessed on 8 June 2018).
95. Bento da Silva, A.; Giacomoni, F.; Pavot, B.; Fillâtre, Y.; Rothwell, J.A.; Sualdea, B.B.; Veyrat, C.; Garcia-Villalba, R.; Gladine, C.; Kopec, R.; et al. PhytoHub V1.4: A new release for the online database dedicated to food phytochemicals and their human metabolites. In Proceedings of the 1st International Conference on Food Bioactivities & Health, Norwich, UK, 13–15 September 2016.

 © 2018 by the authors. Licensee MDPI, Basel, Switzerland. This article is an open access article distributed under the terms and conditions of the Creative Commons Attribution (CC BY) license (http://creativecommons.org/licenses/by/4.0/).

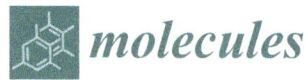

Communication

Comparative Evaluation of Soluble and Insoluble-Bound Phenolics and Antioxidant Activity of Two Chinese Mistletoes

Qing Li [1], Shihua Yang [2], Yongqiang Li [1,*], Xiaofeng Xue [3,*], Yonghua Huang [1], Hengguo Luo [1], Yiming Zhang [1] and Zhichao Lu [1]

[1] College of Food Science and Technology, Yunnan Agricultural University, Kunming 650201, China; 13211674852@163.com (Q.L.); hyh209920@163.com (Y.H.); l15559818968@163.com (H.L.); zym718zhangym@163.com (Y.Z.); luzhichao1s@163.com (Z.L.)
[2] College of Foreign Languages, Yunnan Agricultural University, Kunming 650201, China; yanglifang815@163.com
[3] Institute of Apicultural Research, Chinese Academy of Agricultural Sciences, Beijing 100093, China
* Correspondence: liyongqiang7512@ynau.edu.cn (Y.L.); xue_xiaofeng@126.com (X.X.); Tel.: +86-139-8761-1915 (Y.L.); +86-10-6259-4643 (X.X.)

Received: 31 December 2017; Accepted: 6 February 2018; Published: 8 February 2018

Abstract: Mistletoes are used medicinally in order to treat various human illnesses. Few studies have reported on the phenolic content and antioxidant properties of Chinese mistletoes (CMs). In this work, the total phenolic content (TPC), total flavonoid content (TFC), and antioxidant activities of soluble and insoluble-bound phenolic extracts from CMs hosted by *Camellia assamica* (Mast.) Chang (CMC) and *Pyrus, i, f.* (CMP) were compared. Phenolic compounds in CMC and CMP were identified and quantified using high-performance liquid chromatography (HPLC). The results indicated that the TPC of soluble phenolic extracts was higher than insoluble-bound phenolic counterparts in both CMC and CMP. In addition, the TPC of soluble, insoluble-bound and total phenolic fractions (9.91 ± 0.23, 4.59 ± 0.27 and 14.50 ± 0.35 µmol ferulic acid equivalents per gram (FAE/g) dry sample) extracted from CMP were higher than those extracted from CMC. The soluble phenolic extracts in CMP showed higher antioxidant activities than those in CMC. Eighteen phenolic compounds from soluble and insoluble-bound phenolic extracts from the CMs were identified and quantified by HPLC. This study indicates that CMC and CMP, especially the latter, could be sources of antioxidants in human health care.

Keywords: Chinese mistletoes; phenolics; phenolic contents; antioxidant activity

1. Introduction

Mistletoes belonging to the order Santalales, which comprises Santalaceae, Loranthaceae, and Misodendraceae, are semi-parasites that grow on the Theaceae, Rosaceae, Moraceae and Leguminosae families [1]. Most are distributed in Southern and Central Asia, North-Western Africa, Europe and Eastern Australia [2–4]. Since ancient times, mistletoes have been applied as traditional medicines for the treatment of cancer and some chronic diseases due to their antioxidant and anti-inflammatory activities [3,5–7].

The main phytoconstituents, including proteins, carbohydrates, flavonoids, glycosides, phenolic compounds, tannins and triterpenes, have been identified in mistletoes by their physicochemical properties and spectral analysis [8–10]. In addition, several studies have revealed that mistletoes possess moderate antioxidant capacity due to the presence of phenolic compounds [9–11]. *Viscum articulatum* Burm. f. hosted by *Camellia assamica* (Mast.) Chang (CMC) and *Viscum liquidambaricolum*

Hayata parasitic on *Pyrus, i, f.* (CMP) are two native Chinese mistletoes (CMs). CMC has been commonly used in traditional Chinese medicine for the treatment of hemorrhage, pleurisy, gout, heart disease, epilepsy, arthritis, and hypertension [12]. Previous investigations of CMC have revealed that phenolic glycosides, flavanone glycosides, triterpenoids, organic acids and flavonoids are the major secondary metabolites of this plant [13,14]. A few studies have focused on the phenolic composition and antioxidant activities of soluble phenolic compounds in CMC. However, there has been little research into insoluble-bound phenolic compounds in CMC. Moreover, the phenolic composition and antioxidant activities of CMP are unclear.

Phenolic compounds produced during secondary metabolism are characterized by some phenolic hydroxyl groups in the molecules [15]. These can be divided into several groups, including phenolic acids, flavonoids, stilbenes and lignans, based on the chemical structure of the phenolic compounds [16]. According to their solubility features, phenolics are separated into soluble and insoluble-bound fractions [17–19]. Insoluble-bound phenolics are covalently bound to the cell–wall matrix, including cellulose, arabinoxylans and proteins by ester, ether and carbon–carbon bonds [18]. Organic solvent is used to extract the soluble phenolic compounds, whereas acidic, alkaline or enzymatic hydrolysis are used to release insoluble-bound phenolics [19]. Insoluble-bound phenolics may be slowly and continuously released in the human gastrointestinal tract and during colonic fermentation, which can improve bioaccessibility and potential bioavailability and exert high bioactivity on tissues and cells for a long time [18,20]. However, most studies reported in the literature have ignored insoluble-bound phenolic compounds, and hence have underestimated their phenolic compound content and activities. Phenolic compounds are major sources of dietary antioxidants in the plants [21]. Antioxidants have beneficial health aspects, preventing and scavenging free radicals by means of donating hydrogen atoms to a free radical in order to protect biomolecules, such as proteins, lipids, carbohydrates and DNA [20,22,23], and to alleviate chronic diseases and degenerative ailments [24]. Thus, the beneficial effects of mistletoes may be attributed to their phenolic compounds [21].

The objectives of this study were to quantify the total phenolic and flavonoid contents of soluble and insoluble-bound phenolic extracts and to assess the antioxidant activities of CMC and CMP. The phenolic compounds in these two Chinese mistletoes were identified and quantified by high-performance liquid chromatography (HPLC). Moreover, the content, compositions and antioxidant activities of phenolic extracts in CMC and CMP were compared.

2. Results and Discussion

2.1. Total Phenolic Content (TPC) and Total Flavonoid Content (TFC)

Phenolics are the predominant group of phytochemical compounds, and are widely distributed in flowers, fruits, seeds, roots, stems, leaves of various plants and medicinal herbs [3,25,26]. Figure 1 presents the TPC and TFC of soluble and insoluble-bound phenolic extracts of CMC and CMP. The TPC of soluble, insoluble-bound and total phenolic extracts in CMs ranged from 8.65–9.91 µmol FAE/g DS, 3.95–4.59 µmol FAE/g DS and 12.59–14.50 µmol FAE/g DS, respectively. The TPC of soluble phenolic extracts, either in CMC or in CMP, was significantly higher ($p < 0.05$) than that of insoluble-bound phenolic content. Similar results have been obtained for the TPC of millet, barley, onion and the different parts of *Castanea crenata* [22,26,27]. However, in contrast to the results obtained in the present works, some researchers have found that the TPC of soluble phenolic extracts was lower than insoluble-bound phenolics [28,29], which may be due to the differences of bond strength between phenolic compounds and cell-wall matrix. Moreover, the TPC of soluble, insoluble-bound and total phenolic in extracts of CMP were significantly higher than those in CMC ($p < 0.05$).

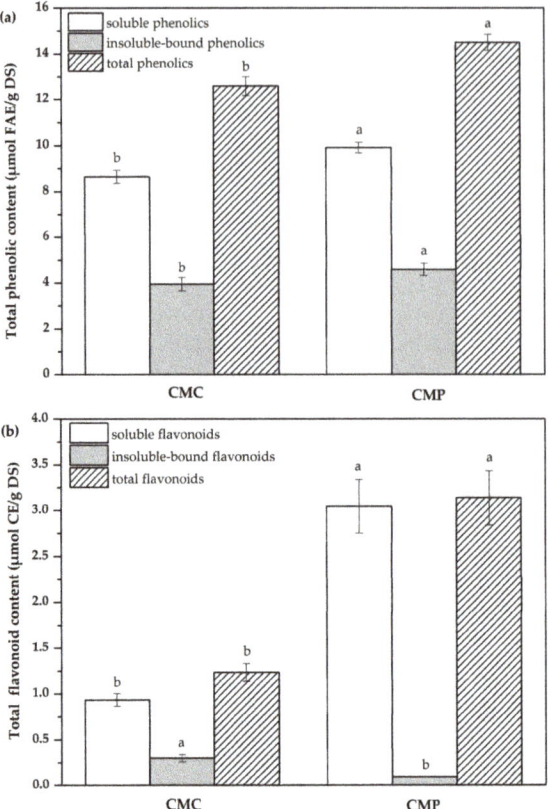

Figure 1. Total phenolic content (**a**) and flavonoid content (**b**) of soluble and insoluble-bound phenolic extracts in the two Chinese mistletoes (CMs). Different letters in each category (soluble, insoluble-bound, and total phenolics) are significantly different ($p < 0.05$). CMC, the Chinese mistletoes hosted by *Camellia assamica* (Mast.) Chang; CMP, the Chinese mistletoes hosted by *Pyrus*, *i*,*f*; FAE, ferulic acid equivalents; CE, catechin equivalents; DS, dry sample.

Flavonoids are phenolic compounds that exhibit various biological activities, such as anti-cancer, anti-allergenic, anti-viral, anti-inflammatory effects, vasodilating actions and gastroprotective properties, as well as having superior antioxidant activities [30]. The TFC of soluble, insoluble-bound and total flavonoids extracts in CMs ranged from 0.93–3.05 μmol CE/g DS, 0.10–0.30 μmol CE/g DS and 1.23–3.14 μmol CE/g DS, respectively. The TFC of the soluble and insoluble-bound flavonoids extracts in CMC and CMP exhibited a similar trend to that of TPC. The results showed that the TFC of the soluble flavonoids fractions in CMs was higher than corresponding insoluble-bound flavonoids. Similar results have been reported in previous studies [22,27]. The TFC of soluble flavonoid extracts in CMP was significantly higher ($p < 0.05$) than that in CMC. However, the TFC of insoluble-bound flavonoids extracts in CMC was significantly higher than that in CMP ($p < 0.05$). This discrepancy may be attributed to majority flavonoids that could bind the proteins and polysaccharides through ether and ester bonds in the CMC [18].

The results of our studies demonstrated that the TPC and TFC of both soluble and insoluble phenolic extracts were different in CMC and CMP. In addition, the TPC and TFC of total soluble phenolics in CMP were higher than those of in CMC.

2.2. Antioxidant Activities In Vitro

The antioxidant capacities of phenolic extracts can be measured in several ways. In this study, four different and complementary methods (ferric reducing antioxidant power (FRAP), hydrogen peroxide scavenging activity (HPSA), DPPH radical scavenging activity (DRSA) and Trolox equivalent antioxidant capacity (TEAC)) were used to describe more fully the antioxidant capacities in vitro. Although these assays are of limited use in predicting health benefits in humans, and extrapolation to an in vivo situation is not possible, they may still be valuable as a screening method for predicting the antioxidant activities of phenolic compounds [31,32].

The antioxidant activities of the soluble and insoluble-bound phenolic compounds extracted in CMC and CMP were detected (Table 1). It has been reported that there is a correlation between antioxidant activities and total phenolic content in many plants [9,15,25,26,33–35]. The FRAP of soluble and insoluble-bound phenolic extracts in CMs ranged from 42.25–44.76 μmol FE/g DS and 8.07–10.31 μmol FE/g DS. The HPSA of two phenolic extracts in CMs were in the range of 1429.34–1431.87 μmol FAE/g DS and 1383.79–1231.67 μmol FAE/g DS. The DRSA and TEAC of soluble phenolic extracts in CMs ranged from 2.19–2.51 μmol FAE/g DS and 81.03–84.92 μmol TE/g DS, and those of insoluble-bound phenolics ranged from 1.51–1.83 μmol FAE/g DS and 5.78–1.40 μmol TE/g DS. The FRAP, HPSA, DRSA and TEAC of the soluble phenolic extracts in CMs were significantly higher than their insoluble-bound phenolic counterparts ($p < 0.05$). The same trends of antioxidant activities were observed in millet, barley and onion [22,27]. In addition, soluble phenolic extracts in CMP had higher antioxidant capacities in terms of FRAP, HPSA, DRSA and TEAC than those in CMC. However, it was found that insoluble-bound phenolic fractions in CMP had significantly higher FRAP and DRSA values than those in CMC ($p < 0.05$). Therefore, our results showed that CMP with higher phenolic and flavonoid contents had stronger antioxidant activities than CMC. Thus, the two CMs might be used as food additives because their phenolic extracts had good antioxidative and radical-scavenging activities.

Table 1. Antioxidant activities of the two Chinese mistletoes.

Plant Material	CMC	CMP
Ferric Reducing Antioxidant Power (μmol FE/g DS)		
Soluble	42.25 ± 1.49a [2]	44.76 ± 0.32a [1]
Insoluble-bound	8.07 ± 0.75b [2]	10.31 ± 0.46b [1]
Hydrogen Peroxide Scavenging Activity (μmol FAE/g DS)		
Soluble	1429.34 ± 7.69a [1]	1431.87 ± 4.16a [1]
Insoluble-bound	1383.79 ± 3.33b [1]	1231.67 ± 12.23b [2]
DPPH Radical Scavenging Activity (μmol FAE/g DS)		
Soluble	2.19 ± 0.11a [2]	2.51 ± 0.04a [1]
Insoluble-bound	1.51 ± 0.07b [2]	1.83 ± 0.09b [1]
Trolox Equivalent Antioxidant Capacity (μmol TE/g DS)		
Soluble	81.03 ± 0.90a [2]	84.92 ± 1.50a [1]
Insoluble-bound	5.78 ± 1.24b [1]	1.40 ± 0.24b [2,*]

* CMC, the Chinese mistletoes hosted by *Camellia assamica* (Mast.) Chang; CMP, the Chinese mistletoes hosted by *Pyrus, i, f.*; FE, Fe^{2+} equivalents; FAE, ferulic acid equivalents; TE, Trolox equivalents; DS, dry sample. Values are mean ± standard deviation ($n = 5$); Values in each row having the different superscripts are significantly different ($p < 0.05$); values in each column having the different letter values are significantly different ($p < 0.05$).

2.3. Identification and Quantification of the Two Chinese Mistletoe (CM) Extracts by High-Performance Liquid Chromatography (HPLC)

The HPLC chromatograms of soluble and insoluble-bound phenolic compounds in CMC and CMP extracts are presented in Figures 2 and 3. The main classes of phenolic compounds identified in CMC and CMP were hydroxybenzoic acids, hydroxycinnamic acids and flavonoids.

The phenolic compounds of soluble phenolic extracts are shown in Table 2. Several hydroxybenzoic acids, including gallic acid, protocatechuic acid, *p*-hydroxybenzoic acid, vanillic acid, syringic acid and vanillin, were identified in CMC and CMP by comparison of their retention time (RT) with those of the available standards (Figure S1). Our results showed that the RT of phenolic compounds of hydroxybenzoic acids in CMP were 1.95–5.88 times higher than those in CMC, except for vanillic acid and syringic acid. The major hydroxycinnamic acids identified were chlorogenic acid, caffeic acid, *p*-coumaric acid, ferulic acid and *trans*-cinnamic acid. In general, the RT of caffeic acid, *p*-coumaric acid and *trans*-cinnamic acid in CMP were 1.12, 9.64 and 2.54 times higher than those in CMC. Flavonoids, namely catechin hydrate, epicatechin, (−)-epigallocatechin, myricetin, quercetin, kaempferol and apigenin were determined. Flavonoids are a large family of compounds in plants [30]. The content of all six phenolic compounds in CMP was higher than those in CMC. In addition, our results showed that myricetin (2209.79 ± 1476.96 µg/g) and epicatechin (238.18 ± 79.30 µg/g) were the most abundant in CMP and CMC, respectively. Previous research has shown that quercetin was the most abundant among five Polish *Viscum album* [9]. The difference between Polish *Viscum album* and CMs may be due to the varieties and the growth conditions of the plants. In addition, flavonoids constituted a substantial content of total phenolic compounds and individually contributed to 24.55% and 60.94% of the content in CMC and CMP, respectively. Vanillic acid (1325.77 ± 23.34 µg/g) and myricetin (2209.79 ± 1476.96 µg/g) might be characteristic phenolic compounds in CMC and CMP, respectively, due to their high contents. Most of the eighteen phenolic compounds were also found in different mistletoes [9,14,36]. Furthermore, myricetin had been recognized as a source that could limit type 2 diabetes mellitus [37]. Hence, the phenolic compounds of CMs have potential to be researched further. The insoluble-bound phenolic profiles are given in Table 3. Eighteen phenolic compounds subdivided into hydroxybenzoic acids, hydroxycinnamic acid and flavonoids, were also identified and quantified by HPLC. Moreover, *p*-coumaric acid (206.97 ± 21.39 µg/g) and (−)-epigallocatechin (223.32 ± 24.87 µg/g) might be characteristic phenolic compounds in insoluble-bound phenolic extracts of CMC and CMP, respectively.

Table 2. Individual soluble phenolic compounds in the two Chinese mistletoes (µg/g DS sample).

Phenolic Compounds	CMC	CMP
Hydroxybenzoic Acids		
Gallic acid	67.51 ± 12.21	172.65 ± 4.34
Protocatechuic acid	39.65 ± 9.27	203.23 ± 12.89
p-Hydroxybenzoic acid	133.88 ± 116.31	787.95 ± 138.89
Vanillic acid	1325.77 ± 23.34	408.82 ± 29.21
Syringic acid	432.33 ± 370.24	66.68 ± 27.90
Vanillin	70.08 ± 36.40	136.92 ± 130.03
Total	2069.23	1776.25
Hydroxycinnamic Acids		
Chlorogenic acid	93.36 ± 50.71	68.85 ± 27.70
Caffeic acid	105.59 ± 12.03	119.18 ± 16.77
p-Coumaric acid	85.05 ± 70.36	820.10 ± 355.68
Ferulic acid	560.48 ± 25.71	248.82 ± 101.63
trans-Cinnamic acid	67.80 ± 9.00	172.60 ± 1.93
Total	912.28	1429.55
Flavonoids		
Catechin hydrate	188.60 ± 138.25	200.51 ± 150.87
Epicatechin	238.18 ± 79.30	569.53 ± 67.92
(−)-Epigallocatechin	237.03 ± 8.36	542.10 ± 23.71
Myricetin	154.88 ± 62.10	2209.79 ± 1476.96
Quercetin	85.22 ± 28.75	834.71 ± 543.19
Kaemferol	40.48 ± 10.23	197.63 ± 157.76
Apigenin	25.50 ± 5.66	447.18 ± 3.32
Total	969.89	5001.44 *

* CMC: the Chinese mistletoes hosted by *Camellia assamica* (Mast.) Chang; CMP: the Chinese mistletoes hosted by *Pyrus, i, f.*; Values are mean ± standard deviation (*n* = 3).

Table 3. Individual insoluble-bound phenolic compounds in the two Chinese mistletoes (μg/g DS sample).

Phenolic Compounds	CMC	CMP
Hydroxybenzoic Acids		
Gallic acid	6.34 ± 0.56	21.41 ± 0.92
Protocatechuic acid	27.43 ± 1.73	23.24 ± 4.45
p-Hydroxybenzoic acid	48.02 ± 22.44	55.20 ± 42.12
Vanillic acid	52.73 ± 8.40	37.40 ± 25.69
Syringic acid	6.39 ± 1.14	10.45 ± 6.34
Vanillin	13.18 ± 7.35	39.69 ± 2.06
Total	154.08	187.40
Hydroxycinnamic Acids		
Chlorogenic acid	12.28 ± 2.43	22.21 ± 12.98
Caffeic acid	49.88 ± 2.41	28.20 ± 1.19
p-Coumaric acid	206.97 ± 21.39	14.26 ± 13.13
Ferulic acid	97.94 ± 4.63	171.18 ± 4.88
trans-Cinnamic acid	43.06 ± 1.02	124.38 ± 2.31
Total	410.12	360.23
Flavonoids		
Catechin hydrate	129.17 ± 32.41	92.21 ± 2.78
Epicatechin	11.21 ± 9.76	26.34 ± 12.67
(−)-Epigallocatechin	14.63 ± 10.29	223.32 ± 24.87
Myricetin	33.14 ± 19.55	75.23 ± 49.31
Quercetin	41.44 ± 11.71	62.30 ± 31.66
Kaemferol	18.15 ± 12.05	99.40 ± 69.46
Apigenin	10.35 ± 9.34	9.33 ± 6.64
Total	258.10	588.13 *

* CMC: the Chinese mistletoes hosted by *Camellia assamica* (Mast.) Chang; CMP: the Chinese mistletoes hosted by *Pyrus, i, f.*; Values are mean ± standard deviation (*n* = 3).

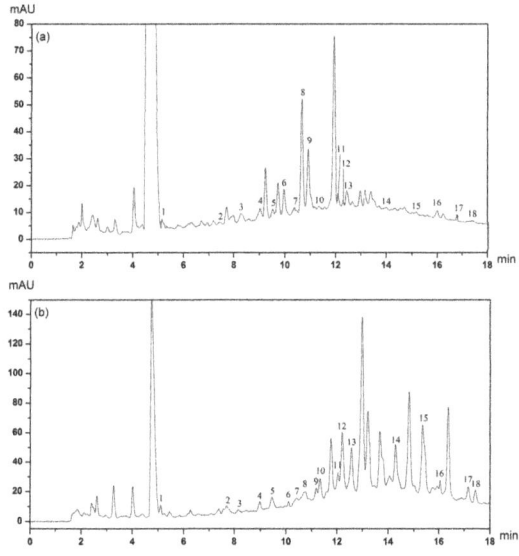

Figure 2. HPLC chromatograms of soluble phenolic extracts of the Chinese mistletoes hosted by *Camellia assamica* (Mast.) Chang (CMC) (**a**) and *Pyrus, i, f.* (CMP) (**b**). The identified compounds: 1, Gallic acid; 2, Protocatechuic acid; 3, Catechin hydrate; 4, Chlorogenic acid; 5, p-Hydroxybenzoic acid; 6, Epicatechin; 7, Caffeic acid; 8, Vanillic acid; 9, Syringic acid; 10 Vanillin; 11, (−)-Epigallocatechin; 12, p-Coumaric acid; 13, Ferulic acid; 14, Myricetin; 15, Quercetin; 16, *trans*-Cinnamic acid; 17, Kaempferol; 18, Apigenin.

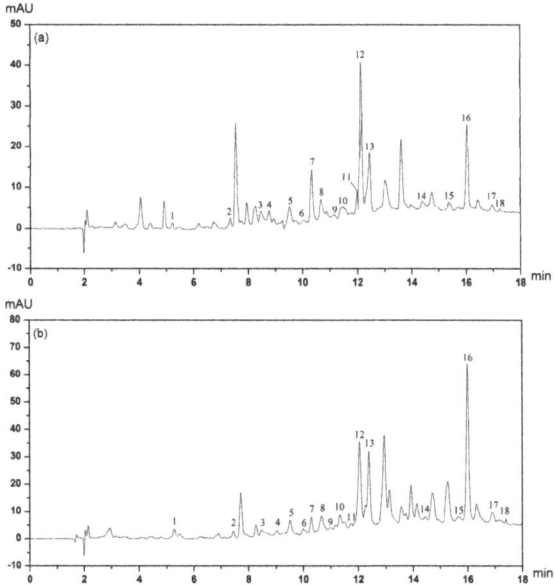

Figure 3. HPLC chromatograms of insoluble-bound phenolic extracts of the Chinese mistletoes hosted by *Camellia assamica* (Mast.) Chang (CMC) (**a**) and *Pyrus, i, f.* (CMP) (**b**). The identified compounds: 1, Gallic acid; 2, Protocatechuic acid; 3, Catechin hydrate; 4, Chlorogenic acid; 5, *p*-Hydroxybenzoic acid; 6, Epicatechin; 7, Caffeic acid; 8, Vanillic acid; 9, Syringic acid; 10 Vanillin; 11, (−)-Epigallocatechin; 12, *p*-Coumaric acid; 13, Ferulic acid; 14, Myricetin; 15, Quercetin; 16, *trans*-Cinnamic acid; 17, Kaempferol; 18, Apigenin.

3. Materials and Methods

3.1. Materials and Chemical Reagent

Viscum articulatum Burm. f. (CMC) and *Viscum liquidambaricolum* Hayata (CMP) were purchased from Pu'er, Yunnan province, China in 2016. Standard phenolic compounds (gallic acid, protocatechuic acid, chlorogenic acid, caffeic acid, *p*-coumaric acid, (−)-epigallocatechin, myricetin, kaempferol, apigenin, epicatechin, quercetin, vanillic acid, syringic acid, *trans*-cinnamic acid, catechin, ferulic acid, *p*-hydroxybenzoic acid and vanillin) were purchased from Beijing Beina Chuanglian Biotechnology Institute (Beijing, China). Folin-Ciocalteu phenol reagent, 6-hydroxy-2,5,7,8-tetramethylchroman-2-carboxylic acid (Trolox), 2,2-diphenyl-1-picrylhydrazyl (DPPH) were obtained from Sigma-Aldrich (St. Louis, MO, USA). 2,4,6-Tripyridyl-s-triazine (TPTZ), 2,2'-azinobis (3-ethylbenzothiazoline-6-sulfonic acid) (ABTS), trichloroacetic acid, ferric chloride, ascorbic acid, ferrous sulfate, potassium ferricyanide, sodium phosphate dibasic, sodium phosphate monobasic dihydrate, H_2O_2, aluminum chloride and potassium persulfate were purchased from Aladdin Industrial Corporation (Shanghai, China). HPLC-grade methanol and formic acid were purchased from Merck (Darmstadt, Germany). All chemicals used in the experiments were of analytical grade.

3.2. Separation of Phenolic Compounds

The soluble and insoluble-bound phenolic compounds from the two CMs were prepared using the methods reported in literature [20,38] with slight modifications. The mistletoes were ground to a fine powder with a Wiley mill (1029-A, Yoshida Seisakusho Co., Tokyo, Japan) for herbal medicine, and screened through a 50-mesh sieve. After the powder was freeze-dried with a vacuum freeze dryer (LGJ-12, Zhengzhou Nanbei Instrument Equipment Co., Ltd., Zhengzhou, China), 40 mL of 70% (v/v) acetone was added to 2.0 g of the dried powder, and then samples were shaken in an ultrasonic bath (SB-3200D, Ningbo Xinzhi biological Polytron Technologies Inc. 300 W, Ningbo, China) at room temperature for 15 min. The mixture was centrifuged at 4000× g for 10 min at 4 °C (TGL20M, Hunan Xiang Li Scientific Instrument Co., Ltd. Hunan, China). The upper layer was collected, and the extractions were repeated twice. The supernatants were combined and evaporated under reduced pressure at 30 °C (RE-52 AA, Shanghai Yarong biochemical instrument factory, Shanghai, China). This extract solution was analyzed as soluble phenolic extract.

The residues were used to extract the insoluble-bound phenolics. The samples were subsequently hydrolyzed with 40 mL NaOH (4 mol/L) at ambient temperature under nitrogen gas for 4 h. The resultant hydrolysate was acidified to pH 2 using HCl (6 mol/L) and then centrifuged at 4000× g for 10 min at 4 °C. The supernatants were combined and extracted 3 times with an equal volume of diethyl ether and ethyl acetate at 1:1 (v/v), and then evaporated under reduced pressure (30 °C). The insoluble-bound phenolic compounds were obtained. All samples were dissolved in 25 mL of HPLC grade methanol, and stored at −20 °C under nitrogen gas and covered with aluminum foil until used.

3.3. Determination of TPC

The TPC was determined using Folin–Ciocalteu phenol reagent, followed by the Chandrasekara and Shahidi [20] and Singleton and Rossi [39] methods, with slight modifications. Briefly, 500 µL of each phenolic extract was added to 0.5 mL Folin–Ciocalteu phenol reagent (2 mol/L) and 1 mL of saturated sodium carbonate (75 g/L). After adding distilled water (to a total volume of 10 mL) and thorough mixing, the mixture was allowed to stand at ambient temperature in the dark for 35 min and centrifuged at 4000× g for 10 min at 4 °C. The absorbance of this solution versus a prepared blank was measured at 760 nm. The content of total phenolics in each sample was determined using a standard curve prepared for ferulic acid and expressed as micromoles (µmol) of ferulic acid equivalents (FAE) per gram of dry sample (DS) (µmol FAE/g DS).

3.4. Determination of TFC

The TFC was measured using the aluminum chloride colorimetric method as described by Kern et al. [40] and Chandrasekara and Shahidi [41], with slight modifications. Briefly, 2 mL of each phenolic extract was added to 4 mL of distilled water and 0.3 mL of 5% $NaNO_2$. Five minutes later, 0.3 mL of 10% $AlCl_3$ was added to the reaction mixture and allowed to react for 1 min. Finally, 2 mL of 1 mol/L NaOH and 1.4 mL of distilled water were added and mixed as quickly as possible. The mixture was centrifuged at 4000× g for 5 min at 4 °C after incubation at ambient temperature in the dark for 15 min. The absorbance of this solution versus a prepared blank was measured at 510 nm. Catechin was used as a reference standard, and the results were expressed as µmol of catechin equivalents (CE) per gram of dry sample (µmol CE/g DS).

3.5. Determination of Ferric Reducing Antioxidant Power (FRAP)

The FRAP method was based on the procedure described by Benzie and Strain [42] and Villanueva-Carvajal et al. [43], with slight modifications. Briefly, the FRAP working solution was prepared from acetate buffer (300 mmol/L, pH 3.6), $FeCl_3$ solution (20 mmol/L), and 2,4,6-tripyridyl-s-triazine (10 mmol/L) in a volume ratio of 1:1:1. The phenolic extracts (100 µL) were mixed with 3 mL of the FRAP working solution and incubated at 37 °C in the dark for 4 min. The absorbance of the solution was measured at 539 nm. Ferrous sulfate was used as a reference standard, and the FRAP was expressed as µmol of Fe^{2+} equivalents (FE) per gram of dry sample (µmol FE/g DS).

3.6. Determination of H_2O_2 Scavenging Activity (HPSA)

The HPSA was measured by using the method described by Wettasinghe and Shahidi [44] and Chandrasekara et al. [41], with slight modifications. Briefly, the phenolic extracts (600 µL) mixed with

0.9 mL of H_2O_2 (40 mmol/L) and 1.5 mL of sodium phosphate buffer (45 mmol/L, pH 7.4), and the resulting solution was left to stand at 30 °C in the dark for 40 min. Then, the absorbance of the solution was measured at 230 nm. The HPSA was calculated using the following formula:

$$\text{HPSA (\%)} = [(c - c_b) - (s - s_b)]/(c - c_b) \times 100\% \tag{1}$$

where c is absorbance of the H_2O_2 with the PBS, c_b is absorbance of the PBS, s is absorbance of the sample and the H_2O_2 with the PBS and s_b is absorbance of the sample and the PBS. Ferulic acid dissolved in methanol was used to prepare the standard curve, the HPSA was expressed as μmol of FAE per gram of dry sample (μmol FAE/g DS).

3.7. Determination of DPPH Radical Scavenging Activity (DRSA)

The determination of the effect of extracts on DRSA was based on a procedure as determined by Hatano et al. [45] and Villanueva-Carvajal et al. [43], with slight modifications. Briefly, 1 mL of the phenolic extract was mixed with 4 mL 79 μmol/L methanolic DPPH solution and shaken vigorously. Absorbance was measured at 517 nm after the solution was incubated in the dark at ambient temperature for 10 min. The radical scavenging activity was calculated using the following formula:

$$\text{DRSA (\%)} = [(c - c_b) - (s - s_b)] / (c - c_b) \times 100\% \tag{2}$$

where c is absorbance of the DPPH solution, c_b is absorbance of the methanol, s is absorbance of the DPPH solution with the sample, and s_b is absorbance of the methanol with the sample. The standard curve was prepared using ferulic acid and expressed as μmol of FAE per gram of dry sample (μmol FAE/g DS).

3.8. Determination of Trolox Equivalent Antioxidant Capacity (TEAC)

The TEAC of the extracts was determined as described by Re et al. [46], with slight modifications. Briefly, 100 μL of phenolic extract was mixed in 3.8 mL ABTS working solution (7 mmol/L ABTS mixed with 2.45 mmol/L potassium persulfate in a volume ratio of 1:1). The absorbance at 734 nm was measured in the dark for 6 min. The TEAC was calculated using the following formula:

$$\text{TEAC (\%)} = [(c - c_b) - (s - s_b)]/(c - c_b) \times 100\% \tag{3}$$

where c is absorbance of the ABTS working solution, c_b is absorbance of the ethanol, s is absorbance of the sample with the ABTS working solution, and s_b is absorbance of the sample with the ethanol. Trolox was used as a reference standard, and the TEAC was expressed as μmol of Trolox equivalents (TE) per gram of dry sample (μmol TE/g DS).

3.9. HPLC Analysis

All the phenolic fractions were injected into a high-performance liquid chromatography (HPLC) system (Agilent Technologies, Palo Alto, CA, USA) equipped with a G1315B diode array detector (DAD) and a G1316A column compartment. The separation was performed on a 150 mm × 4.6 mm, 5μm Agilent Zorbax SB-C18 at 30 °C. Its system controller was linked to a ChemStation for LC 3D systems (Agilent Technologies). The mobile phase consisted of methanol (Solvent A) and water with 0.5% formic acid (Solvent B). The flow rate was maintained at 0.8 mL/min. The gradient program was as follows: 0 min, A:B (5:95, v/v); 20 min, A:B (95:5, v/v); 21 min, A:B (5:95, v/v); and 25 min, A:B (5:95, v/v). The detect wavelength was set at 280 nm. Identification and quantification of the 18 phenolic compounds were based on the RT and characteristic absorption spectrum from the DAD with those of their authentic standards. The quantitation of each phenolic compound was carried out using an external standard method. Available pure known compounds as external standards were used for quantifying samples.

3.10. Statistical Analysis

All the analyses were performed, and the results were expressed as the mean ± the standard deviation of three replicates. An independent-sample *t*-test was performed to determine differences between the two kinds of CM extracts at $p < 0.05$. Statistical analysis was undertaken using SPSS version 22.0 software (SPSS Inc., Chicago, IL, USA).

4. Conclusions

The phenolic compounds and antioxidant activities of phenolic extracts in CMP were firstly studied. Moreover, the content, antioxidant activities and phenolic compounds of soluble and insoluble-bound phenolic extracts in CMC and CMP were also compared. The results of this study showed that the TPC and TFC of soluble phenolic extracts were higher than insoluble-bound phenolic extracts in both CMC and CMP. In addition, the TPC of soluble, insoluble-bound and total phenolic compounds in CMP were significantly higher than those in CMC ($p < 0.05$). The soluble phenolic extracts in CMP showed higher antioxidant activities than those in CMC. Eighteen phenolic compounds from phenolic extracts in these two CMs were identified and quantified by HPLC, respectively. Vanillic acid (1325.77 ± 23.34 µg/g) and myricetin (2209.79 ± 1476.96 µg/g) might be characteristic phenolic compounds in soluble phenolic extracts of CMC and CMP. The phenolic compounds of these two CMs represent a potential source of antioxidants. Therefore, CMC and CMP, especially the latter, may play an important role in human health. It is necessary to explore and possibly promote their use as functional food additives.

Supplementary Materials: Supplementary materials are available online. Figure S1. HPLC chromatograms of 18 phenolic standard samples.

Acknowledgments: This project was supported by the National Natural Science Foundation of China (Project No. 31360378, No. 31560428).

Author Contributions: Y.L. and X.X. designed the experiment scheme. Y.H., H.L., Y.Z. and Z.L. performed the experiments. Q.L. analyzed the data and wrote the paper. S.Y. critically revised the manuscript. X.X. was responsible for the analysis of chromatography. All authors made important contributions to the manuscript and approved the final version.

Conflicts of Interest: The authors declare no conflict of interest.

References

1. Nickrent, D.L. Santalales (Including Mistletoes). In *Encyclopedia of Life Sciences*; John Wiley & Sons, Ltd.: Chichester, UK, 2011. [CrossRef]
2. Nazaruk, J.; Orlikowski, P. Phytochemical profile and therapeutic potential of *Viscum album* L. *Nat. Prod. Res.* **2015**, *30*, 373–385. [CrossRef] [PubMed]
3. Simirgiotis, M.J.; Quispe, C.; Areche, C.; Sepúlveda, B. Phenolic Compounds in Chilean Mistletoe (Quintral, *Tristerix tetrandus*) Analyzed by UHPLC-Q/Orbitrap/MS/MS and Its Antioxidant Properties. *Molecules* **2016**, *21*, 245–259. [CrossRef] [PubMed]
4. Molnár, A.; Végvári, Z. Bioclimatic constrains of European Mistletoe *Viscum album* at its southern distribution limit on past and present temporal scales, Pannon region, Hungary. *Clim. Res.* **2017**, *71*, 237–248. [CrossRef]
5. Yoo, J.M.; Yang, J.H.; Kim, Y.S.; Yang, H.J.; Cho, W.K.; Ma, J.Y. Inhibitory Effects of *Viscum coloratum* Extract on IgE/Antigen-Activated Mast Cells and Mast Cell-Derived Inflammatory Mediator-Activated Chondrocytes. *Molecules* **2017**, *22*, 37. [CrossRef] [PubMed]
6. Lim, Y.C.; Rajabalaya, R.; Lee, S.H.F.; Tennakoon, K.U.; Le, Q.V.; Idris, A.; Zulkipli, I.N.; Keasberry, N.; David, S.R. Parasitic Mistletoes of the Genera *Scurrula* and *Viscum*: From Bench to Bedside. *Molecules* **2016**, *21*, 1048–1081. [CrossRef] [PubMed]
7. Ma, Y.H.; Cheng, W.Z.; Gong, F.; Ma, A.L.; Yu, Q.W.; Zhang, J.Y.; Hu, C.Y.; Chen, X.H.; Zhang, D.Q. Active Chinese mistletoe lectin-55 enhances colon cancer surveillance through regulating innate and adaptive immune responses. *World J. Gastroenterol.* **2008**, *14*, 5274–5281. [CrossRef] [PubMed]

8. Patel, B.P.; Singh, P.K. *Viscum articulatum* Burm. f.: A review on its phytochemistry, pharmacology and traditional uses. *J. Pharm. Pharmacol.* **2017**. [CrossRef] [PubMed]
9. Pietrzak, W.; Nowak, R.; Gawlik-Dziki, U.; Lemieszek, M.K.; Rzeski, W. LC-ESI-MS/MS Identification of Biologically Active Phenolic Compounds in Mistletoe Berry Extracts from Different Host Trees. *Molecules* **2017**, *22*, 624. [CrossRef] [PubMed]
10. Luczkiewicz, M.; Cisowski, W.; Kaiser, P.; Ochocka, R.; Piotrowski, A. Comparative analysis of phenolic acids in mistletoe plants from various hosts. *Acta Pol. Pharm.* **2001**, *58*, 373–379. [PubMed]
11. Geetha, K.M.; Bindu, V.; Murugan, V. Antioxidant potential of *Viscum articulatum* burm. *Chron. Young Sci.* **2013**, *4*, 32–35. [CrossRef]
12. Li, H.Z.; Hou, Z.; Li, C.; Zhang, Y.; Shen, T.; Hu, Q.W.; Ren, D.M. Three pairs of diastereoisomeric flavanone glycosides from *Viscum articulatum*. *Fitoterapia* **2015**, *102*, 156–162. [CrossRef] [PubMed]
13. Li, Y.; Zhao, Y.L.; Huang, N.; Zheng, Y.T.; Yang, Y.P.; Li, X.L. Two New Phenolic Glycosides from *Viscum articulatum*. *Molecules* **2008**, *13*, 2500–2508. [CrossRef] [PubMed]
14. Leu, Y.L.; Kuo, S.M.; Hwang, T.L.; Chiu, S.T. The inhibition of superoxide anion generation by neutrophils from *Viscum articulactum*. *Chem. Pharm. Bull.* **2004**, *52*, 858–860. [CrossRef] [PubMed]
15. Wang, Y.K.; Zhang, X.; Chen, G.L.; Yu, J.; Yang, L.Q.; Gao, Y.Q. Antioxidant property and their free, soluble conjugate and insoluble-bound phenolic contents in selected beans. *J. Funct. Foods* **2016**, *24*, 359–372. [CrossRef]
16. Lewandowska, H.; Kalinowska, M.; Lewandowski, W.; Stępkowski, T.M.; Brzóska, K. The role of natural polyphenols in cell signaling and cytoprotection against cancer development. *J. Nutr. Biochem.* **2016**, *32*, 1–19. [CrossRef] [PubMed]
17. Laus, M.N.; Benedetto, N.A.D.; Caporizzi, R.; Tozzi, D.; Soccio, M.; Giuzio, L.; Vita, P.D.; Flagella, Z.; Pastore, D. Evaluation of Phenolic Antioxidant Capacity in Grains of Modern and Old Durum Wheat Genotypes by the Novel QUENCHER$_{ABTS}$ Approach. *Plant Foods Hum. Nutr.* **2015**, *70*, 207–214. [CrossRef] [PubMed]
18. Shahidi, F.; Yeo, J.D. Insoluble-Bound Phenolics in Food. *Molecules* **2016**, *21*, 1216–1237. [CrossRef] [PubMed]
19. Yu, J.; Vasanthan, T.; Temelli, F. Analysis of Phenolic Acids in Barley by High-Performance Liquid Chromatography. *J. Agric. Food Chem.* **2001**, *49*, 4352–4358. [CrossRef] [PubMed]
20. Chandrasekara, A.; Shahidi, F. Content of Insoluble Bound Phenolics in Millets and Their Contribution to Antioxidant Capacity. *J. Agric. Food Chem.* **2010**, *58*, 6706–6714. [CrossRef] [PubMed]
21. Rice-Evans, C.A.; Miller, N.J.; Paganga, G. Antioxidant properties of phenolic compounds. *Trends Plant Sci.* **1997**, *2*, 152–159. [CrossRef]
22. Chandrasekara, A.; Shahidi, F. Inhibitory Activities of Soluble and Bound Millet Seed Phenolics on Free Radicals and Reactive Oxygen Species. *J. Agric. Food Chem.* **2011**, *59*, 428–436. [CrossRef] [PubMed]
23. Köksal, E.; Bursal, E.; Gülçin, İ.; Korkmaz, M.; Çağlayan, C.; Gören, A.C.; Alwasel, S.H. Antioxidant activity and polyphenol content of Turkish thyme (*Thymus vulgaris*) monitored by liquid chromatography and tandem mass spectrometry. *Int. J. Food Prop.* **2017**, *20*, 514–525. [CrossRef]
24. Al-Rimawi, F.; Rishmawi, S.; Ariqat, S.H.; Khalid, M.F.; Warad, I.; Salah, Z. Anticancer Activity, Antioxidant Activity, and Phenolic and Flavonoids Content of Wild *Tragopogon porrifolius* Plant Extracts. *Evid.-Based Complement. Altern. Med.* **2016**, *2016*. [CrossRef] [PubMed]
25. Yuyen, P.T.; Xuan, T.D.; Khang, D.T.; Ahmad, A.; Quan, N.V.; Anh, T.T.A.; Anh, L.H.; Minh, T.N. Phenolic Compositions and Antioxidant Properties in Bark, Flower, Inner Skin, Kernel and Leaf Extracts of *Castanea crenata* Sieb. et Zucc. *Antioxidants* **2017**, *6*, 31. [CrossRef]
26. Song, F.L.; Gan, R.Y.; Zhang, Y.; Xiao, Q.; Kuang, L.; Li, H.B. Total Phenolic Contents and Antioxidant Capacities of Selected Chinese Medicinal Plants. *Int. J. Mol. Sci.* **2010**, *11*, 2362–2372. [CrossRef] [PubMed]
27. Albishi, T.; John, J.A.; Al-Khalifa, A.S.; Shahidi, F. Antioxidative phenolic constituents of skins of onion varieties and their activities. *J. Funct. Foods* **2013**, *5*, 1191–1203. [CrossRef]
28. Minh, T.N.; Khang, D.T.; Tuyen, P.H.; Minh, L.T.; Anh, L.H.; Quan, N.V.; Ha, P.T.T.; Quan, N.T.; Toan, N.P.; Elzaawely, A.A.; et al. Phenolic Compounds and Antioxidant Activity of Phalaenopsis Orchid Hybrids. *Antioxidants* **2016**, *5*, 31–42. [CrossRef] [PubMed]
29. Minh, T.N.; Tuyen, P.T.; Khang, D.T.; Quan, N.V.; Ha, P.T.T.; Quan, N.T.; Andriana, Y.; Fan, X.; Van, T.M.; Khanh, T.D.; et al. Potential Use of Plant Waste from the Moth Orchid (*Phalaenopsis* Sogo Yukidian "V3") as an Antioxidant Source. *Foods* **2017**, *6*, 85. [CrossRef] [PubMed]

30. Issaad, F.Z.; Fernandes, I.P.G.; Enache, T.A.; Mouats, C.; Rodrigues, I.A.; Oliveira-Brett, A.M. Flavonoids in Selected Mediterranean Fruits: Extraction, Electrochemical Detection and Total Antioxidant Capacity Evaluation. *Electroanalysis* **2016**, *29*, 358–366. [CrossRef]
31. Hermans, N.; Cos, P.; Maes, L.; De, B.T.; Vanden, B.D.; Vlietinck, A.J.; Pieters, L. Challenges and Pitfalls in Antioxidant Research. *Curr. Med. Chem.* **2007**, *14*, 417–430. [CrossRef] [PubMed]
32. Herrera, E.; Jiménez, R.; Aruoma, O.I.; Hercberg, S.; Sánchez-garcía, I.; Fraga, C.; Serramajem, L.; Ngo, J.; Aranceta, J.; Solomons, N.W. Aspects of antioxidant foods and supplements in health and disease. *Nutr. Rev.* **2009**, *67*, S140–S144. [CrossRef] [PubMed]
33. Lou, S.N.; Lin, Y.S.; Hsu, Y.S.; Chiu, E.M.; Ho, C.T. Soluble and insoluble phenolic compounds and antioxidant activity of immature calamondin affected by solvents and heat treatment. *Food Chem.* **2014**, *161*, 246–253. [CrossRef] [PubMed]
34. Kumar, K.N.S.; Saraswathy, A.; Amerjothy, S.; Susan, T.; Ravishankar, B. Total Phenol Content and In Vitro Antioxidant Potential of *Helicanthus elastica* (Desr.) Danser-A Less-explored Indian Mango Mistletoe. *J. Tradit. Complement. Med.* **2014**, *4*, 285–288. [CrossRef] [PubMed]
35. Sulaiman, C.T.; Balachandran, I. Total Phenolics and Total Flavonoids in Selected Indian Medicinal Plants. *Indian J. Pharm. Sci.* **2012**, *74*, 254–258. [CrossRef] [PubMed]
36. Rahmawati, S.I.; Ishimaru, K.; Hou, D.X.; Hayashi, N. Antioxidant Activity and Phenolic Content of Mistletoe Extracts Following High-Temperature Batch Extraction. *Food Sci. Technol. Res.* **2014**, *20*, 201–206. [CrossRef]
37. Meng, Y.; Su, A.; Yuan, S.; Zhao, H.; Tan, S.; Hu, C.; Deng, H.; Guo, Y. Evaluation of Total Flavonoids, Myricetin, and Quercetin from *Hovenia dulcis* Thunb. As Inhibitors of α-Amylase and α-Glucosidase. *Plant Foods Hum. Nutr.* **2016**, *71*, 444–449. [CrossRef] [PubMed]
38. Chandrasekara, A.; Shahidi, F. Determination of antioxidant activity in free and hydrolyzed fractions of millet grains and characterization of their phenolic profiles by HPLC-DAD-ESI-MS^n. *J. Funct. Foods* **2011**, *3*, 144–158. [CrossRef]
39. Singleton, V.L.; Rossi, J.A. Colorimetry of Total Phenolics with Phosphomolybdic-Phosphotungstic Acid Reagents. *Am. J. Enol. Vitic.* **1965**, *16*, 144–158. [CrossRef]
40. Kern, S.M.; Bennett, R.N.; Mellon, F.A.; Kroon, P.A.; Garcia-Conesa, M. Absorption of hydroxycinnamates in humans after high-bran cereal consumption. *J. Agric. Food Chem.* **2003**, *51*, 6050–6055. [CrossRef] [PubMed]
41. Chandrasekara, A.; Naczk, M.; Shahidia, F. Effect of processing on the antioxidant activity of millet grains. *Food Chem.* **2012**, *133*, 1–9. [CrossRef]
42. Benzie, I.F.F.; Strain, J.J. The Ferric Reducing Ability of Plasma (FRAP) as a Measure of "Antioxidant Power": the FRAP Assay. *Anal. Biochem.* **1996**, *239*, 70–76. [CrossRef] [PubMed]
43. Villanueva-Carvajal, A.; Bernal-Martínez, L.R.; García-Gasca, M.T.; Dominguez-Lopez, A. In vitro gastrointestinal digestion of *Hibiscus sabdariffa* L.: The use of its natural matrix to improve the concentration of phenolic compounds in gut. *Food Sci. Technol.* **2013**, *51*, 260–265. [CrossRef]
44. Wettasinghe, M.; Shahidi, F. Scavenging of reactive-oxygen species and DPPH free radicals by extracts of borage and evening primrose meals. *Food Chem.* **2000**, *70*, 17–26. [CrossRef]
45. Hatano, T.; Kagawa, H.; Yasuhara, T.; Okuda, T. Two new flavonoids and other constituents in licorice root: Their relative astringency and radical scavenging effects. *Chem. Pharm. Bull.* **1988**, *36*, 2090–2097. [CrossRef] [PubMed]
46. Re, R.; Pellegrini, N.; Proteggente, A.; Pannala, A.; Yang, M.; Riceevans, C. Antioxidant activity applying an improved ABTS radical cation decolorization assay. *Free Radic. Biol. Med.* **1999**, *26*, 1231–1237. [CrossRef]

Sample Availability: Samples of the plant materials and extracts are available from the authors.

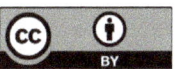

© 2018 by the authors. Licensee MDPI, Basel, Switzerland. This article is an open access article distributed under the terms and conditions of the Creative Commons Attribution (CC BY) license (http://creativecommons.org/licenses/by/4.0/).

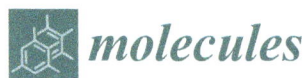

Article

Studies on the Inclusion Complexes of Daidzein with β-Cyclodextrin and Derivatives

Shujing Li [1,2,*], Li Yuan [1], Yong Chen [3], Wei Zhou [1,2] and Xinrui Wang [1,2]

1. Beijing Advanced Innovation Center for Food Nutrition and Human Health, Beijing Technology and Business University, Beijing 100048, China; 10011316015@st.btbu.edu.cn (L.Y.); zhouw@th.btbu.edu.cn (W.Z.); wangxinrui@th.btbu.edu.cn (X.W.)
2. Department of Chemistry, School of Science, Beijing Technology and Business University, Beijing 100048, China
3. Key Laboratory of Photochemical Conversion and Optoelectronic Materials, Technical Institute of Physics and Chemistry, Chinese Academy of Sciences, Beijing 100190, China; chenyong@mail.ipc.ac.cn
* Correspondence: lishujing@mail.ipc.ac.cn; Tel.: +86-10-6898-5573

Received: 31 October 2017; Accepted: 5 December 2017; Published: 8 December 2017

Abstract: The inclusion complexes between daidzein and three cyclodextrins (CDs), namely β-cyclodextrin (β-CD), methyl-β-cyclodextrin (Me-β-CD, DS = 12.5) and (2-hydroxy) propyl-β-cyclodextrin (HP-β-CD, DS = 4.2) were prepared. The effects of the inclusion behavior of daidzein with three kinds of cyclodextrins were investigated in both solution and solid state by methods of phase-solubility, XRD, DSC, SEM, ^{1}H-NMR and 2D ROESY methods. Furthermore, the antioxidant activities of daidzein and daidzein-CDs inclusion complexes were determined by the 1,1-diphenyl-2-picryl-hydrazyl (DPPH) method. The results showed that daidzein formed a 1:1 stoichiometric inclusion complex with β-CD, Me-β-CD and HP-β-CD. The results also showed that the solubility of daidzein was improved after encapsulating by CDs. ^{1}H-NMR and 2D ROESY analyses show that the B ring of daidzein was the part of the molecule that was most likely inserted into the cavity of CDs, thus forming an inclusion complex. Antioxidant activity studies showed that the antioxidant performance of the inclusion complexes was enhanced in comparison to the native daidzein. It could be a potentially promising way to develop a new formulation of daidzein for herbal medicine or healthcare products.

Keywords: daidzein; cyclodextrin; inclusion complex; antioxidant activity

1. Introduction

Daidzein (Figure 1) is one of the major isoflavone compounds and exists widely in soybeans [1]. The present study shows that daidzein possesses multiple biological and pharmacological properties such as antioxidant [2,3], anticancer [4,5], anti-inflammatory [6,7], neuroprotective [8], protective treatment of cardiovascular diseases [9], and autoimmune diseases [10]. However, its use in medicines and in functional food ingredients is limited because of its poor solubility and low bioavailability. Various techniques, such as incorporation into a hydrophilic vehicle [11], phosphorylated daidzein [12], and glycosylation [13], etc., have been developed to improve its water solubility and stability. The formation of an inclusion complex with cyclodextrins (CDs) is another promising way to solve this problem.

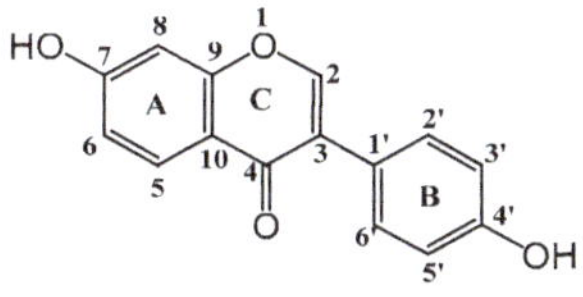

Figure 1. Chemical structure of daidzein.

Cyclodextrins (CDs) are cyclic oligosaccharides built up from glucopyranose units linked by α-1,4 bonds, thus forming a truncated cone. There are three principal types of natural CDs, also known as first-generation CDs: α-CD, β-CD, and γ-CD. These CDs consist of six, seven, and eight glucopyranose units, respectively. β-CD is the most commonly used in pharmaceutical formulations due to its non-toxicity, biodegradability, and its reasonable cost [14]. However, the application of unmodified β-CD is limited, owing to its poor water solubility. Accordingly, modified β-CDs have been synthesized and used, such as methylated-β-cyclodextrin (Me-β-CD) and (2-hydroxy)propyl-β-cyclodextrin (HP-β-CD) [15,16]. The special cone-shaped structure of CDs enables them to enclose the hydrophobic molecules that form the inclusion complexes. As a result of the preparation of the inclusion compound, multiple modifications are gained in the properties of guest molecules, such as improvement of the dissolution of insoluble substances [17,18], stabilization of photosensitive substances [19], and a controlled release of drugs [20,21]. The CDs and their inclusion complexes are used as additives in the drug, food, packaging, cosmetics, and textile industries [22,23].

Some studies have evaluated the improvement of daidzein and genistein solubility by a complexation with HP-β-CD at different host–guest molar ratios [24]. Later, Yatsu [25] reported on the multiple complexations of CDs with soy isoflavones, present in an enriched fraction. Although these studies have demonstrated the feasibility of obtaining inclusion complexes with daidzein, none of them evaluated the inclusion behavior of daidzein with different CDs. Therefore, in this present work, we evaluate the inclusion behavior of daidzein with β-CD, Me-β-CD, and HP-β-CD. The stoichiometric ratios and stability constants describing the extent of formation of the complexes were determined by phase-solubility measurements and Job's method. The inclusion complexes were prepared by the freeze-drying method and were further characterized by X-ray diffraction (XRD), thermogravimetric (TG), differential scanning calorimetry (DSC), scanning electron microscopy (SEM), 1H-nuclear magnetic resonance spectroscopy (^{1}H-NMR) and two-dimensional rotational frame nuclear overhauser effect spectroscopy (2D ROESY). Meanwhile, the antioxidant activities of daidzein and the inclusion complexes were also investigated by the 1,1-diphenyl-2-picrylhydrazyl (DPPH) radical scavenging activity assay.

2. Results and Discussion

2.1. Phase-Solubility Study

Phase-solubility analysis of daidzein with β-CD, Me-β-CD, and HP-β-CD was studied by the method of Higuchi and Connors [26] in an aqueous solution at 25 °C. The phase-solubility diagram is a widely useful method for the evaluation of the inclusion interaction of CDs complexation with poorly water-soluble molecules, as well as the determination of the stability constants (Ks) in the complexes formation. As shown in Figure 2, the aqueous solubility of daidzein increased linearly with the increasing CDs concentration within the studied concentration range. Based on Higuchi and Connors's theory, these three linear host–guest correlations could be classified as A_L type, indicating that a 1:1 stoichiometry of the complexes exists between daidzein and the three different CDs studied. The calculated apparent stability constant (Ks, M^{-1}) of daidzein-β-CD, daidzein-Me-β-CD and daidzein-HP-β-CD, was 776 M^{-1}, 1418 M^{-1}, and 1802 M^{-1}, respectively. The higher apparent stability constants of daidzein-Me-β-CD and daidzein-HP-β-CD can be attributed to the opening enlargement of native β-CD and the destruction of the strong intramolecular hydrogen bond network by the methyl and hydroxypropyl substitutions.

This destruction causes guest molecules to easily access the CD's cavity and give a higher stability constant. The finding that Me-β-CD or HP-β-CD increases the binding capacity for flavonoids has been previously reported [27,28]. Additionally, the solubility of daidzein was significantly increased (4.8-fold, 8.1-fold, and 9.7-fold at 5 mM of β-CD, Me-β-CD, and HP-β-CD) compared to the absence of CDs, which indicated the solubilizing potential for daidzein by CDs.

The stoichiometry of the complex formation between daidzein and CDs was also determined by Job's method (see Supplementary data Figures S1–S3). As shown in the figures, the maximum peak was observed at R = 0.5, which indicates the formation of 1:1 inclusion complexes between daidzein and β-CD, Me-β-CD or HP-β-CD, in accordance with the phase solubility study.

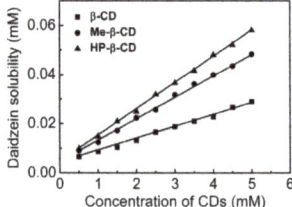

Figure 2. Phase-solubility diagrams of daidzein with β-cyclodextrin (β-CD), methyl-β-cyclodextrin (Me-β-CD), or (2-hydroxy)propyl-β-cyclodextrin (HP-β-CD) at 25 °C.

2.2. XRD Studies

The powder X-ray diffraction patterns (XRD) is an effective method for the analysis of CDs and their inclusion complexes in the powder or microcrystalline state [29,30]. The formation of an inclusion complex between CDs and a crystalline guest means that the latter would no longer exist in the crystalline state and consequently, the diffraction pattern of the complex would not be a simple superposition of those of the two components. As indicated in Figure 3, the XRD patterns of daidzein and β-CD displayed numerous sharp peaks, characteristic of its crystallinity, whereas that of Me-β-CD and HP-β-CD showed two broad peaks, consistent with its amorphous nature. The XRD of the physical mixture of daidzein and CDs was a superposition of the patterns of the components, confirming that no chemical association had occurred between daidzein and CDs. In addition, both kept their original physical characteristics. In contrast, the XRD spectra of daidzein-β-CD, daidzein-Me-β-CD, and daidzein-HP-β-CD inclusion complexes are amorphous and show halo patterns, indicating the formation of an inclusion complex between β-CD (or Me-β-CD, HP-β-CD) and daidzein.

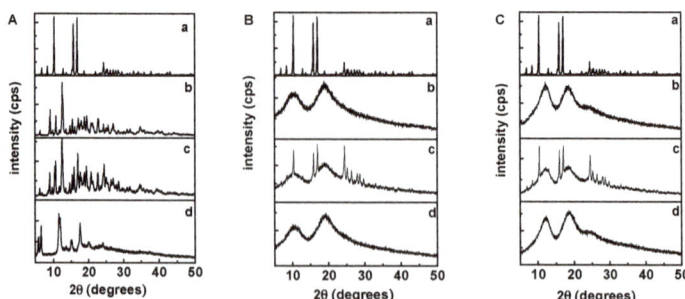

Figure 3. XRD patterns: (**A**) (a) daidzein, (b) β-CD, (c) daidzein/β-CD physical mixture, (d) daidzein-β-CD inclusion complex; (**B**) (a) daidzein, (b) Me-β-CD, (c) daidzein/Me-β-CD physical mixture, (d) daidzein-Me-β-CD inclusion complex; (**C**) (a) daidzein, (b) HP-β-CD, (c) daidzein/HP-β-CD physical mixture, (d) daidzein-HP-β-CD inclusion complex.

2.3. Thermal Analysis

The thermal properties of daidzein, CDs, and daidzein-CDs inclusion complexes were studied by thermogravimetric (TG) methods (see Supplementary data Figures S4–S6). A systematic analysis of the TG curves showed that daidzein decomposed at ca. 315 °C, β-CD at ca. 298 °C, Me-β-CD at ca. 290 °C, and HP-β-CD at ca. 300 °C. In contrast, the decomposition temperature of the daidzein-β-CD, daidzein-Me-β-CD, and the daidzein-HP-β-CD inclusion complex was ca. 296 °C, 292 °C and 299 °C. These results indicate that the daidzein-CDs inclusion complexes were formed [31].

The differential scanning calorimetry (DSC) thermogram provided further information about the thermal properties of daidzein-β-CD, daidzein-Me-β-CD, and the daidzein-HP-β-CD inclusion complex [28]. As shown in Figure 4, daidzein displayed one sharp endothermic peak at 339 °C. In contrast, the DSC curves of β-CD, Me-β-CD, and HP-β-CD had an endothermic peak at 331 °C, 349 °C and 355 °C, respectively. The DSC thermogram of the physical mixture is basically a combination of two components, with the daidzein peaks being only faintly observable due to the lower proportions that it had in the physical mixture. However, in the DSC curves of daidzein-β-CD, daidzein-Me-β-CD, and daidzein-HP-β-CD inclusion complexes, the endothermic peaks were shifted to 345 °C, 368 °C and 380 °C, suggesting that an inclusion structure was formed between the host–guest molecules. These results further confirmed the formation of an inclusion complex between daidzein and CDs.

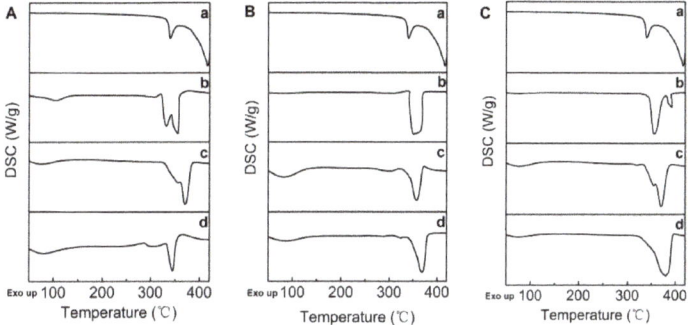

Figure 4. DSC thermograms: (**A**) (a) daidzein, (b) β-CD, (c) daidzein/β-CD physical mixture, (d) daidzein-β-CD inclusion complex; (**B**) (a) daidzein, (b) Me-β-CD, (c) daidzein/Me-β-CD physical mixture, (d) daidzein-Me-β-CD inclusion complex; (**C**) (a) daidzein, (b) HP-β-CD, (c) daidzein/HP-β-CD physical mixture, (d) daidzein-HP-β-CD inclusion complex.

2.4. SEM Studies

Scanning electron microscopy was also a useful method to study the structure of the materials [32,33]. Figure 5 shows the SEM photographs of daidzein, HP-β-CD, their physical mixture, and their inclusion complex. Pure daidzein existed in columnar crystal with medium dimensions and HP-β-CD appeared as a spherical shape with cavity structures. The physical mixture of daidzein with CDs revealed that the characteristic crystals of daidzein and the spheres of HP-β-CD both existed separately, indicating that the two components existed in their original individual forms. In contrast, the daidzein-CDs inclusion complexes appeared as a plate-like crystal structure and were quite different from the sizes and shapes of daidzein and CDs. This observation confirmed the formation of the inclusion complex between daidzein and HP-β-CD. In a similar test, the daidzein-β-CD and daidzein-Me-β-CD appeared to be quite different from the sizes and shapes of β-CD, Me-β-CD and daidzein, respectively, which is a strong indication of an inclusion complex formation (see in the Supplementary data Figures S7 and S8).

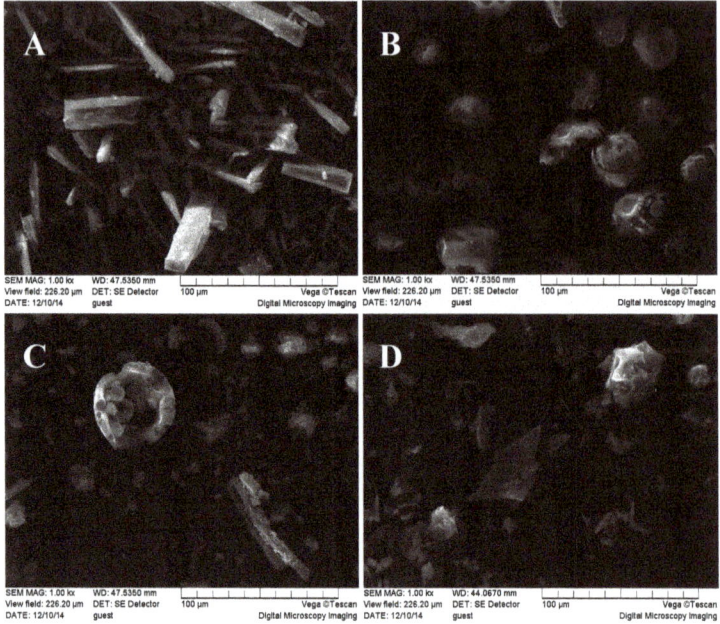

Figure 5. Scanning electron microphotographs: (**A**) daidzein; (**B**) HP-β-CD; (**C**) daidzein/HP-β-CD physical mixture; (**D**) daidzein-HP-β-CD inclusion complex.

2.5. ^{1}H-NMR and 2D NMR

Further evidence supporting the formation of the inclusion complex was obtained by ^{1}H-NMR, which has proved to be the most direct evidence in explaining the host–guest interaction of CDs and guest molecules [18,27]. The ^{1}H-NMR of daidzein has a very low resolved spectrum in D$_2$O due to its poor water solubility. We measured the ^{1}H-NMR spectra of the CDs and the inclusion complexes of daidzein-β-CD, daidzein-Me-β-CD, and daidzein-HP-β-CD in D$_2$O (see Supplementary data Figures S9–S14). The ^{1}H-NMR spectra of the inclusion complexes showed all of the expected proton signals of daidzein and CDs, in agreement with significant solubilization.

To understand the detailed inclusion fashion of daidzein-β-CD, daidzein-Me-β-CD, and daidzein-HP-β-CD, 2D ROESY NMR spectra were also measured. As shown in Figure 6A, the 2D ROESY NMR spectra of daidzein-HP-β-CD showed strong correlation signals between the inner H-3 and H-5 protons of the HP-β-CD and the daidzein protons. The spectra exhibited strong correlation signals between the H-3 protons in the HP-β-CD and the H-2',6' and H-3',5' protons in daidzein and between the H-5 protons in the HP-β-CD and the H-3',5' protons in daidzein, respectively. However, the spectra did not show any significant correlation signals between the H-3 proton in the HP-β-CD and the H-3',5' protons of daidzein. These data indicate that the HP-β-CD selectively includes the daidzein from the wide rim side to form the inclusion complex. It was also shown that daidzein should be encapsulated in the β-CD and Me-β-CD cavities in a similar way (see Supplementary data Figures S15 and S16). A study reported by Borghetti et al. [34] indicated that the formation of the inclusion complex between daidzein with CDs also occurred through the insertion of the B rings of daidzein into the CDs cavity, which is similar to our findings.

Based on these observations, together with the 1:1 stoichiometry, we deduced the possible inclusion modes of daidzein with CDs, as illustrated in Figure 6B.

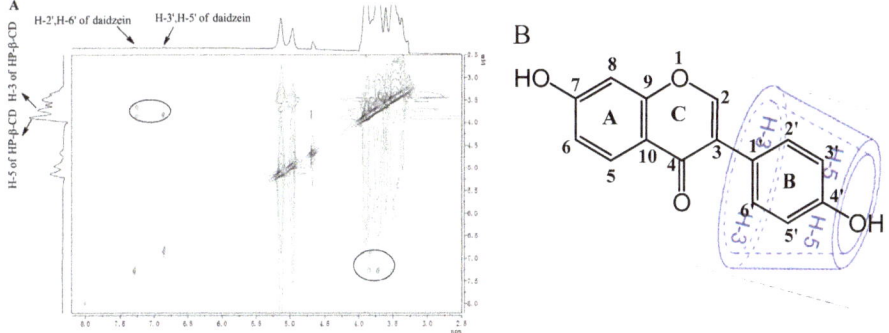

Figure 6. (**A**) ROESY spectrum of the daidzein-HP-β-CD inclusion complex in D$_2$O at 25 °C; (**B**) Possible inclusion mode of the daidzein-HP-β-CD inclusion complex.

2.6. Antioxidant Activity of Daidzein in Free and Complex Form

The evaluation of DPPH scavenging capacity was one of the most general methods to determine the antioxidant activities of different compounds [35,36]. DPPH had a strong absorbance at 517 nm due to the unpaired electron of nitrogen atom, which can accept an electron donated by the antioxidant compound. In this process, the DPPH was decolorized from purple to yellow which can be spectrophotometrically monitored from the changes to absorbance at 517 nm.

Figure 7 showed a comparison of the DPPH radical-scavenging activity of daidzein, daidzein-β-CD, daidzein-Me-β-CD, and daidzein-HP-β-CD complexes. As shown in our findings, after complexation with CDs had occurred, the scavenging capability of daidzein increased significantly. The order was daidzein-HP-β-CD > daidzein-Me-β-CD > daidzein-β-CD, which indicates that the daidzein-CDs complexes have stronger DPPH radical-scavenging ability than the native daidzein have. The DPPH scavenging capacity of the antioxidant is closely related to its hydrogen-donating ability [37–39]. The increasing DPPH scavenging ability of daidzein could be attributed to the enhancement of its hydrogen-donating ability, caused by the complexation of CDs. When daidzein is complexed with CDs, one or more intermolecular hydrogen bonds form between daidzein and the CDs. This weakens the intramolecular hydrogen bonds of daidzein. Ultimately, the hydrogen-donating ability of daidzein is improved.

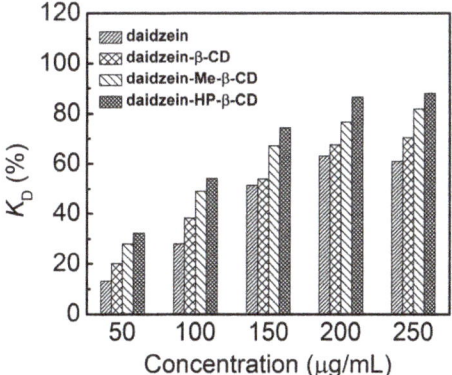

Figure 7. 1,1-diphenyl-2-picryl-hydrazyl (DPPH) radical scavenging activities of the daidzein, daidzein-β-CD, daidzein-Me-β-CD, and daidzein-HP-β-CD inclusion complex.

The stronger interaction between daidzein and HP-β-CD weakened the covalent bonds between hydrogen and oxygen in the hydroxyl groups, which in turn improved the hydrogen donation of the hydroxyl groups of daidzein. In contrast, the multiple methyl group substitutions of Me-β-CD impaired the hydrogen-bonding interaction between daidzein and Me-β-CD. This is unfavorable to the hydrogen-donating ability of daidzein. Ultimately, the DPPH scavenging ability of daidzein-HP-β-CD is stronger than that of daidzein-Me-β-CD, which is consistent with the binding ability of the three CDs. Therefore, we can conclude that the antioxidant property of daidzein-CDs is closely related their mode of binding.

3. Materials and Methods

3.1. Materials

Daidzein (>99%) was obtained from Aladdin Industrial Corporation (Beijing, China); β-cyclodextrin (β-CD, Mw = 1135 g/mol), (2-hydroxy)propyl-β-cyclodextrin (HP-β-CD, Mw = 1380 g/mol, average degree of substitution (DS) = 4.2), methyl-β-cyclodextrin (Me-β-CD, Mw = 1310 g/mol, average degree of substitution (DS) = 12.5) were purchased from Seebio Biotech, Inc. (Shanghai, China).

3.2. Methods

3.2.1. Preparation of Daidzein/β-CD, Daidzein/Me-β-CD and Daidzein/HP-β-CD Inclusion Complexes

Daidzein (0.6 mmol, 127 mg) was dissolved in 20 mL ethanol. CDs (β-CD, Me-β-CD, HP-β-CD, 0.3 mmol) were dissolved in 80 mL water, and then the CDs solutions were added to the daidzein solutions respectively. The mixture was sealed and stirred for 48 h. After evaporating the ethanol from the reaction mixture, the uncomplexed daidzein was filtered. The filtrate was frozen at −40 °C for 24 h and then lyophilized. The resultant powers were collected as the daidzein-CDs complexes.

3.2.2. Preparation of Daidzein/β-CD, Daidzein/Me-β-CD and Daidzein/HP-β-CD Physical Mixture

The physical mixture was prepared by mixing the powders in a 1:1 molar ratio of daidzein and CDs in an agate mortar.

3.2.3. Phase-Solubility Study

Phase-solubility studies were performed according to the method reported by Higuchi and Connors [26]. An excess amount of daidzein was added to 10 mL of aqueous solution containing different concentrations of β-CD, Me-β-CD, and HP-β-CD (from 0 mM to 5.0 mM). The mixtures were vigorously shaken with a shaking rate at 120 rpm in a water bath for 72 h at 25 °C. After reaching equilibrium, the samples were filtered through a 0.45 m hydrophilic membrane filter. All samples were prepared in triplicate. The concentration of daidzein in the filtrate was determined by a CARY-60 spectrophotometer (Varian, Palo Alto, CA, USA). The phase-solubility profiles were obtained by plotting the solubility of daidzein against the concentration of β-CD, Me-β-CD, or HP-β-CD. The apparent stability constants (Ks) were calculated from phase-solubility diagrams according to the following equation:

$$K_s = \frac{\text{Slope}}{S_0(1 - \text{Slope})} \quad (1)$$

where S_0 is the solubility of daidzein at 25 °C in the absence of cyclodextrins and slope means the corresponding slope of the phase-solubility diagrams.

3.2.4. Stoichiometry Determination: Job's Method

The continuous variation method was performed in order to confirm the stoichiometry of the complex. The sum of the concentration of both components was kept constant ([daidzein] +

[CDs] = 1 × 10^{-4} M) whilst the molar fraction of daidzein (R = [daidzein]/[daidzein] + [CDs]) was varied from 0.0 to 1.0. After stirring for 48 h, the UV-vis spectra were measured and the difference in the absorption between that in the presence (A) and absence of CDs (A$_0$), ΔA = A − A$_0$, was plotted against the molar fraction R. The host–guest ratio of the complex can be determined at the stoichiometric ratio.

3.2.5. Powder X-ray Diffraction (XRD)

Monochromatic Cu Kα radiation (wavelength = 1.54056 Å) was produced by a D/MAX 2500V/PC X-ray diffractometer (Rigaku Americas Corporation, Tokyo, Japan). The powders of samples were packed tightly in a rectangular aluminum cell. The samples were exposed to the X-ray beam. The scanning regions of the diffraction angle, 2θ, were 5–70°. Duplicate measurements were made at ambient temperature. Radiation was detected with a proportional detector.

3.2.6. Thermal Analyses

Thermogravimetric (TG) and differential scanning calorimetry (DSC) measurements were performed with a DTG-60AH (Shimadzu, Kyoto, Japan) instrument, at a heating rate of 10 °C/min from 30 °C to 400 °C in a dynamic nitrogen atmosphere (flow rate = 70 mL/min).

3.2.7. Scanning Electron Microscopy (SEM)

SEM photographs were determined on a TESCAN VEGA II. (Tescan Corportion, Brno, Czekh) The powders were previously fixed on a brass stub using double-sided adhesive tape and then were made electrically conductive by coating, in a vacuum with a thin layer of gold for 30 s and at 20 W.

3.2.8. ^{1}H-NMR and 2D NMR

The ^{1}H-NMR and 2D ROESY was all recorded on a BRUKER AVANCE 600 NMR spectrometer (Bruker Corporation, Karlsruhe, Germany) at 25 °C. Deuterium oxide (D$_2$O) was used as the solvent. Chemical shifts were referenced to the solvent values (4.70 ppm for HOD).

3.2.9. DPPH Radical-Scavenging Capacity

The antioxidant activity was measured by the scavenging of the stable free-radical DPPH, which showed a characteristic absorbance peak at 517 nm in ethanol. The addition of an antioxidant resulted in a decrease in the absorbance proportional to the concentration and antioxidant activity of the compound itself [40,41].

An ethanolic solution of the radical DPPH was prepared and protected from light. Daidzein-β-CD, daidzein-Me-β-CD or daidzein-HP-β-CD samples of different concentrations were added to DPPH ethanolic solution. DPPH free-radical scavenging by the daidzein-CDs inclusion complexes and native daidzein were investigated according to the method of Wang et al. [42]. Briefly, DPPH solutions (2.0 mL) in ethanol (2 × 10^{-4} mol/L) and 2.0 mL of tested samples with various concentrations were mixed in the tubes. Then, the mixture was incubated for 60 min in the dark at 30 ± 1 °C. The absorbance was measured at 517 nm in CARY-60 UV-vis spectrometer (Varian, Palo Alto, CA, USA). The lower absorbance of the reaction mixture indicated higher free radical scavenging activity. The DPPH scavenging effect (K$_D$) was calculated using the following equation:

$$K_D = \left(\frac{A_0 - (A_i - A_j)}{A_0} \right) \times 100\% \quad (2)$$

where A$_0$ A$_i$ was the absorbance in the presence of the samples and A$_j$ was the absorbance of the samples alone.

4. Conclusions

The inclusion complexes of daidzein with β-CD, Me-β-CD and HP-β-CD were prepared and characterized by phase-solubility, XRD, DSC, SEM, and antioxidant studies. The phase-solubility, XRD, DSC and SEM studies confirmed that daidzein can form inclusion complexes with three kinds of CDs, and the ratio between the host–guest molecules is 1:1. Furthermore, the solubility of daidzein was improved due to the formation of the inclusion complex. The 2D ROESY and ^{1}H-NMR analyses show that the B ring of daidzein is the part of the molecule that is most likely inserted into the cavity of HP-β-CD, thus forming an inclusion complex. Antioxidant activity studies showed that the antioxidant performance of the inclusion complexes was better than that of the native daidzein, and the daidzein-HP-β-CD inclusion complex was the most effective form. Given the easy preparation and environmentally friendly process of creating daidzein-CDs inclusion complexes, it is a promising way to design a novel formulation of daidzein for herbal medicine or healthcare products.

Supplementary Materials: Supplementary Materials are available online.

Acknowledgments: The authors are grateful to the National Natural Science Foundation of China (No. 31501445).

Author Contributions: S.L. designed the experiments and wrote the paper; L.Y., Y.C., W.Z. and X.W. performed the experiments and analyzed the data.

Conflicts of Interest: The authors declare no conflict of interest.

References

1. Setchell, K.D.; Cassidy, A. Dietary isoflavones: Biological effects and relevance to human health. *J. Nutr.* **1999**, *129*, 758S–767S. [PubMed]
2. Tikkanen, M.J.; Wahala, K.; Ojala, S.; Vihma, V.; Adlercreutz, H. Effect of soybean phytoestrogen intake on low density lipoprotein oxidation resistance. *Proc. Natl. Acad. Sci. USA* **1998**, *95*, 3106–3110. [CrossRef] [PubMed]
3. Kerry, N.; Abbey, M. The isoflavone genistein inhibits copper and peroxyl radical mediated low density lipoprotein oxidation in vitro. *Atherosclerosis* **1998**, *140*, 341–347. [CrossRef]
4. Wada, K.; Nakamura, K.; Tamai, Y.; Tsuji, M.; Kawachi, T.; Hori, A.; Takeyama, N.; Tanabashi, S.; Matsushita, S.; Tokimitsu, N.; et al. Soy isoflavone intake and breast cancer risk in Japan: From the Takayama study. *Int. J. Cancer* **2013**, *133*, 952–960. [CrossRef] [PubMed]
5. Su, S.J.; Traiming, Y.; Lei, H.Y.; Nanhaw, C. The potential of soybean foods as a chemoprevention approach for human urinary tract cancer. *Clin. Cancer Res.* **2000**, *6*, 230–236. [PubMed]
6. Chacko, B.K.; Chandler, R.T.; D'Alessandro, T.L.; Mundhekar, A.; Khoo, N.K.; Botting, N.; Barnes, S.; Patel, P.R. Anti-inflammatory effects of isoflavones are dependent on flow and human endothelial cell ppargamma. *J. Nutr.* **2007**, *137*, 351–356. [PubMed]
7. Widyarini, S.; Spinks, N.; Husband, A.J.; Reeve, V.E. Isoflavonoid compounds from red clover (*Trifolium pratense*) protect from inflammation and immune suppression induced by UV radiation. *Photochem. Photobiol.* **2001**, *74*, 465–470. [CrossRef]
8. Marotta, F.; Mao, G.S.; Liu, T.; Chui, D.H.; Lorenzetti, A.; Xiao, Y. Marandola, P. Anti-inflammatory and neuroprotective effect of a phytoestrogen compound on rat microglia. *Ann. N. Y. Acad. Sci.* **2006**, *1089*, 276–281. [CrossRef] [PubMed]
9. Clarkson, T. Soy, soy phytoestrogens and cardiovascular disease. *J. Nutr.* **2002**, *132*, 566S–569S. [PubMed]
10. Barnes, S. Evolution of the health benefits of soy isoflavones. *Proc. Soc. Exp. Biol. Med.* **1998**, *217*, 386–392. [CrossRef] [PubMed]
11. Huang, Z.R.; Hung, C.F.; Lin, Y.K.; Fang, J.Y. In vitro and in vivo evaluation of topical delivery and potential dermal use of soy isoflavones genistein and daidzein. *Int. J. Pharm.* **2008**, *364*, 36–44. [CrossRef] [PubMed]
12. Xiao, Y.M.; Yang, L.G.; Mao, P.; Yuan, J.W.; Deng, Y.X.; Qu, L.B. Inclusion complexes of phosphorylated daidzein derivatives with β-cyclodextrin: Preparation and inclusion behavior study. *Spectrochim. Acta Part A* **2012**, *85*, 298–302. [CrossRef] [PubMed]
13. Shimoda, K.; Hamada, H. Synthesis of β-Maltooligosaccharides of Glycitein and Daidzein and their anti-oxidant and anti-allergic activities. *Molecules* **2010**, *15*, 5153–5161. [CrossRef] [PubMed]

14. Szejtli, J. Introduction and general overview of cyclodextrin chemistry. *Chem. Rev.* **1998**, *98*, 1743–1753. [CrossRef] [PubMed]
15. Stella, V.J.; Rajewski, R.A. Cyclodextrins: Their future in drug formulation and delivery. *Pharm. Res.* **1997**, *14*, 556–567. [CrossRef] [PubMed]
16. Tablet, C.; Minea, L.; Dumitrache, L.; Hillebrand, M. Experimental and theoretical study of the inclusion complexes of 3-carboxycoumarin acid with β- and 2-hydroxypropyl-β-cyclodextrins. *Spectrochim. Acta Part A* **2012**, *92*, 56–63. [CrossRef] [PubMed]
17. Yang, L.J.; Ma, S.X.; Zhou, S.Y.; Chen, W.; Yuan, M.W.; Yin, Y.Q.; Yang, X.D. Preparation and characterization of inclusion complexes of naringenin with β-cyclodextrin or its derivative. *Carbohydr. Polym.* **2013**, *98*, 861–869. [CrossRef] [PubMed]
18. Xiao, C.F.; Li, K.; Huang, R.; He, G.J.; Zhang, J.Q.; Zhu, L.; Yang, Q.Y.; Jiang, K.M.; Jin, Y.; Lin, J. Investigation of inclusion complex of epothilone A with cyclodextrins. *Carbohydr. Polym.* **2014**, *102*, 297–305. [CrossRef] [PubMed]
19. Blanch, G.P.; Ruiz del Castillo, M.L.; Caja, M.M.; Perez-Mendez, M.; Sanchez-Cortes, S. Stabilization of all-trans-lycopene from tomato by encapsulation using cyclodextrins. *Food Chem.* **2007**, *105*, 1335–1341. [CrossRef]
20. Gallegoyerga, L.; Lomazzi, M.; Sansone, F.; Ortiz, M.C.; Casnati, A.; García Fernández, J.M. Glycoligand-targeted core-shell nanospheres with tunable drug release profiles from calixarene-cyclodextrin heterodimers. *Chem. Commun.* **2014**, *50*, 7440–7443. [CrossRef] [PubMed]
21. Wang, K.; Liu, Y.; Li, C.; Cheng, S.X.; Zhuo, R.X.; Zhang, X.Z. Cyclodextrin-responsive micelles based on poly(ethylene glycol)-polypeptide hybrid copolymers as drug carriers. *ACS Macro Lett.* **2013**, *2*, 201–205. [CrossRef]
22. Marques, H.M.C. A review on cyclodextrin encapsulation of essential oils and volatiles. *Flavour Fragr. J.* **2010**, *25*, 313–326. [CrossRef]
23. Valle, E.M.M.D. Cyclodextrins and their uses: A review. *Process Biochem.* **2004**, *39*, 1033–1046. [CrossRef]
24. Stancanelli, R.; Mazzaglia, A.; Tommasini, S.; Calabrò, M.L.; Villari, V.; Guardo, M.; Ficarra, P.; Ficarra, R. The enhancement of isoflavones water solubility by complexation with modified cyclodextrins: A spectroscopic investigation with implications in the pharmaceutical analysis. *J. Pharm. Biomed. Anal.* **2007**, *44*, 980–984. [CrossRef] [PubMed]
25. Yatsua, F.K.J.; Koestera, L.S.; Lula, I.; Passosb, J.J.; Sinisterra, R.; Bassania, V.L. Multiple complexation of cyclodextrin with soy isoflavones present in an enriched fraction. *Carbohydr. Polym.* **2013**, *98*, 726–735. [CrossRef] [PubMed]
26. Higuchi, T.; Connors, K.A. Phase solubility techniques. *Adv. Anal. Chem. Instrum.* **1965**, *4*, 117–212.
27. Nguyen, T.A.; Liu, B.G.; Zhao, J.; Thomas, D.S.; Hook, J.M. An investigation into the supramolecular structure, solubility, stability and antioxidant activity of rutin/cyclodextrin inclusion complex. *Food Chem.* **2013**, *136*, 186–192. [CrossRef] [PubMed]
28. Yao, Y.S.; Xie, Y.; Hong, C.; Li, G.W.; Shen, H.Y.; Ji, G. Development of a myricetin/hydroxypropyl-β-cyclodextrin inclusion complex: Preparation, characterization, and evaluation. *Carbohydr. Polym.* **2014**, *110*, 329–337. [CrossRef] [PubMed]
29. Celebioglu, A.; Uyar, T. Antioxidant vitamin E/cyclodextrin inclusion complex electrospun nanofibers: Enhanced water solubility, prolonged shelf life, and photostability of vitamin E. *J. Agric. Food Chem.* **2017**, *65*, 5404–5412. [CrossRef] [PubMed]
30. Aytac, Z.; Ipek, S.; Durgun, E.; Tekinay, T.; Uyar, T. Antibacterial electrospun zein nanofibrous web encapsulating thymol/cyclodextrin-inclusion complex for food packaging. *Food Chem.* **2017**, *233*, 117–124. [CrossRef] [PubMed]
31. Kringel, D.H.; Antunes, M.D.; Klein, B.; Crizel, R.L.; Wagner, R.; de Oliveira, R.P.; Dias, A.R.G.; Zavareze, E.D.R. Production, characterization, and stability of orange or eucalyptus essential oil/β-Cyclodextrin inclusion complex. *J. Food Sci.* **2017**, *82*, 2598–2605. [CrossRef] [PubMed]
32. Wei, Y.Q.; Zhang, J.; Zhou, Y.; Bei, W.Y.; Li, Y.; Yuan, Q.P.; Liang, H. Characterization of glabridin/hydroxypropyl-β-cyclodextrin inclusion complex with robust solubility and enhanced bioactivity. *Carbohydr. Polym.* **2017**, *159*, 152–160. [CrossRef] [PubMed]

33. Raza, A.; Sun, H.F.; Bano, S.; Zhao, Y.Y.; Xu, X.Q.; Tang, J. Preparation, characterization, and in vitro anti-inflammatory evaluation of novel water soluble kamebakaurin/hydroxypropyl-β-cyclodextrin inclusion complex. *J. Mol. Struct.* **2017**, *1130*, 319–326. [CrossRef]
34. Borghetti, G.B.; Pinto, A.P.; Lula, I.S.; Sinisterra, R.D.; Teixeira, H.F.; Bassani, V.L. Daidzein/cyclodextrin/ hydrophilic polymer ternary systems. *Drug Dev. Ind. Pharm.* **2011**, *37*, 886–893. [CrossRef] [PubMed]
35. Yuan, C.; Du, L.; Jin, Z.; Xu, X. Storage stability and antioxidant activity of complex of astaxanthin with hydroxypropyl-β-cyclodextrin. *Carbohydr. Polym.* **2013**, *91*, 385–389. [CrossRef] [PubMed]
36. Gharibzahedi, S.M.T.; Razavi, S.H.; Mousavi, M. Characterizing the natural canthaxanthin/ 2-hydroxypropyl-β-cyclodextrin inclusion complex. *Carbohydr. Polym.* **2014**, *101*, 1147–1153. [CrossRef] [PubMed]
37. Yang, J.; Guo, J.; Yuan, J. In vitro antioxidant properties of rutin. *LWT Food Sci. Technol.* **2008**, *41*, 1060–1066. [CrossRef]
38. Jullian, C.; Orosteguis, T.; Pérez-Cruz, F.; Sánchez, P.; Mendizabal, F.; Olea-Azar, C. Complexation of morin with three kinds of cyclodextrin: A thermodynamic and reactivity study. *Spectrochim. Acta Part A* **2008**, *71*, 269–275. [CrossRef] [PubMed]
39. Strazisar, M.; Andrensek, S.; Smidovnik, A. Effect of β-cyclodextrin on antioxidant activity of coumaric acids. *Food Chem.* **2008**, *110*, 636–642. [CrossRef]
40. Liu, M.; Dong, L.N.; Chen, A.J.; Zhang, Y.; Sun, D.Z.; Wang, X.; Wang, B.Q. Inclusion complexes of quercetin with three β-cyclodextrins derivatives at physiological pH: Spectroscopic study and antioxidant activity. *Spectrochim. Acta Part A* **2013**, *115*, 854–860. [CrossRef] [PubMed]
41. Jullian, C.; Cifuentes, C.; Alfaro, M.; Miranda, S.; Barriga, G.; Olea-Azar, C. Spectroscopic characterization of the inclusion complexes of luteolin with native and derivatized β-cyclodextrin. *Bioorg. Med. Chem.* **2010**, *18*, 5025–5031. [CrossRef] [PubMed]
42. Wang, B.S.; Li, B.S.; Zeng, Q.X.; Liu, H.X. Antioxidant and free radical scavenging activities of pigments extracted from molasses alcohol waste water. *Food Chem.* **2008**, *107*, 1198–1204. [CrossRef]

Sample Availability: Samples of the compounds are available from the authors.

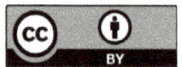

© 2017 by the authors. Licensee MDPI, Basel, Switzerland. This article is an open access article distributed under the terms and conditions of the Creative Commons Attribution (CC BY) license (http://creativecommons.org/licenses/by/4.0/).

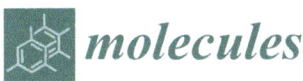

Article

Studies on the Anti-Oxidative Function of *trans*-Cinnamaldehyde-Included β-Cyclodextrin Complex

Munkhtugs Davaatseren [1,†], Yeon-Ji Jo [2,†], Geun-Pyo Hong [3,*], Haeng Jeon Hur [4], Sujin Park [4] and Mi-Jung Choi [5,*]

1. Department of Food Science and Technology, Chung-ang University, Gyeonggi-do 17546, Korea; munkhtugs@hotmail.com
2. Institute of Process Engineering in Life Science, Section I: Food Process Engineering, Karlsruhe Institute of Technology, 76131 Karlsruhe, Germany; jo.yeonji.1986@gmail.com
3. Department of Food Science and Biotechnology, Sejong University, 209 Neungdong-ro, Seoul 05006, Korea
4. Division of Metabolism and Functionality Research, Korea Food Research Institute, 1201-62 Anyangpangyo-ro, Bundang-gu, Seongnam-si, Gyeonggi-do 13539, Korea; mistletoe@kfri.re.kr (H.J.H.); parksj83@naver.com (S.P.)
5. Department of Food Science and Biotechnology of Animal Resources, Konkuk University, 120 Neungdong-ro, Seoul 05029, Korea
* Correspondence: gphong@sejong.ac.kr (G.-P.H.); choimj@konkuk.ac.kr (M.-J.C.); Tel.: +82-2-3408-2914 (G.-P.H.); +82-2-450-3048 (M.-J.C.)
† These authors contributed equally to this article.

Received: 31 October 2017; Accepted: 16 December 2017; Published: 19 December 2017

Abstract: *trans*-Cinnamaldehyde (*t*CIN), an active compound found in cinnamon, is well known for its antioxidant, anticancer, and anti-inflammatory activities. The β-cyclodextrin (β-CD) oligomer has been used for a variety of applications in nanotechnology, including pharmaceutical and cosmetic applications. Here, we aimed to evaluate the anti-inflammatory and antioxidant effects of *t*CIN self-included in β-CD complexes (CIs) in lipopolysaccharide (LPS)-treated murine RAW 264.7 macrophages. RAW 264.7 macrophages were treated with increasing concentrations of β-CD, *t*CIN, or CIs for different times. β-CD alone did not affect the production of nitric oxide (NO) or reactive oxygen species (ROS). However, both *t*CIN and CI significantly reduced NO and ROS production. Thus, CIs may have strong anti-inflammatory and antioxidant effects, similar to those of *t*CIN when used alone.

Keywords: *trans*-cinnamaldehyde; β-cyclodextrin; self-inclusion; anti-inflammation; antioxidant

---

1. Introduction

Cinnamon is commonly used in cosmetics and foods [1], and cinnamon oil is frequently used in the food and beverage industry because of its unique aroma [2]. Several studies have reported that cinnamon and its extracts and active compounds have beneficial biological effects, including antidiabetic effects [1,3], and antibacterial, antifungal, and anticancer activities [2,4]. Moreover, these products inhibit neuroinflammation [5] and reduce oxidative stress [6,7].

The compound *trans*-cinnamaldehyde (*t*CIN) is a key flavor component of cinnamon essential oil [8] that has relatively low toxicity, aside from inducing skin irritation at high doses [9]. Several reports have suggested that *t*CIN has anti-inflammatory effects in macrophages [10,11]. Moreover, *t*CIN has anticancer activity, induces apoptosis [8], inhibits cell proliferation [12], and is beneficial for the management of obesity and diabetes [13]. However, the application of *t*CIN is limited by its insolubility in water; therefore, overcoming this issue could have a major impact on the functionality of *t*CIN. In addition, microencapsulated *t*CIN has no carcinogenic or toxic effects in rodent models [14]. However, the oral absorption of high amounts of cinnamon into the human body is likely to cause side effects such as hyperkeratosis and gastritis [15]. Therefore, the cytotoxicity of *t*CIN should be carefully examined.

Cyclodextrins (CDs) are toroidal-shaped, biocompatible, relatively non-toxic, cyclic oligomers [16]. In aqueous solutions, CDs can incorporate geometrically and polarity-compatible target compounds to improve their stability [17], increase their solubility [18], and enhance their bioavailability [19]. This increases the applicability of CDs in many fields, including pharmaceutics [16,20], cosmetics [17], and food technology [21,22]. Therefore, many researchers have deemed CDs as potential specific drug carriers or nano-inclusion agents with the ability to reduce the toxicity of target compounds, after numerous modifications [23]. CDs are thought to be suitable for use in several pharmacological and biological approaches, helping to address the challenges faced during product formulation. CD encapsulation usually affects the physicochemical properties of bioactive compounds and specific drugs [17,24]. However, few studies have examined *t*CIN and CD inclusion complexes, and most studies have focused only on their applications in nanotechnology. In particular, researchers are interested in elucidating the functionality of these molecules using cell-based experiments; additionally, more in-depth studies are needed to uncover the potential applications of these compounds. Because *t*CIN is a major component of cinnamon and generally considered as a food, *t*CIN could be applied as a functional food with numerous beneficial effects after modification by nanotechnology. Here, we evaluated the physicochemical properties of the β-CD and *t*CIN inclusion complexes (CIs), and determined their anti-inflammatory and antioxidant effects on lipopolysaccharide (LPS)-treated RAW 264.7 murine macrophages.

2. Results and Discussion

2.1. Thermal Properties

Differential scanning colorimetric (DSC) was performed to investigate the formation of complexes between the β-CD polymer and *t*CIN. Figure 1 shows the DSC results for β-CD, *t*CIN, the β-CD-*t*CIN physical mixture, and the CIs. Pure β-CD and pure *t*CIN showed endothermic peaks at 205.5 °C and 292.7 °C, respectively, which correspond to their melting points. The β-CD-*t*CIN physical mixture had two endothermic peaks. The first (at 183.7 °C) was nearly identical to that of pure β-CD, while the second (at 292.4 °C) corresponded to that of *t*CIN. The melting temperature of β-CD alone was higher than that of the CIs. Interaction of the guest with β-CD provides somewhat broader, so that a difference in phase transition temperature is observed [25]. The thermal transition of the CIs occurred at 175.8 °C, along with the endothermic peak. The CIs did not show the *t*CIN melting peak, which was clear evidence of the formation of a complex between the β-CD and *t*CIN. Similar to our results, Seo et al. [25] previously reported that the disappearance of the endothermic peak of eugenol was obvious evidence of the formation of an inclusion complex between eugenol and β-CD.

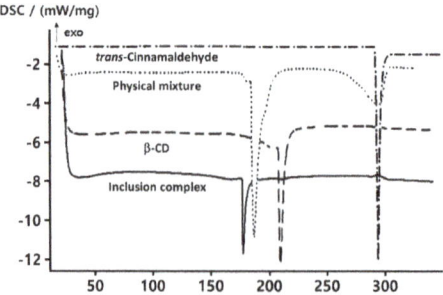

Figure 1. Thermal analysis of *trans*-cinnamaldehyde (*t*CIN) and β-cyclodextrin (β-CD) inclusion complexes (CIs). The CIs were obtained by the molecular inclusion of *t*CIN and β-CD at a molar ratio of 1:1. The physical mixture was obtained by pulverizing the two components in a glass mortar and mixing them accurately in a molar ratio of 1:1.

2.2. Encapsulation Efficiency and Release Characteristics of the CIs

Cinnamon essential oil and tCIN have antibacterial and antifungal effects [2], and have been shown to be promising agents in the treatment of cancer [4]. Despite the beneficial effects of cinnamon, its efficacy and bioavailability are quite low because it is used in low doses for oral absorption in the human body [26]. Thus, the encapsulation efficiency of CIs with different molar ratios of β-CD and tCIN was measured before evaluating the tCIN release rate. The encapsulation efficiency of CI decreased from 90% to 62%, with increasing tCIN concentrations in the CIs. The encapsulation efficiency when the molar ratio of the two components was 1:1, was 85% (Figure 2A). Similar observations were reported in previous studies, with encapsulation efficiencies ranging from 70% to 95% after the preparation of CIs with various concentrations of wall and core materials [27]. Hill, Gomes, and Taylor [27] found that the encapsulation efficiency for tCIN in β-CD inclusion complexes was 85% when the inclusion complexes were prepared at a molar ratio of 1:1, similar to our current results. Many studies have shown that the type of material used for preparing the wall, the ratio of the materials used for the core and the wall, the encapsulation technique, and the physicochemical properties of capsules affect the encapsulation efficiency value [28–31]. In particular, the CI technique is effective for encapsulating highly lipophilic oils with high encapsulation efficiency when prepared such that the molar ratio of the materials used for the core and wall is 1:1. In contrast, in our study, at a 1:1 molar ratio of CI and tCIN, the CI had the lowest encapsulation efficiency.

The release profiles of tCIN from CIs were observed to determine the stability of the CIs at 4, 25, and 37 °C over a period of 7 days (Figure 2B–D). The tCIN release rate tended to increase over time as the tCIN concentration increased. The CIs at a 0.5:1 molar ratio of tCIN and β-CD were more stable than those at a 1:1 and a 2:1 molar ratio. Especially, the release rate of tCIN from CI dynamically increased at a 2:1 molar ratio of tCIN and β-CD, to up to about 40%, regardless of the temperature.

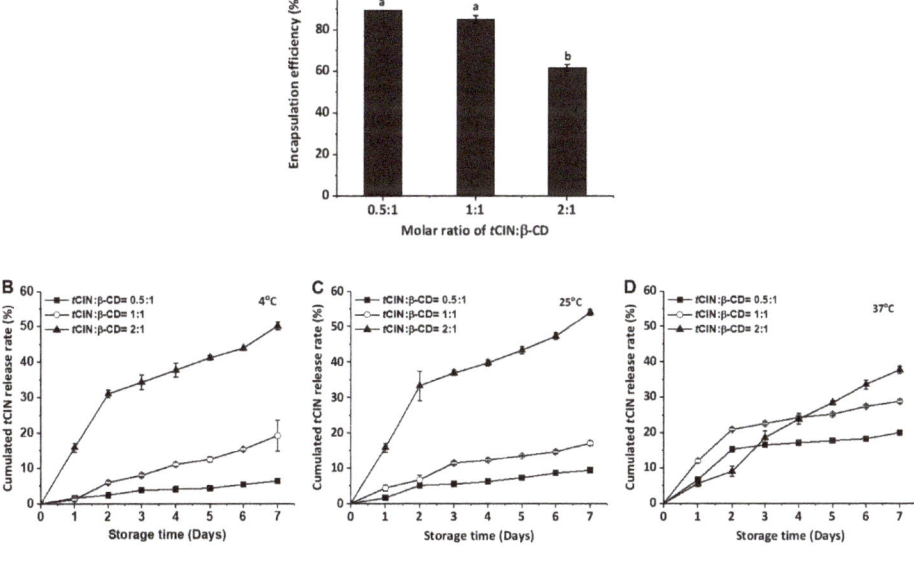

Figure 2. Encapsulation efficiency (**A**) and release amount (**B–D**) of the inclusion complex (CI) with different ratios of *trans*-cinnamaldehyde (tCIN) and β-cyclodextrin (β-CD). The release amount was measured at different storage temperatures, i.e., 4 °C (**B**), 25 °C (**C**), and 37 °C (**D**), for 7 days and expressed as a percentage (%).

In general, the storage temperature had a pronounced effect on the release rate of tCIN from CIs. At 4 °C and 25 °C, tCIN release from CIs did not differ significantly with storage temperature ($p > 0.05$) in our study. However, tCIN release from CIs was more affected by storage temperature at 37 °C than at the other storage temperatures, even though the concentration was low. tCIN release from CIs at the molar ratios of 0.5:1 and 1:1, and a 2:1 molar ratio of tCIN and β-CD, was 20%, 28%, and 37%, respectively. According to a study by Wang et al. [30], the release rate of garlic oil from the inclusion complex, examined at temperatures ranging from 25 to 50 °C, reached 75.8% at 37 °C after incubation for 60 h. Thus, the release profiles of the core materials can be controlled to suit a given application using various types and concentrations of coating materials, different encapsulation techniques, and various extra-environmental conditions, such as temperature, pH, and humidity [32,33]. In this study, functionality evaluation was performed to observe the effects of tCIN release on anti-inflammatory and antioxidant activity.

2.3. Anti-Oxidant Activities of the CIs

Figure 3 shows the antioxidant activity of the CIs over a period of 7 days, as measured by the 1,1-diphenyl-2-picrylhydrazyl (DPPH) (Figure 3A) and 2,20-azino-bis(3-ethylbenzothiazoline-6-sulphonic) acod (ABTS) (Figure 3B) radical-scavenging activity assays. These antioxidant activities were investigated to evaluate the storage stability of CI-containing antioxidants, such as tCIN. In our study, The CIs were obtained by molecular inclusion at 1:1 molar ratio of tCIN and β-CD. Free β-CD did not show any antioxidant activity on its own when tested at the same concentration range as carvacrol and its inclusion complexes (data not shown). Free tCIN did not show any antioxidant activity because of its instability in distilled water. However, tCIN is well-known for its high antioxidant activity in previous studies [6,7]. In the DPPH and ABTS radical-scavenging assay, the antioxidant activity of the CIs significantly increased after 3 days compared with that of the CIs at day 0 (initial CIs). The results of the ABTS assay also showed that the antioxidant activity of the CIs increased with increasing storage temperature and time. In general, the inclusion of tCIN with β-CD makes it difficult to react with free radicals. However, tCIN is released from CIs, and this free tCIN reacts with free radicals, eventually increasing the antioxidant activity [34]. This could be also explained with the results of release rate (%) presented in Figure 2B–D; after 7 days, tCIN release from CIs at 4 °C, 25 °C, and 37 °C was up to 19%, 17% and 30%, respectively. The ABTS radical-scavenging activity of CIs at 4 °C, 25 °C, and 37 °C was 0.88%, 1.18%, and 2.43%, respectively. Therefore, we suggest that the increase in the antioxidant activity was most likely related to the free tCIN concentration, because an increased release of tCIN was observed with increasing storage temperatures.

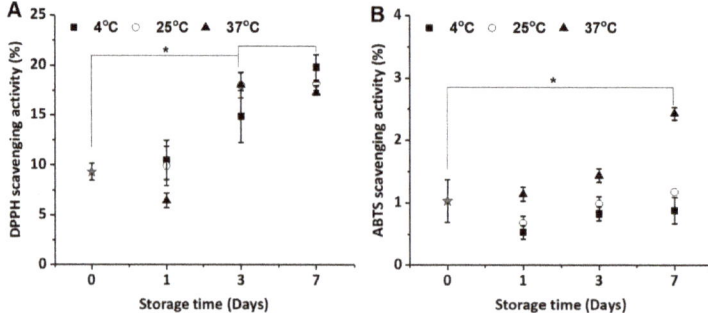

Figure 3. Antioxidant activity of *trans*-cinnamaldehyde (tCIN) and β-cyclodextrin (β-CD) inclusion complex (CI). (**A**) DPPH and (**B**) ABTS radical-scavenging activities were measured at different storage temperatures (4 °C, 25 °C and 37 °C) for 7 days. The CIs were obtained by molecular inclusion at 1:1 molar ratio of tCIN and β-CD. Data are the mean ± standard deviation (SD). * $p < 0.05$ versus the radical-scavenging ability of the CIs at day 0 (initial CIs). DPPH, 1,1-diphenyl-2-picrylhydrazyl; ABTS, 2,20-azino-bis(3-ethylbenzothiazoline-6-sulphonic) acid.

2.4. Cell Viability

In order to determine whether the storage time of the CIs affected their influence on cell viability, CIs were prepared in a culture medium and stored at 4 °C, and cell viability was determined before and after 3 weeks of storage. According to the MTT assay data, β-CD exhibited no significant cytotoxicity at a concentration of 500 µM, whereas tCIN and CI exhibited no significant cytotoxicity up to a concentration of 100 µM in RAW 264.7 macrophages (Figure 4). Interestingly, a 3-week storage (Figure 4B) slightly increased the cytotoxicity of tCIN, when compared to that observed before storage (Figure 4A); this could be caused by the oxidation of tCIN during storage. However, 3 weeks of storage of the CIs in a culture medium at 4 °C had no notable effect on cell viability. This result supported the findings of a previous report by Yang et al. [35], who demonstrated that the cytotoxicity of a target compound decreased after β-CD inclusion. Therefore, the tCIN and β-CD inclusion complex may have an important role in maintaining the stability of functional foods.

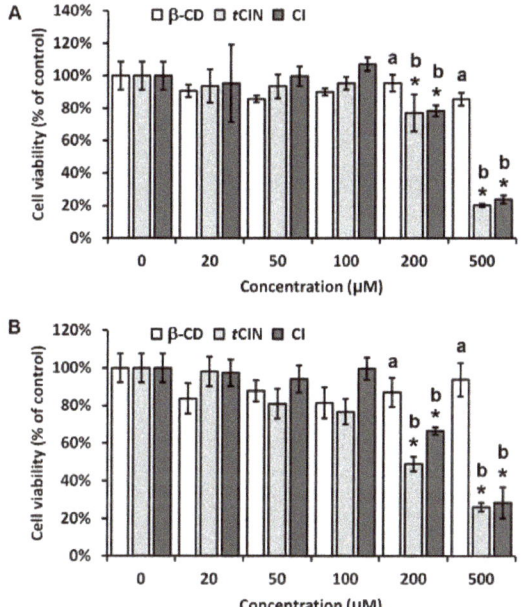

Figure 4. Cell viability. RAW 264.7 macrophages were seeded in 96-well plates for 24 h, followed by 18 h of starvation. Cells were treated with increasing concentrations of β-CD, tCIN, and CIs for 24 h. Cell viability was measured using the MTT assay, and quantified as a percentage (%) of the control. MTT assays were performed at (**A**) week 0 and (**B**) after 3 weeks of storage at 4 °C to evaluate the stability of CI and the effects of storage on CI. The CI was obtained by molecular inclusion at a 1:1 molar ratio of tCIN and β-CD. Data are the mean ± standard deviation (SD). * $p < 0.05$ versus the control. The different letters indicate $p < 0.05$ at the same treatment concentration. β-CD, β-cyclodextrin; tCIN, trans-cinnamaldehyde; CI, tCIN and β-CD inclusion complexes; MTT, 3-(4,5-dimethylthiazol-2-yl)-2,5-diphenyltetrazolium bromide.

2.5. Inhibition of NO Production

LPS, which is a cell wall component of Gram-negative bacteria, activates macrophages and triggers inflammatory responses by producing pro-inflammatory cytokines and mediators. These mediators, including inducible nitric oxide synthase (iNOS), cyclooxygenase (COX)-2, tumor necrosis factor (TNF)-α, and interleukin (IL)-1β, can be released by various cells, including murine RAW 264.7 macrophages. Alternatively, iNOS expression and NO production are known to be beneficial in both acute and chronic inflammation [36]. According to Lee and Choi [29], cinnamon extracts significantly inhibit NO production. Ho et al. [5] reported that among the major components of cinnamon, tCIN shows the highest inhibition of NO production and iNOS expression at both the protein and mRNA levels, at concentrations of 25–100 µM. We evaluated the effects of CIs on NO production in LPS-induced RAW264.7 macrophages. The NO production assays were performed to determine whether storage affected the stability of the CIs. The CIs were prepared in a culture medium and stored at 4 °C, and the production of NO was determined before and after 3 weeks of storage. We evaluated whether the storage time affected NO reduction. For this, CIs were prepared in a culture medium and stored at 4 °C, and the production of NO was determined before and after 3 weeks of storage. We found that treatment with β-CD alone had no effect on NO production induced by LPS in RAW macrophages. In contrast, treatment with only tCIN significantly reduced NO production. Interestingly, CI treatment had effects similar to that of treatment with tCIN alone; it resulted in reduced NO production, even after storage of samples for 3 weeks at 4 °C (Figure 5).

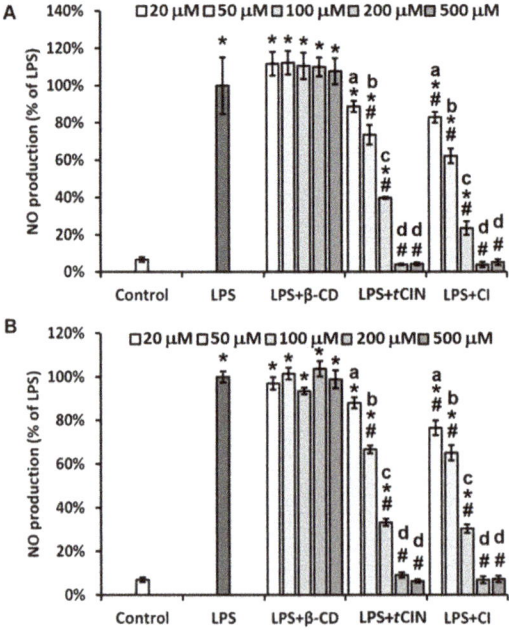

Figure 5. Inhibition of nitric oxide (NO) production by the *trans*-cinnamaldehyde (tCIN) and β-cyclodextrin (β-CD) inclusion complex (CI). RAW 264.7 macrophages were seeded in 96-well plates for 24 h, followed by 18 h of starvation. Cells were treated with increasing concentrations of β-CD, tCIN, and CIs for 30 min, and were then treated with LPS for 24 h. NO production was determined using an NO detection kit, according to the manufacturer's protocol. NO production was determined at (**A**) week 0 and (**B**) after 3 weeks of storage at 4 °C to evaluate the stability and effects of storage on CIs. The CI was obtained by molecular inclusion at a 1:1 molar ratio of tCIN and β-CD. Data are the mean ± standard deviation (SD). * $p < 0.05$ versus the control, # $p < 0.05$ versus LPS. The different letters indicate $p < 0.05$ within the same treatment group. LPS, lipopolysaccharide.

2.6. ROS Suppression

To evaluate the antioxidant effects of the CIs, the levels of ROS were determined in LPS-treated RAW 264.7 macrophages using 2′,7′-dichlorodihydrofluorescein diacetate (H2DCFDA, D-399). The LPS-treated cells showed significantly higher levels of fluorescence than the untreated control, and tCIN significantly reduced this effect (Figure 6). This result is similar to that reported by

Lee et al. [11], wherein *t*CIN was shown to inhibit LPS-induced ROS generation in J774A.1 macrophages. Interestingly, as shown in Figure 6B, *t*CIN self-inclusion in β-CD improved the ROS-reduction effect in LPS-treated RAW 264.7 cells. At *t*CIN and CI concentrations above 100 µM, the LPS-induced ROS level was reduced by approximately 5-fold (Figure 6A), indicating that CIs could be used as potential antioxidant agents. However, additional in vitro and in vivo studies of the effects of CIs on inflammation and oxidative stress are required. In addition, its underlying mechanisms need to be studied further for a better understanding and elucidation of its beneficial effects.

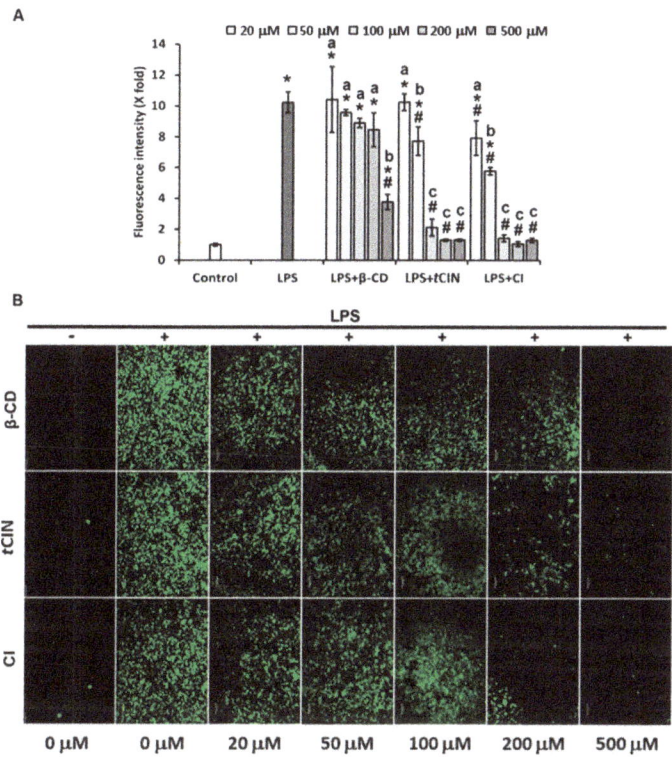

Figure 6. Inhibition of reactive oxygen species (ROS) production by the *trans*-cinnamaldehyde (*t*CIN) and β-cyclodextrin (β-CD) inclusion complexes (CIs). RAW 264.7 macrophages were seeded in 96-well plates with black walls and transparent bottoms for 24 h, and then subjected to starvation for 18 h. Cells were treated with increasing concentrations of β-CD, *t*CIN, and CIs for 30 min, and then treated with LPS for 24 h. ROS levels were determined using H2DCFDA, according to the manufacturer's protocol. (**A**) The fluorescence intensity was measured using a fluorescent microplate reader, and quantified as fold change compared to that of the control group; (**B**) Intensity was visualized using a fluorescence microscope at 100× magnification. The CIs were obtained by molecular inclusion at a 1:1 molar ratio of *t*CIN and β-CD. Data are the mean ± standard deviation (SD). * $p < 0.05$ versus the control, # $p < 0.05$ versus LPS. The different letters indicate $p < 0.05$ within the same treatment group. LPS, lipopolysaccharide; H2DCFDA, 2′,7′-dichlorodihydrofluorescein diacetate.

3. Materials and Methods

3.1. Materials

Murine RAW264.7 macrophages were purchased from the American Type Culture Collection (ATCC TIB-71; ATCC, Manassas, VA, USA). Dulbecco's modified Eagle's medium (DMEM; low glucose,

1000 mg/L; phenol red, LM 001-11) and fetal bovine serum (FBS; S 001-07) were purchased from Welgene Inc. (Daegu, Korea). LPS (cat. no. L6529), tCIN (cat. no. C80687), vitamin C (cat. no. A0278), 1,1-diphenyl-2-picrylhydrazyl (DPPH; cat. no. D9132), and 2,2′-azino-bis (3-ethylbenzothiazoline-6-sulfonic acid) diammonium salt (ABTS; cat. no. A1888) were purchased from Sigma-Aldrich (St. Louis, MO, USA). β-CD (cat. no. 030-08342) was purchased from Wako Pure Chemical Industries, Ltd. (Osaka, Japan). The nitric oxide (NO) detection kit (cat. no. ADI-917-010) was purchased from Enzo Life Sciences (Farmingdale, NY, USA).

3.2. Sample Preparation

For in vitro experiments, tCIN, β-CD, and CI samples were prepared in distilled water (for test of encapsulation efficiency, release study, and anti-oxidant activity) or cell culture medium (for test of cell viability, NO production, and ROS determination). 1 mM each of β-CD (pure powder) and tCIN (predissolved in dimethyl sulfoxide [DMSO]) were dissolved in distilled water or culture medium using a shaking incubator at 200 rpm. For CI preparation, 1 mM β-CD (pure powder) was dissolved in distilled water or culture medium in a shaking incubator at 200 rpm for 30 min, and tCIN was then added to the solution at the molar ratios of 0.5:1, 1:1, 1:2. The mixture was then placed in a shaking incubator at 200 rpm and 55 °C for 6 h for encapsulation by self-assembling aggregation. The CI samples were stored at 4 °C. The physical mixture was obtained by pulverizing the two components in a glass mortar, and mixing accurately weighed (1:1 molar ratio) amounts of tCIN and β-CD.

3.3. DSC Measurement

Differential scanning colorimetric (DSC) studies were performed using a DSC 200F3 apparatus (Netzsch-Geraetebau GmbH, Selb, Germany) to confirm the formation of the CIs. β-CD, tCIN, the β-CD-tCIN physical mixture, and CIs were analyzed. The β-CD-tCIN physical mixture was prepared. The temperature was calibrated using indium. The samples were weighed with an accuracy of 3 ± 0.01 mg and hermetically sealed in an aluminum pan. Each sample was scanned from 20 to 300 °C, with the heating set at 10 °C/min under nitrogen gas injection.

3.4. Encapsulation Efficiency and Release Study

The encapsulation efficiency (EE%) of tCIN was determined using a UV/VIS spectrophotometer (OPTIZEN, Mecasys Co., Daejeon, Korea). To extract free tCIN, n-hexane (9 mL) and the CIs (1 mL) were mixed together and centrifuged at 4000 rpm for 10 min. The extracted free tCIN in the supernatant of n-hexane was determined using an ultraviolet (UV)/visible (VIS) spectrophotometer at 285 nm. The EE% was indirectly calculated using a calibration curve constructed from the values of a series of tCIN solutions in n-hexane with standard concentrations. The EE% was then obtained as a percentage from the following equation:

$$\text{Encapsulation efficiency (\%)} = \frac{\text{Total amount of } t\text{CIN [g]} - \text{Free amount of } t\text{CIN [g]}}{\text{Total amount of } t\text{CIN [g]}} \quad (1)$$

The CIs were stored at different temperatures to determine the amount of tCIN released. The tCIN released from the CIs was determined at intervals using a UV/VIS spectrophotometer, according to the protocol followed by Chun et al. [37], with modifications. The CIs were stored at 4 °C in a refrigerator and at 25 and 37 °C in an incubator. A 1-mL aliquot of the tCIN emulsion was withdrawn at week 4, and the amount of tCIN extracted was measured as described above. The amount of tCIN released was expressed as a percentage of the initial total amount of tCIN.

3.5. Anti-Oxidative Activity

The antioxidant capacity of the CIs was measured using the DPPH free radical-scavenging and ABTS radical-scavenging capacity methods according to Brand-Williams et al. [38], and Re, et al. [39], respectively. Vitamin C (ascorbic acid, 1 mg/mL) was used as a positive control, and the free radical-scavenging capacity was expressed as a percentage. All determinations were performed at least in triplicate.

3.6. Cell Culture

Murine RAW264.7 macrophages were subcultured to 70–80% confluence every 2–3 days in 100-mm dishes (Falcon, Bedford, MA, USA) in DMEM supplemented with 10% FBS, and were incubated in a humidified atmosphere containing 5% CO_2 and 95% air at 37 °C. For the experiments, the cells were seeded in 96-well plates for cell cytotoxicity, reactive oxygen species (ROS), and nitric oxide (NO) determination in DMEM containing 10% FBS for 24 h. The day before treatments, all cells were starved in DMEM containing 1% FBS overnight, and then treated with β-CD, *t*CIN, or CIs with or without 1 μg/mL LPS for further experiments.

3.7. Cell Viability

The protective effects of *t*CIN and β-CD CIs were evaluated in LPS-treated RAW cells using a 3-(4,5-dimethylthiazol-2-yl)-2,5-diphenyltetrazolium bromide (MTT) assay. The β-CD, *t*CIN, and CI samples were prepared and stored at 4 °C for 3 weeks to evaluate the effect of their stability on cell viability. Cell viability experiments were performed using fresh samples and samples stored for 3 weeks. RAW cells (4×10^4 cells/well) were seeded in 96-well plates for 24 h and then starved in DMEM supplemented with 1% FBS overnight before treatment. The cells were treated with different concentrations of β-CD, *t*CIN, and CIs for 24 h, and cell viability was assessed using the MTT assay. The absorbance was measured using an enzyme-linked immunosorbent assay (ELISA) plate reader (Thermo Scientific Multiskan GO microplate spectrophotometer; Thermo Scientific, Lafayette, CO, USA) at 540 nm, and cell viability was determined as a percentage of the control cells.

3.8. NO Production

The cells were prepared as described for the MTT assay. RAW264.7 macrophages (4×10^4 cells/well) were seeded in 96-well plates for 24 h and then starved in DMEM supplemented with 1% FBS overnight before treatment. After starvation, the cells were pre-incubated with different concentrations of β-CD, *t*CIN, and CIs for 30 min, and then stimulated with LPS (1 μg/mL). After 24 h, the supernatant was collected, and NO production was determined using an NO detection kit, according to the manufacturer's protocol.

3.9. ROS Determination

The level of intracellular ROS induced by LPS was determined using 2′,7′-dichloro-dihydrofluorescein diacetate (H2DCFDA, D-399), also known as dichlorofluorescin diacetate (Life Technologies Korea LLC, Seoul, Korea), according to the manufacturer's protocol. Briefly, RAW cells were seeded in black-walled, transparent-bottom 96-well plates (Thermo Scientific Nunc, Rochester, NY, USA) for 24 h and starved overnight before treatment, as described above. The cells were treated with 20 μM H2DCFDA for 1 h in a humidified cell culture incubator and washed twice with phosphate-buffered saline (PBS). H2DCFDA fluorescence was analyzed using a Spectra Max M2e spectrophotometer (Molecular Devices, Bath, UK), at an excitation wavelength of 485 nm, and the fluorescein signal was detected at an emission wavelength of 535 nm. The relative ratio of each sample intensity was calculated as a percentage of the control group value. Fluorescence images were obtained using a Nikon Eclipse Ti fluorescent microscope (Nikon Inc., Tokyo, Japan) at 100× magnification.

3.10. Statistical Analysis

Data are presented as the mean ± standard deviation (SD). The significance of differences between groups was assessed using multiple comparisons and analysis of variance (ANOVA), followed by the Tukey honest significant difference (HSD) test. Differences with P values of less than 0.05 were considered statistically significant.

4. Conclusions

In this study, tCIN was solubilized by formulating it as an inclusion complex with β-CD polymer using molecular inclusion techniques. The encapsulation efficiency was confirmed to be 85%, and high retention of tCIN was maintained for 4 weeks. In addition, tCIN self-inclusion in the β-CD polymer did not elevate the toxicity to more than that of tCIN alone. In fact, the CIs appeared to prevent the oxidation of tCIN during prolonged storage. NO assays revealed that the β-CD self-inclusion method did not affect the NO-reducing effects of tCIN, even after 3 weeks of storage. Furthermore, the results of DPPH and ABTS radical-scavenging activity assay, and the DCF-DA assay showed that β-CD self-inclusion had no negative effects on the anti-oxidative properties of tCIN. Collectively, these results indicated that tCIN self-inclusion in β-CD could play an important role in developing nano-functional food applications.

Acknowledgments: This research was supported by Basic Science Program through the National Research Foundation of Korea (NRF) funded by the Ministry of Science, ICT and Future Planning (No. 2014M3A7B4051898).

Author Contributions: Munkhtugs Davaatseren and Yeon-Ji Jo performed experiments and data analysis, and contributed to the preparation of this manuscript. Haeng Jeon Hur and Sujin Park performed some experiments and analyzed the data. Geun-pyo Hong and Mi-Jung Choi were responsible for the conception and design of the study, data presentation and manuscript preparation. All the authors read and approved the final manuscript.

Conflicts of Interest: The authors declare no conflict of interest.

References

1. Lee, R.; Balick, M.J. Sweet wood-cinnamon and its importance as a spice and medicine. *J. Sci. Heal.* **2005**, *1*, 61–64. [CrossRef] [PubMed]
2. Chang, S.T.; Chen, P.F.; Chang, S.C. Antibacterial activity of leaf essential oils and their constituents from *Cinnamomum osmophloeum*. *J. Ethnopharmacol.* **2001**, *77*, 123–127. [CrossRef]
3. Sartorius, T.; Peter, A.; Schulz, N.; Drescher, A.; Bergheim, I.; Machann, J.; Schick, F.; Siegel-Axel, D.; Schürmann, A.; Weigert, C.; et al. Cinnamon extract improves insulin sensitivity in the brain and lowers liver fat in mouse models of obesity. *PLoS ONE* **2014**, *9*, e92358. [CrossRef] [PubMed]
4. Kwon, H.K.; Hwang, J.S.; So, J.S.; Lee, C.G.; Sahoo, A.; Ryu, J.H.; Jeon, W.K.; Ko, B.S.; Im, C.R.; Lee, S.J.; et al. Cinnamon extract induces tumor cell death through inhibition of NFκB and AP1. *BMC Cancer* **2010**, *10*, 392–402. [CrossRef] [PubMed]
5. Ho, S.C.; Chang, K.S.; Chang, P.W. Inhibition of neuroinflammation by cinnamon and its main components. *Food Chem.* **2013**, *138*, 2275–2282. [CrossRef] [PubMed]
6. Mathew, S.; Abraham, T.E. Studies on the antioxidant activities of cinnamon (*Cinnamomum verum*) bark extracts, through various in vitro models. *Food Chem.* **2006**, *94*, 520–528. [CrossRef]
7. Prasad, K.N.; Yang, B.; Dong, X.; Jiang, G.; Zhang, H.; Xie, H.; Jiang, Y. Flavonoid contents and antioxidant activities from *Cinnamomum* species. *Innov. Food Sci. Emerg. Technol.* **2009**, *10*, 627–632. [CrossRef]
8. Cabello, C.M.; Bair, W.B.; Lamore, S.D.; Ley, S.; Bause, A.S.; Azimian, S.; Wondrak, G.T. The cinnamon-derived Michael acceptor cinnamic aldehyde impairs melanoma cell proliferation, invasiveness, and tumor growth. *Free Radic. Biol. Med.* **2009**, *46*, 220–231. [CrossRef] [PubMed]
9. Zhang, J.H.; Liu, L.Q.; He, Y.L.; Kong, W.J.; Huang, S.A. Cytotoxic effect of *trans*-cinnamaldehyde on human leukemia K562 cells. *Acta Pharmacol. Sin.* **2010**, *31*, 861–866. [CrossRef] [PubMed]
10. Chao, L.K.; Hua, K.F.; Hsu, H.Y.; Cheng, S.S.; Lin, I.F.; Chen, C.J.; Chen, S.T.; Chang, S.T. Cinnamaldehyde inhibits pro-inflammatory cytokines secretion from monocytes/macrophages through suppression of intracellular signaling. *Food Chem. Toxicol.* **2008**, *46*, 220–231. [CrossRef] [PubMed]
11. Lee, S.H.; Lee, S.Y.; Son, D.J.; Lee, H.; Yoo, H.S.; Song, S.; Oh, K.W.; Han, D.C.; Kwon, B.M.; Hong, J.T. Inhibitory effect of 2′-hydroxycinnamaldehyde on nitric oxide production through inhibition of NF-κB activation in RAW 264.7 cells. *Biochem. Pharmacol.* **2005**, *69*, 791–799. [CrossRef] [PubMed]

12. Chuang, L.Y.; Guh, J.Y.; Chao, L.K.; Lu, Y.C.; Hwang, J.Y.; Yang, Y.L.; Cheng, T.H.; Yang, W.Y.; Chien, Y.J.; Huang, J.S. Anti-proliferative effects of cinnamaldehyde on human hepatoma cell lines. *Food Chem.* **2012**, *133*, 1603–1610. [CrossRef]
13. El-Bassossy, H.M.; Fahmy, A.; Badawy, D. Cinnamaldehyde protects from the hypertension associated with diabetes. *Food Chem. Toxicol.* **2011**, *49*, 3007–3012. [CrossRef] [PubMed]
14. Hooth, M.J.; Sills, R.C.; Burka, L.T.; Haseman, J.K.; Witt, K.L.; Orzech, D.P.; Fuciarelli, A.F.; Graves, S.W.; Johnson, J.D.; Bucher, J.R. Toxicology and carcinogenesis studies of microencapsulated *trans*-cinnamaldehyde in rats and mice. *Food Chem. Toxicol.* **2004**, *42*, 1757–1768. [CrossRef] [PubMed]
15. Bickers, D.; Calow, P.; Greim, H.; Hanifin, J.M.; Rogers, A.E.; Saurat, J.H.; Sipes, I.G.; Smith, R.L.; Tagami, H. A toxicologic and dermatologic assessment of cinnamyl alcohol, cinnamaldehyde and cinnamic acid when used as fragrance ingredients. *Food Chem. Toxicol.* **2005**, *43*, 799–836. [CrossRef] [PubMed]
16. Radi, A.E.; Eissa, S. Electrochemistry of cyclodextrin inclusion complexes of pharmaceutical compounds. *Open Chem. Biomed. Methods J.* **2010**, *3*, 74–85. [CrossRef]
17. Al-Rawashdeh, N.A.; Al-Sadeh, K.S.; Al-Bitar, M.B. Inclusion complexes of sunscreen agents with β-cyclodextrin: Spectroscopic and molecular modeling studies. *J. Spectrosc.* **2013**, *2013*, 841409–841420. [CrossRef]
18. Marangoci, N.; Mares, M.; Silion, M.; Fifere, A.; Varganici, C.; Nicolescu, A.; Deleanu, C.; Coroaba, A.; Pinteala, M.; Simionescu, B.C. Inclusion complex of a new propiconazole derivative with β-cyclodextrin: NMR, ESI–MS and preliminary pharmacological studies. *Results Pharm. Sci.* **2011**, *1*, 27–37. [CrossRef] [PubMed]
19. Auda, S.H. Nimesulide/Methyl β-cyclodextrin inclusion complexes: Physicochemical characterization, solubility, dissolution, and biological studies. *Drug Dev. Res.* **2014**, *75*, 68–75. [CrossRef] [PubMed]
20. Nicolescu, C.; Arama, C.; Monciu, C.M. Preparation and characterization of inclusion complexes between repaglinide and β-cyclodextrin, 2-hydroxypropyl-β-cyclodextrin and randomly methylated β-cyclodextrin. *Farmacia* **2010**, *58*, 78–88.
21. Astray, G.; Gonzalez-Barreiro, C.; Mejuto, J.C.; Rial-Otero, R.; Simal-Gándara, J. A review on the use of cyclodextrins in foods. *Food Hydrocoll.* **2009**, *23*, 1631–1640. [CrossRef]
22. Cravotto, G.; Binello, A.; Baranelli, E.; Carraro, P.; Trotta, F. Cyclodextrins as food additives and in food processing. *Curr. Nutr. Food Sci.* **2006**, *2*, 343–350. [CrossRef]
23. Trotta, F.; Zanetti, M.; Cavalli, R. Cyclodextrin-based nanosponges as drug carriers. *Beilstein J. Org. Chem.* **2012**, *8*, 2091–2099. [CrossRef] [PubMed]
24. García, A.; Leonardi, D.; Salazar, M.O.; Lamas, M.C. Modified β-cyclodextrin inclusion complex to improve the physicochemical properties of albendazole. Complete in vitro evaluation and characterization. *PLoS ONE* **2014**, *9*, e88234. [CrossRef] [PubMed]
25. Seo, E.J.; Min, S.G.; Choi, M.J. Release characteristics of freeze-dried eugenol encapsulated with β-cyclodextrin by molecular inclusion method. *J. Microencapsul.* **2010**, *27*, 496–505. [CrossRef] [PubMed]
26. Cheng, D.M.; Kuhn, P.; Poulev, A.; Rojo, L.E.; Lila, M.A.; Raskin, I. In vivo and in vitro antidiabetic effects of aqueous cinnamon extract and cinnamon polyphenol-enhanced food matrix. *Food Chem.* **2012**, *135*, 2994–3002. [CrossRef] [PubMed]
27. Hill, L.E.; Gomes, C.; Taylor, T.M. Characterization of beta-cyclodextrin inclusion complexes containing essential oils (*trans*-cinnamaldehyde, eugenol, cinnamon bark, and clove bud extracts) for antimicrobial delivery applications. *LWT Food Sci. Technol.* **2013**, *51*, 86–93. [CrossRef]
28. Choi, M.J.; Ruktanonchai, U.; Soottitantawat, A.; Min, S.G. Morphological characterization of encapsulated fish oil with β-cyclodextrin and polycaprolactone. *Food Res. Int.* **2009**, *42*, 989–997. [CrossRef]
29. Lee, K.H.; Choi, E.M. Stimulatory effects of extract prepared from the bark of *Cinnamomum cassia blume* on the function of osteoblastic MC3T3-E1 cells. *Phytother. Res.* **2006**, *20*, 952–960. [CrossRef] [PubMed]
30. Wang, J.; Cao, Y.; Sun, B.; Wang, C. Physicochemical and release characterisation of garlic oil-β-cyclodextrin inclusion complexes. *Food Chem.* **2011**, *127*, 1680–1685. [CrossRef]
31. Zuidam, N.J.; Nedovic, V.A. *Encapsulation Technologies for Active Food Ingredients and Food Processing*; Springer: London, UK, 2010; pp. 127–1160. ISBN 9781441910073.
32. Lakkis, J.M. *Encapsulation and Controlled Release Technologies in Food Systems*; Blackwell Publishing: Oxford, UK, 2007; pp. 13–40. ISBN 9780470277881.

33. Lu, Z.; Cheng, B.; Hu, Y.; Zhang, Y.; Zou, G. Complexation of resveratrol with cyclodextrins: Solubility and antioxidant activity. *Food Chem.* **2009**, *113*, 17–20. [CrossRef]
34. Yang, J.; Guo, J.; Yuan, J. In vitro antioxidant properties of rutin. *LWT Food Sci. Technol.* **2008**, *41*, 1060–1066. [CrossRef]
35. Yang, R.; Chen, J.B.; Xiao, C.F.; Liu, Z.C.; Gao, Z.Y.; Yan, S.J.; Zhang, J.H.; Zhang, H.B.; Lin, J. Inclusion complex of GA-13316 with β-cyclodextrin: Preparation, characterization, molecular modeling, and in vitro evaluation. *Carbohydr. Polym.* **2014**, *111*, 655–662. [CrossRef] [PubMed]
36. Sung, M.J.; Davaatseren, M.; Kim, W.; Park, S.K.; Kim, S.H.; Hur, H.J.; Kim, M.S.; Kim, Y.S.; Kwon, D.Y. Vitisin A suppresses LPS-induced NO production by inhibiting ERK, p38, and NF-κB activation in RAW 264.7 cells. *Int. Immunopharmacol.* **2009**, *9*, 319–323. [CrossRef] [PubMed]
37. Chun, J.Y.; Jo, Y.J.; Bjrapha, P.; Choi, M.J.; Min, S.G. Antimicrobial effect of α- or β-cyclodextrin complexes with *trans*-cinnamaldehyde against *staphylococcus aureus* and *Escherichia coli*. *Dry. Technol.* **2015**, *33*, 377–383. [CrossRef]
38. Brand-Williams, W.; Cuvelier, M.; Berset, C. Use of a free radical method to evaluate antioxidant activity. *LWT Food Sci. Technol.* **1995**, *28*, 25–30. [CrossRef]
39. Re, R.; Pellegrini, N.; Proteggente, A.; Pannala, A.; Yang, M.; Rice-Evans, C. Antioxidant activity applying an improved ABTS radical cation decolorization assay. *Free Radic. Biol. Med.* **1999**, *26*, 1231–1237. [CrossRef]

Sample Availability: Samples of the compounds are available from the authors.

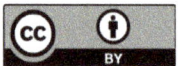

© 2017 by the authors. Licensee MDPI, Basel, Switzerland. This article is an open access article distributed under the terms and conditions of the Creative Commons Attribution (CC BY) license (http://creativecommons.org/licenses/by/4.0/).

MDPI
St. Alban-Anlage 66
4052 Basel
Switzerland
Tel. +41 61 683 77 34
Fax +41 61 302 89 18
www.mdpi.com

Molecules Editorial Office
E-mail: molecules@mdpi.com
www.mdpi.com/journal/molecules

www.ingramcontent.com/pod-product-compliance
Lightning Source LLC
LaVergne TN
LVHW071943080526
838202LV00064B/6666